Springer Series in Pharmaceutical Statistics

Recent advances in statistics have led to new concepts and solutions in different areas of pharmaceutical research and development. "Springer Series in Pharmaceutical Statistics" focuses on developments in pharmaceutical statistics and their practical applications in the industry. The main target groups are researchers in the pharmaceutical industry, regulatory agencies and members of the academic community working in the field of pharmaceutical statistics. In order to encourage exchanges between experts in the pharma industry working on the same problems from different perspectives, an additional goal of the series is to provide reference material for non-statisticians. The volumes will include the results of recent research conducted by the authors and adhere to high scholarly standards. Volumes focusing on software implementation (e.g. in SAS or R) are especially welcome. The book series covers different aspects of pharmaceutical research, such as drug discovery, development and production.

Jiawei Wei • Leslie Meng • Frank Bretz
Feng Chen • Jun Wang
Editors

Estimands in Clinical Trials

A Practical Guide

Springer

Editors
Jiawei Wei
Novartis
Shanghai, China

Leslie Meng
Boehringer-Ingelheim
Ulm, Germany

Frank Bretz
Novartis
Basel, Switzerland

Feng Chen
Nanjing Medical University
Nanjing, China

Jun Wang
National Medical Products Administration
Beijing, China

ISSN 2366-8695 ISSN 2366-8709 (electronic)
Springer Series in Pharmaceutical Statistics
ISBN 978-3-032-02191-5 ISBN 978-3-032-02192-2 (eBook)
https://doi.org/10.1007/978-3-032-02192-2

This Springer imprint is published by the registered company Springer Nature Switzerland AG
The registered company address is: Gewerbestrasse 11, 6330 Cham, Switzerland

Foreword: Toward a Future Where Clinical Trials Address the Right Questions for Decision-Making

As noted in the 2014 concept paper for the addendum to the ICH E9 guideline (ICH, 2014), despite the fact that clinical trials have been used to support regulatory decision-making for decades, there was no harmonized agreement on the precise question that a given clinical trial should try to answer about an experimental medicinal product. The concept paper was written at a time when there was controversy over the suitability of prevailing methods of statistical analysis, specifically methods assuming that missing or unwanted data were "missing at random." This lack of clarity meant that some discussions on statistical methods were held in a vacuum, without the reference point of a clear and agreed question of interest.

The ICH E9(R1) guideline, the addendum to ICH E9 on estimands and sensitivity analysis in clinical trials, was written as a basis to formulate, discuss, and agree questions of interest that should be addressed in clinical trials to support regulatory decision-making (ICH, 2019). The guidance gives a basis for sponsors and regulators to discuss estimands for a given clinical trial and their consequences for choices in respect of trial design and analysis. The guidance does not seek to dictate questions of interest across the spectrum of experimental settings, nor does it directly promote or critique specific analytical approaches. In a very real sense, the guidance promotes discussion on the questions of interest for drug developers, regulators, prescribers, patients, and other stakeholders and how to approach statistical analysis so that it aligns to an agreed question of interest.

Now, approximately 5 years after adoption of the final guidance and 10 years after the initial concept paper, this book has managed to capture and collate those discussions in the most comprehensive presentation of thinking and writing relating to estimands of which I am aware. It provides a nose to tail summary, covering not only the ICH guidance itself but also the extensive discussions, activities, and literature arising therefrom, both on estimands and on consequent issues relating to statistical analysis. In fact, seeing all of the discussion topics, working groups, regulatory guidelines, and published literature documented in one place is quite remarkable. The authors and editors have managed to provide a reference book that is, to date, complete on this important topic, and it is my privilege to offer a few thoughts by way of introduction and endorsement.

Everyone involved in clinical trials is taught early in their career that "statistical significance does not equate to clinical relevance." While providing evidence that a beneficial effect exists is a pre-requisite to a medicine being approved, the decisions of regulators and of other stakeholders also require an understanding of the magnitudes of benefits and risks that might be derived from a particular treatment. Indeed, how else to make a benefit–risk trade-off other than to quantify not only the existence but also the magnitudes of each? The ICH E9(R1) guideline recognizes that there are multiple treatment effects that can be identified in respect of each efficacy, or safety, outcome and provides a framework and language to discuss which questions can be formulated, which are meaningful in a given context and, ultimately, which of those should be prioritized so that evidence can be generated accordingly. Deriving an estimand centers around five strategies that could be used to frame different scientific questions of interest in respect of each identified intercurrent event. [For any readers unfamiliar with the terminology, all will become clear in Chap. 2 of this book and, as an aside, please note that I elect to avoid the word "handle" in this context: It makes sense that we handle data, and handle missing data—which is the context in which that particular word appears, just twice, in the ICH E9(R1) guideline—but it is a potentially confusing term in respect of framing a clinical question of interest in respect of intercurrent events.] These five strategies represent the conceivable questions of interest that might be considered in relation to primary, secondary, or exploratory trial objectives. In addition, listing these strategies in the E9(R1) guideline facilitated the ability to highlight issues with certain prevailing, and concerning, analytical practices. For example, analyses based on subgroups defined based on post-randomization outcomes or analyses using follow-up restricted to the period while a patient was receiving treatment or was on trial. The strategies provide the basis to formulate relevant clinical questions of interest that, as outlined in Chap. 5, identify an effect that is causal in nature, that is, an effect attributable to (the difference between) treatment (conditions). This is a critical point to understand when developing an estimand. A related sentence in E9(R1) that is important, but has perhaps gone largely unappreciated, is:

"When defining a treatment effect of interest, it is important to ensure that the definition identifies an effect due to treatment and not due to potential confounders such as differences in duration of observation or patient characteristics."

This is an important principle to keep in mind while reading this book and while engaging in estimand discussions.

The content of this book is detailed and does not shy away from the more complex discussions in this field but is presented in an attractively accessible manner with plentiful use of case studies, making it appropriate reading for those who are new to the topic, those wishing to develop their understanding, and those seeking to become expert. I encourage readers to consider the case studies as illustrations of the processes of thinking and documentation around estimands and not as conclusions for which strategies and estimands are somehow correct or agreed in a given setting. Indeed, I would certainly contest some of the justifications from sponsors and regulators that are presented in the case studies but that is, after all, precisely the discussion promoted by the E9(R1) guideline. One justification of particular interest is the argument in favor of a treatment-policy question because the intercurrent event and its consequences reflect clinical practice. At first reading this seems logical, trivial even. Indeed, such a justification seems straightforward to accept where the intercurrent event is "treatment discontinuation due to toxicity": Why should we be interested in anything other than the effect of treatment reflecting that such discontinuations occur (outside the uncommon, though not unheard of, scenario that a prevention of particular adverse events is developed after the confirmatory trial has been completed)? It is more complicated, however, to follow that logic where the intercurrent event is "use of rescue medication," in particular where the clinical question of interest relates to quantifying the effect of the administration of the drug itself, rather than the effect of comparing two treatment strategies that might eventually be used in clinical practice. That, as I understand it, is often the precise purpose of undertaking a placebo-controlled trial. Regardless, the extensive range of case studies presented provides an extremely useful resource in itself, illustrating a wide range of intercurrent events, a wide range of strategies used to frame clinical questions of interest in respect of those intercurrent events, a wide range of considerations and justifications for preferring one framing of a clinical question (strategy) over another and, beyond that, illustrations of the consequences for trial design, data collection, and statistical analysis. The case studies illustrate not only questions of potential primary importance but questions of potential secondary importance, such as the nice examples of seeking to understand the impact of the treatment effect of a biological medicine from the development of anti-drug antibodies or whether a treatment is truly a disease modifier in multiple sclerosis. They also illustrate areas where analysis aligned with a causal estimand offers a potential improvement over existing practice, such as the example of analyses presently used to support demonstration and quantification of vaccine efficacy. This book goes on from the case studies to reflect further on consequences for statistical analysis, for each type of variable (continuous, binary, time to event, etc.), in respect of each of the five estimand strategies—a particularly useful resource for colleagues, mostly statisticians, charged with aligning the analysis to the estimand. Related to this, one particular consequence of discussions around estimands is the access to methodological thinking and techniques to which those involved in clinical drug development have not usually been exposed, notably the discipline referred to as causal inference, and these are also highlighted in this book.

The ICH E9(R1) guideline has certainly changed drug development, in particular for confirmatory trials, though not—at least, not yet—in a transformative way. Arguably, the biggest change has been improving the alignment of a main, or primary, statistical analysis with a stated estimand, with a consequent shift in both the data used for analysis (data are no longer ignored for estimation unless agreed as being irrelevant to the research question) and the approaches used for statistical analysis, in particular relating to the handling of missing data. Looking ahead, there remains a presently untapped potential for greater use of well-informed, multidisciplinary discussions to determine appropriate clinical questions of interest that, once agreed, are used to drive considerations relating to trial design and analysis. Evolution in the use and in the usefulness of estimands will be accelerated by making these discussions available to a wider audience, based on resources such as this.

Indeed, there are many interesting discussions to continue, in particular around which strategies reflect clinical questions of greatest interest for regulatory, physician, and patient decision-making. The ICH E9(R1) guideline highlights that "treatment-policy" questions might be more generally acceptable to support regulatory decision-making. Sometimes, this will be because that strategy reflects the question of greatest interest in respect of one or more intercurrent events. Other times, it will be because the type or extent of assumptions associated with analytical approaches to answering other questions is deemed to introduce too much uncertainty. However, and as reflected through this book content, this text in the ICH E9(R1) guideline should not, and has not, dissuaded the discussion of alternatives. Indeed, it is readily easy to think of circumstances where each of the five strategies outlined in the E9(R1) guideline can reflect a question of interest in respect of certain intercurrent events that could be important for regulatory decision-making. Although such questions move further away from strict adherence to the intention-to-treat principle of including patients and follow-up regardless of adherence to the planned course of treatment, this should not be understood as under-estimating the importance of randomization in experimental design. At least I consider that randomization is both vitally important and universally helpful for estimation regardless of the clinical questions of interest posed. Still, this exemplifies the main areas, at the time of writing, where discussions on estimands are still to evolve. First, there is a need for greater engagement of disciplines beyond clinical trial statisticians into the conversation of which clinical questions of interest (treatment effects) should be quantified to best inform the decision-making of all different stakeholders—with that conversation based first and foremost on clinical rather than statistical considerations. Second, the need to characterize instances where "treatment-policy" questions might not be "more generally acceptable." This might arise because the more informative clinical question of interest relates to an individual treatment, rather than a treatment sequence. Alternatively, it might arise because there are particular challenges to conducting a clinical trial in a given therapeutic setting. For example, where it is not possible to use one clear and identifiable treatment sequence in the control arm through the course of a trial due to changing clinical practice, or where intercurrent events would occur in a trial that would not occur in clinical practice.

Third, if questions of putative importance would best be addressed using methods of statistical analysis with which the community is less familiar or which require (at least, which appear based on contemporaneous thinking to require) more, or stronger, assumptions. Work is needed in respect of those alternative approaches to address how sponsors, regulators, and others should best investigate those assumptions to become comfortable that those analyses are sufficiently reliable for decision-making. These are substantial challenges and are more likely to be addressed as more people get more familiarity with the issues, based on resources such as this.

Once again, I congratulate the authors, contributors, and editors for this high quality and comprehensive piece of work that I hope serves as an education and resource for all.

London, UK
April 2025

Robert Hemmings

Preface

Since its release in 2019, the ICH E9(R1) guideline on estimands and sensitivity analysis has led to a significant shift in the design, conduct, analysis, and interpretation of clinical trials. At its core, the estimand framework provides a structured approach to explicitly aligning the clinical question of interest with the trial objectives. It does so while taking into account intercurrent events—events that occur after randomization or treatment initiation and either preclude the observation of a variable or affects its interpretation. By clearly defining what we aim to estimate and how such intercurrent events are addressed, the framework enhances the transparency and interpretability of trial results. Over the past 6 years, the adoption of the estimand framework has supported improved regulatory and scientific dialogue, more targeted trial designs, and a better understanding of treatment effects across drug development programs.

This book offers a comprehensive, up-to-date, and practical introduction to the estimand framework and its application in clinical trials. Building on the earlier work by Mallinckrodt, Molenberghs, Lipkovich, and Ratitch (2020), it reflects both the conceptual underpinnings of the framework and the growing body of experience gained by the scientific and regulatory community since the release of the ICH E9(R1) guideline. In particular, this volume provides practical guidance on implementing the estimand framework in diverse clinical settings. It introduces the core concepts of the framework and offers a detailed direction on how to define and describe estimands in clinical trial protocols and related documents. To support practical implementation, this book includes a wide range of case studies from various therapeutic areas, along with summaries of estimand-related content from regulatory guidelines for specific indications. It also presents statistical analysis methods and approaches for handling missing data across continuous, binary, recurrent, and time-to-event endpoints—always within the estimand framework and tailored to different trial contexts.

How This Book Came About

The origins of this book trace back to 2017, shortly after the release of the draft ICH E9(R1) guideline. In response to the paradigm shift introduced by this draft guideline, a group of industry professionals from the China Clinical Trial Statistics (CCTS) and the Drug Information Association (DIA) Statistics Community established the DIA-CCTS Estimand Working Group (DC-EWG). Their goal was to foster a better understanding of the estimand framework, resolve key questions, and develop strategies for its practical implementation in clinical trials. In 2021, building on several years of collaborative effort, the group initiated the development of a comprehensive guidance document in Chinese—informally known as the "Bluebook" and led by two of us (J.W. and L.M.). This early publication compiled case studies across therapeutic areas, interpretations of disease-specific guidelines, and insights into applying the estimand framework across diverse trial settings.

This book builds on the foundation laid by the Chinese Bluebook and represents a natural progression from regional exploration to global application. It reflects a truly collaborative and international effort, drawing on the expertise of more than 70 contributors from over 40 academic, regulatory, and industry institutions worldwide. This diverse authorship brings together a broad spectrum of experiences and perspectives, enriching the content and ensuring its relevance across a wide range of clinical trial contexts. This book has undergone a rigorous peer-review process involving more than 40 experts, whose careful evaluation has contributed to the consistency, clarity, and scientific quality of the chapters.

How to Read This Book

The content of this book is organized into five parts, each focusing on a key dimension of the estimand framework and its implementation in clinical trials. Part I introduces the estimand framework, establishing the core concepts and terminology. It discusses the alignment of trial objectives with study design, conduct, analysis, and interpretation and provides essential background on estimands, estimators, and estimates. Additional topics include the importance of cross-functional collaboration, documentation and reporting principles, causal inference considerations, and a summary of international initiatives since the release of ICH E9(R1). Part II presents case studies across a variety of therapeutic areas, including oncology, hematology, immunology, infectious diseases, neuroscience, cardiology, and respiratory diseases. These examples illustrate the flexibility and breadth of the estimand framework in clinical trial contexts and provide practical insights into its application across different clinical challenges. Part III focuses on the intersection between the estimand framework and regulatory guidance. It illustrates how the framework has been adopted by guidelines from the International Council for Harmonisation (ICH) and various regulatory agencies, including the European Medicines Agency

(EMA), the U.S. Food and Drug Administration (FDA), and the National Medical Products Administration (NMPA) of China. Part IV covers statistical methodologies for analysis under the estimand framework. It includes methods tailored to a variety of endpoint types—continuous, binary, time-to-event, and recurrent events—and addresses topics, such as covariate adjustment and principal stratification. Finally, Part V explores the use of the estimand framework in diverse clinical trial settings, including early-phase drug development, safety and benefit–risk assessments, health technology assessments, bioequivalence and non-inferiority studies, complex innovative designs, multi-regional clinical trials, decentralized trials, and clinical trial disruptions, such as the COVID-19 pandemic.

Who Should Read This Book

The scope and structure of this book are designed to support readers in applying the estimand framework thoughtfully and effectively. It is intended for a broad audience of professionals and students involved in clinical research—particularly those engaged in the design, conduct, and analysis of clinical trials across the drug development lifecycle. For those new to the field, this book offers a structured introduction to the estimand framework and its practical applications. For experienced professionals, it serves as a reference guide, providing an extensive collection of case studies, summaries of disease-specific regulatory guidelines, and detailed discussions of statistical methodologies tailored to the estimand framework. In addition, this book may be of value to teachers and students in statistics or related disciplines, whether in dedicated courses on clinical trial methodology or broader curricula in biostatistics or pharmaceutical sciences.

Shanghai, China — Jiawei Wei
Ulm, Germany — Leslie Meng
Basel, Switzerland — Frank Bretz
Nanjing, China — Feng Chen
Beijing, China — Jun Wang
April 2025

Acknowledgments

As a collaborative effort, this book would not have been possible without the generous contributions and support of many individuals. We are particularly grateful to our colleagues who contributed to the original Chinese Bluebook, many of whom also played a key role in shaping this volume—either as authors, reviewers, or both. We especially thank Tian Hong, Yuxiu Liu, James Pan, Shuhang Wang, Naiqing Zhao, and Jiangxiu Zhou for their support and guidance during the development of the Bluebook, which laid the foundation for this work. We are also indebted to the many colleagues who contributed their time and expertise in reviewing individual chapters of this volume. Their thoughtful feedback and scientific rigor greatly enhanced the quality and consistency of this book. In particular, we thank Mouna Akacha, Jonathan Bartlett, James Bell, Björn Bornkamp, Francesca Callegari, James Carpenter, Gang Chen, Olivier Collignon, Richard Cook, Qiqi Deng, Evgeny Degtyarev, Bharani Dharan, Vlad Dragalin, Stefan Englert, Chrissie Fletcher, Margaret Gamalo, Lorenzo Guizzaro, Eva Hua, Bo Huang, Shuping Jiang, Brennan Kahan, Oliver Keene, Ray Lin, Xinxu Li, Ilya Lipkovich, Helle Lynggaard, Tianmeng Lyu, Dominic Magirr, Devan Mehrotra, Marian Mitroiu, Tim Morris, Tobias Mütze, Michael O'Kelly, Camilla Olarte Parra, Elena Polverejan, Yongming Qu, James Roger, Steve Ruberg, Kaspar Rufibach, Satoru Tsuchiya, Kelly Van Lancker, Wei Wang, William Wang, David Wright, Dong Xi, Marcel Wolbers, and Emmanuel Zuber for their generous and constructive input. Finally, we extend our sincere thanks to our publisher for their support throughout the development of this book. In particular, we are grateful to Eva Hiripi (Editorial Manager) and Daniel Jagadisan (Production Editor) for their patience, professionalism, and continued commitment in guiding this project to completion.

Contents

Part I
Introduction to the Estimand Framework

This opening part of the book provides a comprehensive introduction to the estimand framework, according to the ICH E9(R1) guideline. It describes the role of estimands in the planning, design, conduct, analysis, and interpretation of clinical trials. It also establishes a foundational understanding of the distinctions and interrelationships among estimands, estimators, and estimates, which will be referenced throughout the remainder of this book. In addition, this part offers a step-by-step introduction to the estimand thinking process, including strategies for effective collaborations within multidisciplinary clinical teams. Moreover, a detailed discussion on the documentation of estimands is included, highlighting best practices for transparent reporting and presentation across clinical trial documents. This part of the book also includes an introduction to the principles of causal inference, illustrating how these concepts support the formulation of meaningful clinical questions about causal relationships between an intervention and its effects. Finally, key initiatives and collaborative efforts that have emerged after the release of the ICH E9(R1) guideline are reviewed.

Chapter 1
Aligning Trial Planning, Design, Conduct, Analysis, and Interpretation

Yankun Gong, James Bell, and Jiayu Fu

Abstract Clinical trials are interventional studies that investigate specific health questions in human participants, often studying an investigational treatment in a specific patient population. In 2019, the International Council for Harmonisation of Technical Requirements for Pharmaceuticals for Human Use (ICH) released the E9(R1) guideline for precisely describing treatment effects corresponding to clinical questions of interest in clinical trials. Before the release of the ICH E9(R1) guideline, treatment effects were often ambiguously defined, and descriptions of the clinical questions of interest were usually missing in the protocol, potentially leading to problems with the interpretation of the reported treatment effects. In this introductory chapter, we provide a clinical trial example where the absence of an agreed definition of treatment effect (or estimand, i.e., "what is to be estimated") led to a disagreement between the sponsor and the regulator regarding the clinical question of interest, which impacted the approvability of the drug. Motivated by examples like this, the ICH E9(R1) guideline proposed a structured framework to strengthen the dialogue between disciplines involved in the formulation of clinical trial objectives, design, conduct, analysis, and interpretation, as well as between the sponsor and the regulator regarding the treatment effect(s) of interest that a clinical trial should address. The use of a structed framework formalizes the entire thinking process and communication among different stakeholders. By adopting it, the dilemma in the motivating example could have been avoided.

Y. Gong (✉)
GB&DM, Pfizer (China) Research & Development Co., Ltd, Shanghai, China
e-mail: yankun.gong@pfizer.com

J. Bell
Clinical Operation, Elderbrook Solutions GmbH, High Wycombe, UK
e-mail: james.bell@cantab.net

J. Fu
Biostatistics, Zai Lab (Shanghai) Co., Ltd., Beijing, China
e-mail: jiayu.fu@zailaboratory.com

J. Wei et al. (eds.), *Estimands in Clinical Trials*, Springer Series in Pharmaceutical Statistics, https://doi.org/10.1007/978-3-032-02192-2_1

1.1 Introduction

Clinical trials are prospective research studies on human participants, designed to answer specific health questions. Clinical trials in drug development are usually classified into four phases: Phase I clinical trials are often conducted in healthy volunteers and aim to study the safety, tolerability, and pharmacokinetics of a prospective drug. The questions of interest can be the following: What is the maximum tolerated dose in controlling the dose-limiting toxicity? How and where does the drug distribute within the body? Phase II clinical trials try to provide early evidence of the clinical efficacy of the drug in a targeted population of patients. The questions of interest can include the following: Is there evidence of the drug being effective? What is the optimal dose of the drug? Phase III clinical trials are conducted with the dual purposes of confirming the efficacy and safety of the drug in the specific patient population of interest and, typically, of supporting the regulatory approval of the drug. The questions of interest can include the following: What is the clinical efficacy of the drug? What is the safety profile of the drug? Can the efficacy and safety results from earlier clinical trials be confirmed in a relatively large population? Phase IV clinical trials are generally carried out after the drug has been approved by health authorities to obtain further information about its risks and benefits. The question of interest can be the following: How does the drug work in large, diverse populations over long periods of time? It is important to design the right clinical trials with the right objectives to address the different clinical questions of interest from many key stakeholders, including regulators, sponsors, investigators, patients, and so on.

The International Council for Harmonisation of Technical Requirements for Pharmaceuticals for Human Use (ICH) is unique in bringing together regulatory authorities and the pharmaceutical industry to harmonize technical requirements for medical products, discuss scientific and technical aspects of pharmaceuticals, and develop ICH guidelines. In 2019, the ICH released the E9(R1) guideline on estimands and sensitivity analysis in clinical trials (ICH, 2019) for precisely describing the treatment effect corresponding to a clinical question of interest. Before the release of the ICH E9(R1) guideline, clinical trial protocols already contained statements of the trial objectives, design, procedures, and data analysis plan. However, clear descriptions of the clinical questions of interest were usually missing, sometimes leading to misunderstandings between sponsors and regulators regarding what was being estimated in the clinical trials. In addition, without a clear description of the clinical questions, confusion could also arise as to what data needs to be collected and how to interpret the results. For example, are the data collected relevant to the planned analysis? Do the analysis results precisely answer the clinical questions and thus address the trial objectives?

To address these issues, the ICH E9(R1) guideline presents a structured framework to strengthen the dialogue among different stakeholders regarding the treatment effect of interest that the clinical trial is addressing, as well as the discussions between disciplines involved in the formulation of clinical trial objectives, design, conduct, analysis, and interpretation. In this introductory chapter, we discuss a clinical trial example to further motivate the need for the estimand framework introduced in the ICH E9(R1) guideline.

1.2 Motivating Example

In 2011, the US Food and Drug Administration (FDA) held a public advisory committee meeting (FDA, 2011) on the antidiabetic drug dapagliflozin. It was jointly developed by the pharmaceutical companies AstraZeneca and Bristol Myers Squibb. The primary focus of the meeting was on safety, although one of the FDA statistical reviewers also raised an efficacy issue in their review (Statistical Review and Evaluation of Dapagliflozin, 2014).

The statistical review focused primarily on six clinical trials, all of which had similar designs. Here, we use trial MB102013 (ClinicalTrials.gov identifier: NCT00528372) for illustration purposes. This trial was a multicenter, randomized, double-blind, placebo-controlled, parallel group trial. The aim of the trial was to evaluate the efficacy and safety of dapagliflozin as monotherapy in patients with type 2 diabetes who had inadequate glycemic control with diet and exercise. There was a 24-week short-term, double-blind treatment period and a 78-week long-term, sponsor-open, investigator- and patient-blinded treatment period. The total treatment period in the trial was 102 weeks, but the trial primarily evaluated the treatment effect of dapagliflozin after 24 weeks of double-blind treatment.

Patients with a lack of glycemic control after Week 4 were eligible to receive open-label rescue medication according to the predefined criteria. This was an approved oral antihyperglycemic agent, used according to conventional standards of care. It was used to treat hyperglycemia to reduce the risk of complications. This was both an ethical necessity and a means to help patients remain in the trial. The rescue medication provided by the sponsor in this trial was metformin.

The primary variable of the trial was the change in glycated hemoglobin A1c (HbA1c) from baseline to Week 24. A higher HbA1c value indicates more glucose in the blood over the past 3 months, which increases the risk of patients developing diabetes complications, such as diabetic retinopathy or peripheral vascular disease.

For the primary analysis, the analysis set included all patients with baseline and at least one post-baseline HbA1c values. An analysis of covariance (ANCOVA) model was used to compare the change from baseline values of HbA1c at Week 24 between the dapagliflozin and placebo arms. HbA1c values observed after receiving rescue medication were set to missing. In case of missing HbA1c data at Week 24 or the exclusion of HbA1c data due to the intake of rescue medication prior to Week 24, the last observation carried forward (LOCF) imputation method was used.

When reviewing the trial results, the FDA statistical reviewers disagreed with the primary analysis approach used by the sponsor and suggested an alternative one. The FDA statistical reviewer commented that while the FDA had implicitly endorsed LOCF imputation for diabetes trials in the past, there was now more awareness in the statistical community of the limitations of this approach. Instead, the reviewer had included a sensitivity analysis in which the primary HbA1c outcomes were used, regardless of the rescue medication, and no statistical adjustment was made for rescue. The reviewer argued that while this approach was also imperfect, it came closer to being an intent-to-treat (ITT) analysis (ICH, 2021). The ITT principle cited here asserts that the effect of a treatment policy can be best assessed by evaluating patients on the basis of the intention to treat the patient (i.e., the planned treatment regimen) rather than the actual treatment given to them. It has the consequence that patients allocated to a treatment group should be followed up, assessed, and analyzed as members of that group, irrespective of their compliance with the planned course of treatment (ICH, 1998).

The dapagliflozin example illustrates the different understanding of the sponsor and the regulator regarding the primary trial objective relating to the treatment effect of interest. Essentially, each stakeholder was answering a different clinical question:

- Sponsor: Compare the treatment effect of dapagliflozin versus placebo had patients not received rescue medication.
- Regulator: Compare the treatment effect of dapagliflozin with the addition of rescue medication (if protocol-specified glycemic criteria were met) versus placebo with the addition of rescue medication (if protocol-specified glycemic criteria were met).

Both clinical questions were aligned with the main objective of the trial, which was ambiguously stated in the protocol as to evaluate the efficacy and safety of dapagliflozin as monotherapy in patients with type 2 diabetes who had inadequate glycemic control with diet and exercise. Without a clearly defined clinical question of interest in the trial protocol, differing interpretations and priorities among stakeholders were not identified and discussed in advance. As a result, the sponsor made decisions on the aspects of trial conduct and analysis that were later challenged by regulators.

The dapagliflozin example highlights how the absence of an agreed estimand (i.e., "what is to be estimated") can result in disagreements between sponsors and regulators about the clinical question of interest. In this case, discussions centered on issues around data collection and analysis methods rather than the underlying clinical question of interest. These discussions occurred at the review stage, potentially impacting the drug's approval. Defining "what is to be estimated" at the trial planning stage by formulating the clinical question of interest and ensuring alignment between the sponsor and the regulator can effectively avoid such situations.

1.3 Toward the Development of the ICH E9(R1) Guideline

The ICH E9 guideline, published in 1998, provides guidance on statistical issues in clinical trials, from trial design, conduct, and analysis to evaluation and reporting (ICH, 1998). Many of the principles outlined in this guideline focus on minimizing bias. Bias is the systematic deviation of an estimate from its true value. In clinical trials, bias for treatment effects can come from the effects of any factors associated with the design, conduct, analysis, and interpretation of the results. Since bias can affect, or even invalidate, the conclusions of clinical trials, it is important to identify potential sources of bias in advance and take measures to reduce them.

According to the ICH E9 guideline, two of the most important design techniques to avoid bias in clinical trials are blinding and randomization. Blinding is intended to limit conscious and unconscious bias in the conduct, outcomes, and interpretation of a clinical trial. This can arise from the influence of patients, investigators, and other people involved in the conduct or analysis of the trial if they know what treatment a patient has received. Randomization helps avoid possible bias in the selection and allocation of patients, arising from the predictability of treatment assignments. Missing data is another potential source of bias. The ICH E9 guideline, therefore, emphasizes the need for prespecifying strategies to minimize the occurrence of missing data. It also states that there is no universal solution for handling missing data, and sensitivity analysis should be performed to explore its impact on the analysis results.

One approach to minimize missing data is to follow up with patients for the duration of the whole trial, irrespective of their compliance with the planned course of treatment. If all patients are followed up throughout the trial and all their primary variables are measured, it will provide the complete data of all patients. This approach aligns with the ITT principle in which randomization is the basis for making inferences about treatment effects. The ICH E9 guideline highlights the importance of randomization in this regard and recommends the ITT principle as a standard for statistical inference. This is consistent with the FDA position in the dapagliflozin example cited previously.

In 2010, the US National Research Council published a report on the prevention and treatment of missing data in clinical trials (National Research Council, 2010). This report brought the term "estimand" to the attention of the clinical trial community, introducing it as follows:

> A clinical trial typically measures outcomes that quantify the impact of the interventions under study for a defined period of time. Inference focuses on summaries of these measures (such as the mean) for the target population of interest. These summary quantities are often called parameters, or estimands.

It also states that the choice of estimand involves both the outcome measure and the population of interest.

The report emphasizes that the estimand should be determined first, followed by the selection of the analysis method. Since missing data may limit the comparability between treatment arms and affect the estimation of treatment effects, the handling of missing data should also be considered after selecting the estimand. As the report primarily focuses on the mechanisms of missing data and providing statistical analysis methods under different missing mechanism assumptions, it unfortunately led some readers to mistakenly equate the topic of estimands with the handling of missing data.

In October 2014, the ICH endorsed the final concept paper for the ICH E9(R1) addendum to the ICH E9 guideline, highlighting the issues arising from the absence of guidance on the primary estimand for a confirmatory clinical trial. It introduces an estimand as the property that is to be estimated in the context of a scientific question of interest.

In August 2017, the ICH endorsed a draft version of the ICH E9(R1) guideline for public consultation. In November 2019, ICH released its final E9(R1) guideline on estimands and sensitivity analysis in clinical trials. Since then, the ICH E9(R1) guideline has been implemented by essentially all regulatory ICH members.

The ICH E9(R1) guideline broadened the scope of the estimand discussion, moving beyond the topic of missing data. It proposed a structured framework for formulating the trial objectives, trial design, data collection, data analysis, and result interpretation. This was aimed at strengthening the dialogue among stakeholders, including between sponsors and regulators, on relevant questions to be addressed by clinical trials. This guideline emphasized the importance of causal treatment effects, defining treatment effects as (ICH, 2019, Section A.3)

> how the outcome of treatment compares to what would have happened to the same subjects under alternative treatment (i.e., had they not received the treatment, or had they received a different treatment).

Such (causal) treatment effects are explicitly caused by the treatment, not by potential confounding factors, such as differences in observation periods or patient characteristics; see Chap. 5 for details.

1.4 A Structured Framework

Building on the ICH E9 guideline, the ICH E9(R1) guideline proposed a structured framework (Fig. 1.1) to facilitate alignment from the initial choice of clinical trial objectives to the interpretation of the analysis results. According to this framework, clear trial objectives should be translated into key clinical questions of interest by defining appropriate estimands, which specify the target of estimation for a given trial objective. Once the estimand is defined, a suitable method of estimation, referred to as the main estimator, can be selected. This estimator relies on specific assumptions that underpin its validity. To ensure the robustness of the results and evaluate how sensitive the conclusions are to deviations from these assumptions, sensitivity analyses targeting the same estimand should be performed. Supplementary analyses can be conducted in addition to the main and sensitivity analysis to provide additional insights when answering the clinical question of interest.

Use of the ICH E9(R1) structured framework formalizes the thinking and communication process around trial design. It also helps strengthen the dialogue between disciplines involved in the formulation of clinical trial objectives, design, conduct, analysis, and interpretation to ensure alignment and clarity throughout the entire process. Effective communication between sponsors and regulators is equally

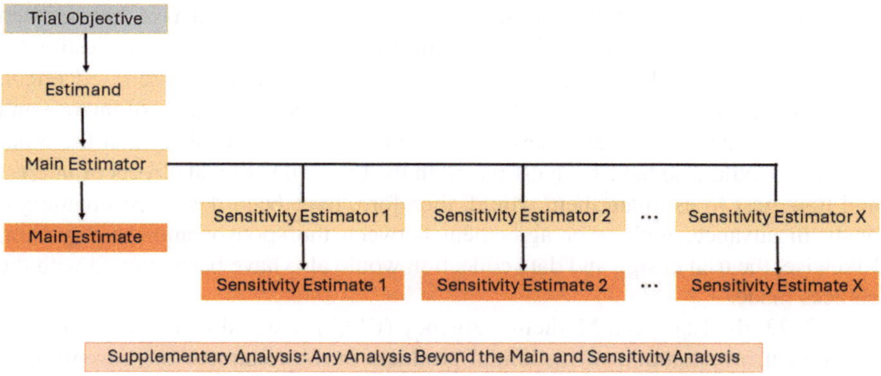

Fig. 1.1 Aligning the target of estimation, method of estimation, and sensitivity analysis for a given trial objective. (This figure is an adaptation of a figure from the ICH E9(R1) guideline (ICH, 2019), modified by adding the boxes to the right and bottom)

critical, particularly regarding the treatment effect(s) a clinical trial is designed to address. The structured framework introduced in the ICH E9(R1) guideline is relevant whenever a treatment effect is estimated or a hypothesis related to a treatment effect is tested, whether related to efficacy or safety. While the main focus of the guideline is on randomized clinical trials, the principles are also applicable for single-arm trials and observational studies.

1.5 Motivating Example Revisited

Having introduced the ICH E9(R1), we now revisit the dapagliflozin example, where there was a disagreement on the clinical question of interest between the sponsor and the regulator. In light of the structured framework, we can now see that the disagreement between the sponsor and the regulator was fundamentally about what was of clinical interest for the treatment effect regarding the use of rescue medication: The sponsor wanted to estimate the treatment effect of dapagliflozin if patients had not taken rescue medication, whereas the FDA wanted to estimate the treatment effect of dapagliflozin with the addition of rescue medication as needed. In other words, they were interested in different estimands but were unable to articulate these differences because the estimand framework was not available at the time. Instead, they discussed the differences in data collection and analysis methods: The sponsor proposed an ANCOVA using the LOCF approach that excluded data after the intake of rescue medication, whereas the regulator preferred an ANCOVA that included data collected after rescue medication.

If the estimand framework had been available during the planning of this trial, the sponsor could have identified at an early stage the importance of rescue medication when describing the clinical question of interest. Discussions, both internally and with the regulator, on the resulting estimand of interest should have then resulted in an agreement on the preferred main estimand, for which an appropriate estimator would have been selected. This may have been the regulator's preferred effect, including the effects of rescue medication. Supplementary estimands of interest and analyses for them would also have been identified, making it likely that the other estimand would also have been estimated in the trial. The clinical effects of interest and how best to estimate them would, therefore, have been described unambiguously in advance, with prior agreement between the sponsor and the regulator. Likewise, the trial design and data collection would also have been aligned with the choices made.

In 2023, the European Medicines Agency (EMA) released its revised guideline on clinical investigation of medicinal products in the treatment or prevention of diabetes mellitus, providing additional insights and advice for constructing appropriate estimands in this therapeutic area (EMA, 2023). This guideline suggests different strategies for handling post-randomization events, such as rescue medication intake and how to handle missing data. It is interesting to note that in the dapagliflozin example, the sponsor implicitly used the same variables and strategies suggested by the EMA (2023) to address rescue medication intake, but a different analysis method was used. Chapter 12 provides more details on the EMA (2023) guideline.

1.6 Concluding Remarks

Clinical trials are planned and conducted to study a treatment's efficacy, safety, and tolerability for a given medical condition. They involve many stakeholders, including trial sponsors, regulators, patients, and investigators. A clear description of the treatment effect of interest is crucial to avoid any misunderstanding of benefits and risks. The ICH E9(R1) guideline provides a structured framework to assist in formulating the clinical questions of interest for clinical trials. This strengthens the dialogue between disciplines involved in the formulation of the clinical trial plan, design, conduct, analysis, and interpretation, as well as between stakeholders regarding the treatment effect(s) of interest that a clinical trial should address. The estimand framework fosters a proactive approach to clearly describing what is to be estimated, a structured language to precisely describe the treatment effect of interest, a collaborative platform for stakeholders to efficiently align on the suitability of clinical trial designs, and the interpretation of clinical trial results.

As stated in the ICH E9(R1) guideline, an estimand is a precise description of the treatment effect, reflecting the clinical question to be addressed by a prespecified clinical trial objective. Five attributes are used to construct an estimand: treatment, population, variable, intercurrent events, and population-level summary. Importantly, the ICH E9(R1) guideline introduces intercurrent events as "events occurring after treatment initiation that affect either the interpretation or the existence of the measurements associated with the clinical question of interest," along with five strategies for addressing them when defining the clinical question of interest (ICH, 2019, Section A.3.1). Chapter 2 provides more details on estimands, intercurrent events, and the five strategies. The implementation of the ICH E9(R1) guideline through the proposed estimand framework is a multidisciplinary effort and helps align the target of estimation, method of estimation, and sensitivity analysis for a given trial; see Chap. 3 for more details. Moreover, it promotes the standardization of clinical trials, which also impacts various aspects of clinical trial operations, including trial design, data collection, statistical analysis, and result interpretation. Chapter 4 provides details on the documentation of estimands and reporting of results.

References

EMA (2023) Guideline on clinical investigation of medicinal products in the treatment or prevention of diabetes mellitus. Available at: https://www.ema.europa.eu/

FDA briefing Document for the July 19, 2011 Meeting of the Endocrinologic and Metabolic Drugs Advisory Committee (2011). Available at: http://web.archive.org/web/20161024142229if_/http://www.fda.gov/downloads/AdvisoryCommittees/CommitteesMeetingMaterials/Drugs/EndocrinologicandMetabolicDrugsAdvisoryCommittee/UCM262994.pdf. Accessed 21 May 2024.

ICH (1998) E9 statistical principles for clinical trials. Step 5 available at https://ich.org/

ICH. (2019). E9(R1) addendum on estimands and sensitivity analysis in clinical trials to the guideline on statistical principles for clinical trials. Step 4 document available at https://ich.org/

ICH (2021) E9(R1) training material. Available at https://ich.org/

National Research Council. (2010). *The prevention and treatment of missing data in clinical trials*. National Academies Press (US). Available at http://www.nap.edu/

Statistical Review and Evaluation of Dapagliflozin (2014). Available at: 202293Orig1s000StatR.pdf (fda.gov) Accessed 21 May 2024.

Chapter 2
Estimands, Estimators, and Estimates

Jiayu Fu, James Bell, Juan Zhang, and Feng Chen

Abstract The International Council for Harmonization (ICH) E9(R1) guideline introduces a structured framework to align planning, design, conduct, analysis, and result interpretation for clinical trials. Defining an estimand is one of the key elements in the framework, connecting the initial choice of clinical objectives and the interpretation of the analysis results. It is a precise description of the treatment effect, reflecting the clinical question of interest. An estimand comprises five attributes, which include the population, variable, treatment, intercurrent events, and population-level summary. Intercurrent events are a new concept proposed in the ICH E9(R1) guideline. They occur during the patients' treatment journey and affect the existence or interpretation of the outcomes. The ICH E9(R1) guideline offers five main strategies to handle intercurrent events. Different strategies reflect different clinical questions of interest and have different impacts on the estimand attributes. For a given estimand, the main estimator provides its main estimate; sensitivity estimator(s) test the robustness of the main estimate to the assumptions for the main estimator. Supplementary analyses are conducted in addition to the main and sensitivity analyses with the intent to provide additional insights into the understanding of the treatment effect. Aligning estimation to specific estimands highlights whether statistical methods assess the same or different clinical questions of interest and links the results of estimation back to whether the trial objectives are met.

J. Fu (✉)
Department of Biostatistics, Zai Lab (Shanghai) Co., Ltd., Beijing, China
e-mail: jiayu.fu@zailaboratory.com

J. Bell
Department of Clinical Operations, Elderbrook Solutions GmbH, High Wycombe, UK
e-mail: james.bell@cantab.net

J. Zhang
Department of Statistics, Beone Medicines (Beijing) Co., Ltd., Beijing, China
e-mail: juan1.zhang@beigene.com

F. Chen
School of Public Health, Nanjing Medical Universtiy, Nanjing, China
e-mail: fengchen@njmu.edu.cn

J. Wei et al. (eds.), *Estimands in Clinical Trials*, Springer Series in Pharmaceutical Statistics, https://doi.org/10.1007/978-3-032-02192-2_2

2.1 Introduction

According to the ICH E9(R1) guideline, estimands are defined as a precise description of the treatment effect, reflecting the clinical question posed by the trial objective (ICH 2019). The structured framework introduced in Chap. 1 (Fig. 1.1) aligns the objectives of a clinical trial with its design, conduct, and analysis methods by constructing the estimand. The purpose of introducing estimands is to precisely and transparently define the target of estimation and separate this clearly from how it is being estimated. Precise description of estimands has implications for trial design, conduct, labeling, and communication with key stakeholders, such as regulators, sponsors, investigators, and patients (Akacha et al. 2017). It also refines the clinical questions of interest, which are aligned with the trial objectives, and provides clarity to the analysis. Previously, the link between what was being estimated and the trial objectives was often unclear, as demonstrated by the dapagliflozin example discussed in Chap. 1. It was also ambiguous about whether alternative statistical analyses aimed at assessing the same or different treatment effects. Such issues could obscure whether the trial objectives were met, even when results were statistically significant.

One key purpose of drug development is to assess both the existence and magnitude of a treatment effect. To achieve this, we must carefully consider what we mean by "treatment effect" and ask ourselves questions such as:

- Which outcomes are we comparing and between which treatments?
- What patients are we targeting?
- How do we summarize the treatment effect?
- How do we handle changes during trial conduct and their effects on outcomes?

Indeed, precisely defining the treatment effect of interest requires specification of the treatments (or treatment regimens) to be compared, the target population, the primary variable of interest, and its population-level summary measure, as well as potential impactful events occurring post-treatment initiation. These events generally include those occurring during the patients' treatment journey, which may impact the definition of treatment effect. These events are referred to as intercurrent events in the ICH E9(R1) guideline.

In this chapter, we describe in more detail the key elements in the structured framework introduced in Chap. 1: estimands, estimators, and estimates. We begin by discussing the new concept of intercurrent events in Sect. 2.2. Their interplay with clinical questions of interest is then explored in Sect. 2.3. In Sect. 2.4, the definitions of estimands are described. Following this, we examine the strategies for addressing intercurrent events and their impacts on estimands in Sect. 2.5. Finally, the estimation of estimands is introduced in Sect. 2.6.

2.2 Intercurrent Events

The ICH E9(R1) guideline introduces the concept of intercurrent events to help with the precise definition of treatment effects in clinical trials. Intercurrent events are defined as events occurring after treatment initiation that affect either the interpretation or the existence of the outcomes associated with the clinical question of interest. They are essential for describing treatment effects as they could represent changes occurring post-treatment initiation and impact outcomes. According to the definition, we recommend considering the intercurrent events from the following three points:

1. It should be an event that occurs after the initiation of the treatment or treatment regimen. For example, events that occurred before the treatment or treatment regimen, such as having previously received a particular intervention, do not fall within the scope of intercurrent events.
2. It would either prevent the outcomes associated with the clinical question of interest from subsequently existing or affect the interpretation of the outcomes. Death, for instance, is a prime example of an intercurrent event that prevents future outcomes from existing, provided that death is not part of the outcome itself. Intercurrent events that affect the interpretation of outcomes relevant to the clinical question often involve a change in patient treatment, either in terms of the investigated treatment(s) or other treatments. For example, initiating additional medication during treatment is typically considered an intercurrent event, as the outcome is likely to vary with or without the additional medication.
3. Missing data itself is not an intercurrent event. However, missing data is frequently associated with intercurrent events. For example, if a patient discontinues study medication because of an adverse event or lack of efficacy (the intercurrent event), then it is not uncommon for the patient to withdraw consent, thus leading to a missing data problem.

Intercurrent events occur during a patient's treatment journey. In a randomized clinical trial, their impact cannot usually be minimized through randomization. Intercurrent events do not always have to be viewed as defects to sidestep in clinical trials, particularly when they are likely to happen in real clinical practice. They are also not the same as protocol deviations, although some protocol deviations are intercurrent events and should be minimized as much as possible.

It is important to thoughtfully evaluate the potential reasons for intercurrent events during trial planning. For example, the intercurrent event of treatment discontinuation can occur for various reasons: a perceived lack of efficacy, adverse events, or patient withdrawal from treatment due to logistical difficulties of remaining in the trial. Understanding these reasons helps in selecting appropriate strategies for addressing intercurrent events, which are introduced in Sect. 2.5.

The expected frequency of intercurrent events is also important. It can depend on the treatment and may affect the choice of strategies. For instance, the intercurrent event of taking rescue medication due to a lack of efficacy may be more likely to occur in the control arm than in the investigational arm, whereas the opposite may hold for discontinuation due to adverse events.

According to the ICH E9(R1) guideline, the description of intercurrent events might theoretically include very specific details of changes occurring post-treatment initiation, such as a single missed dose of a chronic treatment or a dose taken at the wrong time of the day. If such specific criteria are unlikely to affect the interpretation of the outcome, addressing them as intercurrent events may not be necessary. Some events may occur with extremely low frequencies and be deemed negligible. However, this may cause difficulties if such an event does occur but no strategy to handle it has been prespecified. For example, patient death in a clinical trial of a nonfatal condition may be deemed too rare to consider, but it could still happen. More discussion is provided in Sect. 3.4 of Chap. 3 for the identification of intercurrent events.

In summary, we recommend comprehensively anticipating and prospectively considering the reasons, frequencies, relationship to treatment, and relevance to outcomes of intercurrent events when defining estimands.

2.3 Clinical Questions of Interest

The motivation for every clinical trial and its design is described by its objectives (Bell et al. 2021). The clinical question of interest is, therefore, aligned with the defined trial objective. It is common to describe the trial objective based on the target population, the treatments being compared, and the variables of interest, such as the wording of "to assess the superiority of new drug monotherapy versus placebo in symptom reduction in patients with some disease." Before the publication of the ICH E9(R1) guideline, the statement of the clinical question was generally vague and a repetition of the trial objective. The drawbacks of a vague description of the clinical question were gradually revealed with increased debates among stakeholders, just as for the dapagliflozin example mentioned in Chap. 1.

The ICH E9(R1) guideline highlights the importance of concisely defining the treatment effect of interest in the clinical question. Precise specification of the clinical question is, therefore, crucial in clinical research, taking into account not only the population, treatments, and the variable stated in the trial objective but also the intercurrent events. These events can affect the study treatment, the population, and the variable. Constructing the estimand requires careful consideration of the intercurrent events, as different ways of accounting for intercurrent events may result in different clinical questions of interest (Casey et al. 2020). In Sect. 3.5 of Chap. 3, the formulation of clinical questions of interest is discussed more elaborately.

2.4 Estimands and Their Attributes

Estimands precisely describe what is to be estimated in alignment with the clinical question of interest. The ICH E9(R1) guideline outlines the five attributes of estimands.

(a) Population
Population refers to the set of patients targeted by the clinical question. It is the target population for the investigated treatment or treatment regimen. It is the population-level set of patients rather than the sample-level set of patients that are in the trial. In essence, it represents potential patients for whom we infer treatment benefits, not just the actual patients recruited in the clinical trial. In general, the population should be well-defined in terms of indication (e.g., specific type, severity, or degree of progression) and, if applicable, demographics (e.g., age or sex) and treatment status (e.g., previous or current therapies).

(b) Variable
The variable, also referred to as the endpoint, is the patient-level measurement (or derivation thereof) used to assess the treatment effect. The description should include units, time (or time frame), and any requirements for its assessment (e.g., investigator-assessed or independently adjudicated). It is important to avoid describing the variable using summary measures across patients (e.g., the proportion of patients with a response).

(c) Treatment
The treatment attribute should describe the treatments that are under assessment. Along with the specific descriptions of the investigational and potential control treatment(s) under assessment, any required background therapies should also be outlined. Any further concomitant therapies on top of the background therapies for the indication that patients may use should also be covered in the treatment attribute. In other words, it can be characterized as an individual therapy or a series of therapies with or without a predefined sequence.

(d) Intercurrent Events
We provided the definition of intercurrent events and a discussion of their potential interplay with the treatment effect in Sect. 2.2. Different ways of addressing intercurrent events define different treatment effects and, hence, reflect different clinical questions. The ICH E9(R1) guideline proposes five strategies, which account for the interplay of the intercurrent events and other estimand attributes. We further discuss these strategies in Sect. 2.5.

(e) Population-Level Summary
Population-level summary is the description of how the patient-level outcomes will be combined and summarized, both within and between the arms of treatment conditions. For instance, within the arms, binary outcomes might be summarized as proportions and, between arms, as odds ratio, risk ratio, or risk difference. Although summary measures are commonly single numbers, in a broader sense, they may also take the form of functions over time, such as a survival distribution for a time-to-event endpoint.

Precisely specifying these five attributes results in a clear definition of the treatment effect of interest and refines the clinical question of interest. Documentation practice of estimands is introduced in Chap. 4, and case studies illustrating estimands for different therapeutic areas are discussed in Part II of the book. There are some points that warrant special mention.

- For the population attribute, typically, its characteristics align with the trial's main inclusion/exclusion criteria. However, there does not have to be complete correspondence, as some criteria might stem from trial ethics or logistics.
- For the attribute of population-level summary, it is important to ensure that the summary measure is a quantity that exists at the population (rather than the patient) level. For example, the mean of a continuous variable typically exists at a population level (if all population members have a value).
- While we discuss estimands in terms of treatment effects throughout this chapter, the attributes still apply to the single-arm setting. Examples include pharmacokinetic studies in early drug development or single-arm trials involving indirect comparisons against a threshold based on historical data, as introduced in Sects. 21.2 and 21.4 of Chap. 21, respectively.

2.5 Strategies to Address Intercurrent Events

When intercurrent events occur, determining how to address them naturally becomes the next concern. The ICH E9(R1) guideline proposes five main strategies to address intercurrent events and their interplay with other estimand attributes. Additional strategies can be established in principle. Different formulations of the clinical question of interest correspond to different strategies being selected for intercurrent events. In this section, we introduce the five proposed strategies and illustrate them based on a toy example, which was inspired by the dapagliflozin trial discussed in Chap. 1.

2.5.1 An Illustrative Example

The primary objective of our illustrative trial is to assess whether investigational treatment A is superior to standard treatment B in terms of the mean change of glycated hemoglobin (HbA1c) from baseline to Week 24 for a population of patients with type 2 diabetes. HbA1c (in units of mmol/mol) represents how much hemoglobin in the blood has become glycated (chemically bonded with glucose). A high HbA1c indicates higher blood sugar levels and, consequently, a greater likelihood of developing diabetes complications.

The change in HbA1c from baseline to Week 24 is the primary variable of the trial and is measured as a continuous variable. A reduction of the HbA1c value from baseline to Week 24 indicates a risk reduction of macrovascular or microvascular complications (Zoungas et al. 2012), which is a positive outcome. Readers can refer to Sect. 12.2 of Chap. 12 for further discussion on type 2 diabetes.

Eligible patients are randomly assigned to receive either investigational treatment A or standard treatment B. These treatments are administered weekly for at least 24 weeks. Patients' HbA1c values are evaluated at baseline (pretreatment) and every 8 weeks thereafter. During the 24-week treatment period, patients who show a lack of glycemic control may receive rescue medication to treat hyperglycemia, which can affect the primary outcome interpretation. Therefore, the use of rescue medication during study treatment is considered an intercurrent event.

We illustrate the example in Fig. 2.1, where the treatment assignments and changes in HbA1c values for four patients (IDs: A1, A2, B1, and B2) are shown, without loss of generality. Two patients (IDs: B1 and B2) assigned to treatment B experience the intercurrent event. When it occurs, the patient's state transitions from "Treatment B" to "Treatment B with rescue medication." Without the occurrence of the intercurrent event, the values of HbA1c from baseline to Week 24 for patients A1 and A2 are -21 mmol/mol and -19 mmol/mol, respectively. However, the situation is more complex for patients B1 and B2, and we need to discuss the interplay between the use of rescue medication and the clinical question of interest.

2.5.2 *Five Strategies for Addressing Intercurrent Events*

In this subsection, we discuss the five intercurrent event strategies proposed in the ICH E9(R1) guideline.

2.5.2.1 Treatment Policy Strategy

Under a treatment policy strategy, the effects of the intercurrent event are considered and included in the treatment effect, in alignment with the clinical question of interest. This implies that the intercurrent event becomes part of the assessed treatment policy. Consequently, the occurrence of the intercurrent event is important and should not be ignored, as it affects the outcome of interest, and these outcomes are considered relevant. When treatment policy strategy handles all intercurrent events in a randomized controlled trial, the effect of assigning/prescribing patients to one treatment policy versus another is assessed. Treatment policy is, therefore, usually not a direct assessment of the "pure" efficacy of the investigated treatment itself.

In the illustrative example, under this strategy, we are interested in the treatment effect, including the effects of rescue medication use. Specifically, we are comparing two treatment policies: A with rescue medication as needed versus B with rescue medication as needed rather than A versus B. The observed changes in HbA1c from baseline to Week 24 for patients B1 and B2 (i.e., −16 mmol/mol and -14 mmol/

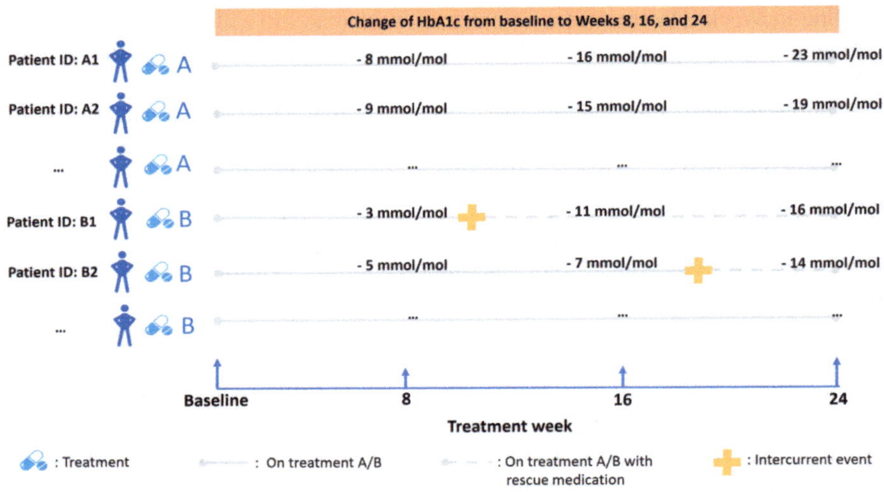

Fig. 2.1 An illustrative example

mol, respectively) are relevant for the primary outcome of interest accordingly. The estimated treatment effect comes not only from the study treatment but also from rescue medication. Thus, the intercurrent event affects the treatment attribute.

The ICH E9(R1) guideline specifically points out that for intercurrent events that transition the patient's state to an absorbing type (such as death), the treatment policy strategy cannot be used because the outcome does not exist after the occurrence of such an intercurrent event.

2.5.2.2 Hypothetical Strategies

When using hypothetical strategies for an intercurrent event, the focus is on a specific hypothetical scenario where the intercurrent event would or would not occur. Different hypothetical scenarios can be envisaged, making the hypothetical strategy a class of potential strategies.

In the illustrative example, if the clinical question of interest is to evaluate the efficacy of the investigated treatment itself, it is conceivable to define the hypothetical scenario of "if the patient does not have access to rescue medication for the 24-week duration."

When adopting a hypothetical strategy, it is crucial to precisely describe and thoroughly justify the hypothetical scenario (FDA 2022). Simply presuming that the intercurrent event would not have occurred in the hypothetical scenario is inadequate; it is also important to contemplate what would have taken place or could realistically take place instead. We recommend fully describing and justifying the hypothetical scenario for both clinical and regulatory purposes. For example, stating "assume patients did not use rescue medication" is not precise enough, as there are at least two possible situations: (1) No rescue medication was available, and (2) the patient was not expected to require it. Different hypothetical scenarios have different clinical meanings and result in different treatment effects.

The alternative scenario under the hypothetical strategy is usually unobserved, which creates missing data issues. Consequently, statistical inference becomes more dependent on missing data assumptions for hypothetical strategies.

2.5.2.3 Composite Variable Strategies

In composite variable strategies, the intercurrent event itself is viewed as part of the variable of interest, and the clinical question of interest encompasses its occurrence. Often, intercurrent events reflect unfavorable outcomes and are defined as such within the variable. This is most common for death (as the intercurrent event) in trials with binary or event-based variables. Composite variable strategies can also be applied to continuous variables, but this requires additional considerations (Permutt and Li 2017; Wang et al. 2018).

In our illustrative example, patients with a lack of glycemic control might receive rescue medication. As rescue medication intake indicates a lack of efficacy of the study treatment, a composite strategy could be adopted whereby an unfavorable outcome is assigned to patients requiring rescue medication. In this context, an outcome value or rank (or an algorithm for determining them) is prespecified as part of the variable definition. For instance, we could prespecify patients B1 and B2's HbA1c value after Week 24 as a number indicating an unfavorable outcome, such as 86 mmol/mol, based on a 10% threshold (Esposito et al. 2011). Their change from baseline, as the primary variable, can then be obtained accordingly.

Under the composite strategy, the intercurrent event affects the variable attribute of the estimand. There are common examples that are often not even recognized as intercurrent events. For instance, in oncology clinical trials, one might define progression-free survival as a variable of interest, where the intercurrent event of death is incorporated into the variable's definition.

2.5.2.4 While on Treatment Strategies

When using while on treatment strategies for the intercurrent event, only the treatment effect before the occurrence of the intercurrent event is considered, and the outcomes after the occurrence of the intercurrent event are considered to be irrelevant for the clinical question of interest.

Under while on treatment strategies, if a clinical trial includes repeated measurements for the same patient, the measurements taken up to the occurrence of the intercurrent event may be used to define the variable quantifying the treatment effect of interest. The variable "area under the curve" is a typical example of this approach. Alternatively, the last observation taken while on treatment may also be used as part of the variable definition, although it is a single measurement.

It is crucial that a patient's measurements relevant to the variable can be defined for all patients, regardless of the time until the intercurrent event; otherwise, the estimand will be undefined. This constraint limits the types of variables that can be used for a while on treatment strategy. For example, a measure for treatment effect at Week 52 would be undefined under this strategy, as some patients will not remain on treatment until then. However, one could define an average measure for treatment effect over time up to Week 52 while on treatment, as the period that they were on treatment can be used.

In the illustrative example, the HbA1c values are repeatedly measured every eight weeks. An average change of HbA1c from baseline may serve to quantify the treatment effect if it answers the clinical question of interest. Consequently, the primary variable transitions from being strictly the "change of HbA1c from baseline to Week 24" to the "average change of HbA1c from baseline to Week 24 or before receiving rescue medication." In this case, the use of this strategy affects the variable attribute of the estimand.

Particular care is required if the occurrence of the intercurrent event differs between the treatments being compared. If the occurrence depends on the treatment, it may not only directly reflect the treatment's tolerability but also indirectly reflect the treatment effect itself, as the need for rescue therapy may indicate a lack of efficacy. In our example, receiving rescue medication is more likely to occur in patients with treatment B. This may supportively indicate that treatment A has a better effect in keeping patients' compliance.

2.5.2.5 Principal Stratum Strategies

The principal stratum strategy focuses on the population of interest, referred to as the principal stratum, comprising patients for whom an intercurrent event would or would not occur, regardless of treatment allocation or if assigned a particular treatment. The treatment effect is assessed within a subset of patients who either would or would not experience the intercurrent event.

We must differentiate between principal stratum strategies and subgroup analysis (Bornkamp et al. 2021; Lipkovich et al. 2022). The principal stratum pertains to a population that would or would not experience intercurrent events in either arm, whereas subgroup analysis is based on the intercurrent events actually experienced in the assigned arm only. In the illustrative example, patients B1 and B2, who receive rescue medication, belong to the subgroup with intercurrent events. They may or may not belong to the principal stratum of interest, which is defined here as the population that would not receive rescue medication regardless of treatment assignment. Using this strategy affects the population attribute of the estimand.

Determining membership in the principal stratum can sometimes be achieved through special trial designs, such as a crossover design, which provides greater opportunities for implementing this strategy because comparisons are made within the same patients (Matthews et al. 2022). More commonly, membership is estimated through statistical techniques from causal inference, as discussed in Chaps. 5 and 19 of this book.

The principal stratum strategy can pose issues of interpretation since any inference may exclude a large proportion of the total population, with usually no a priori means of identifying which patients belong to it. Moreover, there is also an open question regarding whether patients who never experience an intercurrent event actually exist or if their status is at least partially a function of circumstances and/or luck. This uncertainty raises concerns that the underlying population of interest for this estimand may not truly exist.

2.5.3 *Choice of Strategies*

The choice of strategies to address intercurrent events depends on the definitions of the intercurrent event and the clinical questions of interest. We recommend clearly specifying the intercurrent events with the occurrence reason in constructing estimands. For example, knowing the specific reasons for the intercurrent event of an early termination of treatment provides information for determining the strategies. If a patient withdraws treatment due to a lack of efficacy, the composite variable strategy may be used by considering the patient as a nonresponder; if the patient withdraws due to moving, the hypothetical strategy may be used by assuming that the treatment is not discontinued early. For real cases of intercurrent events and addressing strategies, we refer to Part II of the book.

Among the five strategies, three have clear links to specific attributes of the estimand: The treatment policy strategy relates to the treatment attribute, the composite variable strategy to the variable attribute, and the principal stratum strategy to the population attribute. Hypothetical strategies have a more general impact on multiple attributes, depending on the hypothetical scenarios applied. The while on treatment strategy considers the effect up to or at the time of intercurrent events and imposes some strict limitations on the patient-level variable, requiring that the variable exists regardless of when the intercurrent event occurs.

2.5.4 *Combination of Strategies*

Typically, multiple types of intercurrent events occur in a clinical question of interest. It is often desirable to handle these events with different strategies. For example, consider a major treatment change (e.g., dose interruption for more than 1 week due to COVID-19) as another intercurrent event that could impact the interpretation of the outcome in the previous illustrative example. Although this could be handled by the same strategy as that for receiving rescue medication, it may be clinically preferable to take a different approach. A combination of the strategies for the two intercurrent events may need to be considered.

Sometimes, combinations of strategies are straightforward to apply. For instance, the combination of a treatment policy strategy for a major treatment change, with a composite variable strategy for receiving rescue medication, gives the following estimand attributes:

- Treatment: treatments A and B, regardless of major treatment change.
- Variable:
  - change of HbA1c from baseline to 86 mmol/mol in case of rescue medication intake.
  - change of HbA1c from baseline to Week 24 otherwise.

Sometimes, additional attention is required when combining strategies. For example, when using hypothetical and treatment policy strategies for different types of events, it is essential to clarify under the hypothetical scenario whether the other type of intercurrent event may or may not occur. The order of multiple intercurrent events within a patient often matters and requires careful consideration and definition in both estimand construction and subsequent estimation methods.

2.6 Estimators and Estimates

The structured framework (Fig. 1.1) introduced by the ICH E9(R1) guideline also aligns estimands and their estimation for a given trial objective. Matching estimation to specific estimands highlights whether statistical methods assess the same or different quantities. Additionally, it links the results of estimation back to whether the trial objectives were met.

Estimators are the methods used to estimate a given estimand. They are formally defined in the ICH E9(R1) guideline as a method of analysis to compute an estimate of the estimand using clinical trial data. The estimator produces an estimate, a numerical value, to support the interpretation of results and quantify the treatment effect. It also provides confidence or credible intervals to reflect the certainty in those estimates and forms a basis for statistical decision-making. All estimators rely on assumptions, and whether an estimate is interpretable depends on the nature and robustness of the assumptions made in the analysis. Assumptions need to be explicitly stated and justifiable.

Therefore, for each estimand, a main estimator should be defined, along with its clear assumptions. The assumptions should include those relating to the analysis methods for treatment effect estimation and statistical inference. It is particularly important to clarify assumptions regarding the handling of data that are missing either because they were not collected or because they are not used under an intercurrent event strategy.

Consequently, in addition to the main analysis, sensitivity analysis needs to be conducted to test the robustness of the estimates to the assumptions for the main estimator. This may involve changing the type of analysis model, modifying model terms (such as covariates), or, most commonly, introducing different assumptions around the missing data. Since sensitivity analysis is intended to check the impact of the statistical method used on estimation, it inherently targets the same estimand as the main estimator.

For an estimand, there should be one main estimator and one or more sensitivity estimators, resulting in one or more sensitivity estimates. When selecting sensitivity analyses, it is recommended to modify one statistical assumption at a time. Simultaneously, changing multiple aspects of assumptions makes it difficult to determine which specific assumption(s) are responsible for any differences in results.

Supplementary analysis generally refers to an analysis conducted in addition to the main and sensitivity analyses, with the intent of providing additional insights into the treatment effect. It supports the interpretation of trial results based on the main estimator for each agreed estimand, often corresponding to a different estimand than the main estimand. For example, this might involve estimating a hypothetical strategy rather than the treatment policy strategy that was defined as part of the main estimand. Alternatively, it could involve analyzing a dichotomized responder variable rather than the underlying continuous variable in the main estimand. Supplementary analysis is generally used to provide context to the estimates of the main estimand or support its conclusions and is typically considered lower in priority for the evaluation of results.

Sometimes, it is not clear when an analysis is a supplementary analysis of another estimand or a stand-alone estimand in its own right. This is subjective and typically based upon whether the estimand of the supplementary analysis is important enough to stand alone or if it is most useful in supporting another estimand. Therefore, we recommend labeling each analysis as being main, sensitivity, or supplementary to clearly state the purpose of the analysis and identify the estimand it targets. More discussion on the estimation of estimands can be found in Sect. 3.8 of Chap. 3 and Part IV of the book.

2.7 Concluding Remarks

An estimand is the precise definition of the treatment effect to be quantified in order to answer the clinical questions of interest. Intercurrent events, a concept introduced in the ICH E9(R1) guideline, are among the five key attributes of estimands. These events need to be addressed when describing the clinical question of interest and when defining estimands.

For a given estimand, an aligned main estimator should be implemented to provide an estimate for the reliable interpretation of the treatment effect. Sensitivity estimators, based on the same estimand, are selected to evaluate the robustness of the main estimator. Supplementary estimators are always based on different but related estimands and provide additional insights for understanding the treatment effect.

References

Akacha, M., Bretz, F., & Ruberg, S. (2017). Estimands in clinical trials–broadening the perspective. *Statistics in Medicine, 36*, 5–19.

Bell, J., Hamilton, A., Sailer, O., & Voss, F. (2021). The detailed clinical objectives approach to designing clinical trials and choosing estimands. *Pharmaceutical Statistics, 20*(6), 1112–1124.

Bornkamp, B., Rufibach, K., Lin, J., Liu, Y., Mehrotra, D. V., Roychoudhury, S., Schmidli, H., Shentu, Y., & Wolbers, M. (2021). Principal stratum strategy: potential role in drug development. *Pharmaceutical Statistics, 20*(4), 737–751.

Casey, M., Degtyarev, E., Lechuga, M. J., Aimone, P., Ravaud, A., Motzer, R. J., Liu, F., Stalbovskaya, V., Tang, R., Butler, E., Sailer, O., Halabi, S., & George, D. (2020). Estimand framework: Are we asking the right questions? A case study in the solid tumor setting. *Pharmaceutical Statistics., 20*(2), 324–334.

Esposito, K., Chiodini, P., Bellastella, G., Maiorino, M. I., & Giugliano, D. (2011). Proportion of patients at HbA1c target <7% with eight classes of antidiabetic drugs in type 2 diabetes: Systematic review of 218 randomized controlled trials with 78 945 patients. *Diabetes, Obesity and Metabolism, 14*(3), 228–233.

FDA. (2022). *Estimand framework implementation*. Short course SC06 given at RISW 2022.

ICH. (2019). *ICH E9 (R1) addendum on estimands and sensitivity analysis in clinical trials to the guideline on statistical principles for clinical trials*. Step 4 document available at https://ich.org/

Lipkovich, I., Ratitch, B., Qu, Y., Zhang, X., Shan, M., & Mallinckrodt, C. (2022). Using principal stratification in analysis of clinical trials. *Statistics in Medicine, 41*(19), 3837–3877.

Matthews, J., Bazakou, S., Henderson, R., & Sharples, L. (2022). Contrasting principal stratum and hypothetical strategy estimands in multi-period crossover trials with incomplete data. *Biometrics, 79*(3), 1896–1907.

Permutt, T., & Li, F. (2017). Trimmed means for symptom trials with dropouts. *Pharmaceutical Statistics, 16*(1), 20–28.

Wang, M., Liu, J., Molenberghs, G., and Mallinckrodt, CH. (2018). An evaluation of the trimmed mean approach in clinical trials with dropout. Pharmaceutical Statistics 17(3), 278–289.

Zoungas, S., Chalmers, J., Ninomiya, T., Li, Q., Cooper, M. E., Colagiuri, S., Fulcher, G., Galan, G. E., Harrap, S., Hamet, P., Heller, S., MacMahon, S., Marre, M., Poulter, N., Travert, F., Patel, A., Neal, B., & Woodward, M. (2012). Association of HbA1c levels with vascular complications and death in patients with type 2 diabetes: Evidence of glycemic thresholds. *Diabetologia, 55*, 636–643.

Chapter 3
Implementation of the Estimand Thinking Process Through Multidisciplinary Collaborations

Elena Polverejan, Bharani Dharan, and Juan Zhang

Abstract The implementation of the estimand framework can be facilitated effectively by following the steps of an estimand thinking process in line with the principles laid out in the ICH E9(R1) guideline. This process requires collaborative efforts from multidisciplinary teams, including statisticians, clinicians, and professionals from other groups such as regulatory affairs and clinical operations. This chapter describes the seven steps of the estimand thinking process, related to trial objectives, intercurrent events, clinical questions, estimands, trial design, analysis approaches, and documentation. These steps will be illustrated by a practical application from a hypothetical case study on major depressive disorder (MDD). The description of the estimand thinking process and the case study is intended to be a practical aid to clinical trial teams in applying the estimand framework to clinical trials. This chapter also highlights the importance of multidisciplinary collaborations in implementing the estimand thinking process.

3.1 Introduction

As described in Chap. 1, the estimand framework is a structured trial planning framework proposed by ICH (2019) that promotes transparency and dialogue between sponsors and regulators on relevant questions to be addressed by a clinical

E. Polverejan
Quantitative Sciences and Clinical Pharmacology, Johnson & Johnson, Titusville, NJ, USA
e-mail: epolvere@its.jnj.com

B. Dharan
Advanced Quantitative Science, Novartis Pharmaceuticals, East Hanover, USA
e-mail: bharani.bharani-dharan@novartis.com

J. Zhang (✉)
Department of Statistics, Beone Medicines (Beijing) Co., Ltd, Beijing, China
e-mail: juan1.zhang@beonemed.com

J. Wei et al. (eds.), *Estimands in Clinical Trials*, Springer Series in Pharmaceutical Statistics, https://doi.org/10.1007/978-3-032-02192-2_3

trial. This framework ensures the alignment of trial objectives and clinical questions of interest with trial design, data collection, data analysis, and result interpretation.

The implementation of the estimand framework is facilitated by following the steps of an estimand thinking process introduced with the ICH E9(R1) training material (ICH 2021). This process requires collaborative efforts from multidisciplinary teams, including statisticians, clinicians, and professionals from other groups such as regulatory affairs and clinical operations. Their involvement is critical from the planning phase to the conduct and reporting of the trial.

In this chapter, we will first introduce the estimand thinking process in Sect. 3.2. We will then discuss how to implement each step of the estimand thinking process in Sects. 3.3 through 3.9. We will also emphasize the importance of multidisciplinary collaborations in Sect. 3.10.

3.2 Estimand Thinking Process

The concept of the estimand thinking process builds upon the structured framework described in Sect. 1.4 of Chap. 1. In this section, we provide a detailed discussion of this thinking process, outlining a comprehensive approach that encompasses the following seven steps:

1. Define trial objectives: Begin by clearly defining the objectives of the trial, taking into account the therapeutic context and the intended application of the treatment. This foundational step ensures that the trial's direction is firmly rooted in its clinical purpose.
2. Identify intercurrent events: Recognize and catalog potential events that occur after treatment initiation and affect either the interpretation of treatment effect, such as treatment discontinuation or the use of additional therapies, or the existence of the measurements associated with the clinical question of interest. Understanding these events is crucial for the interpretation of the trial's results.
3. Formulate clinical questions: Develop specific, clinically relevant questions that the trial aims to answer, incorporating strategies for managing intercurrent events. This step bridges the gap between clinical objectives and the estimand description.
4. Describe the estimands: Describe the estimands that encapsulate the trial's questions in precise language, ensuring a clear target for the analysis. This critical step translates clinical queries into quantifiable treatment effects.
5. Align trial design choices: Tailor the trial's design and data collection methods to support the estimands, ensuring that every aspect of the trial contributes to answering the key questions.
6. Select suitable analysis approaches: Choose appropriate statistical methods for estimating the defined estimands, including both main analyses and sensitivity analyses. This alignment is essential for drawing valid conclusions from the trial data.

7. Document the chosen estimands: Document the estimands and their underlying rationale, providing a clear roadmap for estimating the defined estimands.

These steps, echoing the framework outlined in the ICH E9(R1) training material (ICH 2021), offer a structured yet flexible approach to trial planning and analysis. While the process is designed to be sequential, it inherently accommodates iteration, allowing for refinement and adaptation as the trial planning progresses and new insights emerge.

In the following sections, we will discuss how to implement each step of this process. A case study will be used to exemplify each step. This case study is based on a hypothetical confirmatory trial for short-term monotherapy treatment in major depressive disorder (MDD). It is detailed in the Estimand 1 example of Polverejan et al. (2023) and used in this chapter with slight modifications.

3.3 Define Trial Objectives

The initial step of the estimand thinking process is to define trial objectives, which support the decision-making of the trial stakeholder(s) and take into account the therapeutic setting and the intent of treatment. A team discussion on the trial objectives can be started by identifying the stakeholder(s) of the trial and what decision(s) they need to make based on the trial. As presented in Polverejan et al. (2023), a health authority agency might need to decide whether a trial contributes substantial evidence of short-term or long-term efficacy for a new treatment to be submitted for approval. A sponsor developing a new drug might, for example, need to determine whether a trial provides enough evidence of efficacy to decide on continuing its development. Payers might need to determine whether the decision to prescribe a new drug is more clinically effective over a long period than the decision to prescribe another well-established drug. Physicians and patients will need enough information to enable their individual decision-making on starting a treatment.

A trial objective includes statement(s) detailing what a stakeholder requires to support their decisions. It can be a statement such as "to assess the superiority of investigational versus alternative treatment on the variable of interest for the target population." Trial objectives tend to be brief, stating what needs to be demonstrated to support the trial stakeholders' decisions. While we recommend several minimal components for trial objectives, they can also be more detailed, as described in Bell et al. (2021). For several examples of trial objectives that support different stakeholders and the decisions they need to make, see the estimand examples from Polverejan et al. (2023). At a minimum, a trial objective should mention the following:

- Target population for treatment.
- Variable of interest.
- Treatment regimens that are being compared or investigated.
- What a trial needs to demonstrate to support the stakeholder's decision-making.

The first three minimal components are also reflected with more details in the clinical questions of interest and in the attributes of the aligned estimands. They are discussed in Chap. 2 and in the upcoming Sect. 3.6. The last component is needed to support the stakeholder's decision-making, as a trial typically needs to demonstrate superiority, non-inferiority, or equivalence versus an alternative treatment (which can also be placebo, corresponding to receiving no active treatment).

Clinical trial teams may consider answering the following questions to facilitate the necessary multidisciplinary collaborations and determine the above components.

Target population for treatment:

- What is the target population for the investigational treatment, including typical comorbidities and behaviors?
- What is the medical need in this population?
- Are there subpopulations that are of more interest than others?

Variable of interest, reflected with more details in the variable attribute of the estimand:

- What are the variables of interest that best reflect a treatment benefit in the target population?
  Treatment regimens that are being compared or investigated:

- How is the treatment regimen defined? A treatment regimen can be monotherapy, add-on therapy to other available treatment(s), or a combination of therapies. It can allow specific rescue or concomitant medications and dose adjustments, or it can involve a complex sequence of interventions, such as induction and maintenance treatment.
- How is the investigational treatment regimen envisioned to be positioned, relative to the existing therapeutic options for the same target population?
- If applicable: What are the appropriate alternative treatments to act as comparators that are pertinent to the same clinical context and target population as the investigational treatment?

Additional questions that can aid a trial team to define trial objectives:

- What is the desired Target Product Profile (TPP) and the intended label for the investigational treatment? According to the World Health Organization (WHO 2024), a TPP outlines the desired 'profile' or characteristics of a target product that is aimed at a particular disease or diseases. TPPs state intended use, target populations and other desired attributes of products, including safety and efficacy-related characteristics.
- How does the trial fit into the development program?
- What are the expected constraints for the trial? They could include timing, cost, planned regulatory interactions, operational challenges, available dosage and formulations for the treatments used in the trial, etc.

3.3.1 Case Study Revisited: Define Trial Objectives

We consider now the case study based on a hypothetical confirmatory trial for short-term monotherapy treatment in MDD. As mentioned above, a trial might have multiple stakeholders. We consider a health authority agency to be one of the main stakeholders for this trial. This agency needs to determine if the trial contributes substantial evidence of short-term efficacy in MDD for a new investigational treatment named Drug X.

The first step of the estimand thinking process is to define a trial objective that supports the stakeholder's decision-making. The trial objective is formulated as follows:

To assess the superiority of Drug X versus placebo in short-term symptom reduction when given as monotherapy treatment in MDD patients.

This objective mentions what the trial needs to demonstrate (superiority of Drug X versus placebo) and the other minimal components: target population for treatment (MDD patients), the variable of interest (short-term MDD symptom reduction), and treatment regimens that are being compared (monotherapy Drug X versus placebo).

3.4 Identify Intercurrent Events

The second step of implementing the estimand thinking process in a trial is to identify the intercurrent events for that trial. Intercurrent events were defined and described in Chaps. 1 and 2. Examples of intercurrent events include treatment discontinuation due to an adverse event, treatment discontinuation due to a lack of efficacy, intake of rescue medication, initiation of subsequent therapy, treatment switch, and death. Intercurrent events need to be identified early in trial planning, as they need to be addressed in the clinical questions of interest and the corresponding estimands, discussed in the upcoming Sects. 3.5 and 3.6.

The clinician along with the statistician should lead the discussion to identify the trial intercurrent events expected from potential patient journeys. This discussion requires a good understanding of potential patient journeys, considering the target population and the type of treatment(s) being investigated or compared. Input from other disciplines might also be needed, such as from regulatory affairs, clinical operations, and pharmacovigilance. As mentioned in Sect. 3.2, the estimand thinking process is initially designed to be sequential, but it inherently accommodates iteration, allowing for adaptation as the trial planning progresses. While many of the intercurrent events can be identified based on potential patient journeys, some might need to be added due to considerations related to trial design (e.g., initiation of only a particular type of rescue medication being allowed in a trial).

Different types of intercurrent events could be initially identified from the team discussion. However, it is recommended to consolidate them into fewer categories of event types. This may involve merging the related events expected to be handled in similar ways. For example, treatment discontinuation due to several reasons might be consolidated into treatment discontinuation due to adverse events, lack of efficacy, or other reasons. Treatment discontinuation could also be considered a single intercurrent event if this can be justified. The consolidation of intercurrent events is important to keep clinical questions of interest and estimand definitions understandable and avoid unnecessary complexity.

It is also recommended to include only relevant intercurrent events rather than listing all possible intercurrent events that might occur, especially if these come with very low frequencies or are not expected to meaningfully impact the treatment effect. For example, in a scenario where only 0.2% of patients are anticipated to start an additional medication to treat the target disease, with such a relatively low frequency, the intercurrent event, "start of an additional medication," may not need to be specified in the clinical question of interest. This avoids unnecessarily complex clinical questions that cannot be easily understood by clinical teams or other relevant stakeholders.

A special case is death, which is always a potential intercurrent event whenever it is not a component of the variable of interest. This is because death affects the existence of the outcome measurements and, therefore, impacts the variable of interest. In nonfatal disease indications, how to address death as an intercurrent event should still be discussed by the trial team. In many circumstances, the team might choose to document in the trial protocol that deaths are generally not expected in the trial due to the disease indication, treatment mechanism, or short duration of the trial.

3.4.1 Case Study Revisited: Identify Intercurrent Events

In the MDD case study, there are two identified intercurrent events: treatment discontinuation and start of other pharmacological treatments for MDD. The clinical question of interest will address how the identified intercurrent events are handled.

3.5 Formulate Clinical Questions of Interest

The third step of implementing the estimand thinking process in a trial is to formulate the clinical questions of interest for that trial. Clinical question(s) of interest need to be defined for each of the defined trial objectives. A clinical question of interest introduces in a concise way the treatment effect of interest to the corresponding trial stakeholder(s). It is best formulated using natural, nontechnical language for easy comprehension to allow multidisciplinary discussions within a clinical trial team and support its communication to stakeholder(s). A clinical question of interest will be paired with a formal, detailed definition of the corresponding estimand (see Sect. 3.6). Clinical trial teams are encouraged to justify how answering the proposed clinical questions of interest would support stakeholder decision-making.

Each clinical question of interest defined for a trial objective incorporates the minimal components of a trial objective (see Sect. 3.3): target population for treatment, variable of interest, and treatment regimens that are compared or investigated. In addition, it needs to address how the intercurrent events (identified in the previous step of the estimand thinking process) are addressed. It is important to provide justification for the clinical question of interest, including the rationale for the selected strategies for addressing intercurrent events.

Different formulations of the clinical question of interest with regard to addressing intercurrent events would imply using different intercurrent event strategies in the estimand definition. Chapter 2 provides a detailed introduction to various types of strategies to handle intercurrent events. Examples of how the treatment effect formulation in a clinical question of interest translates into different intercurrent event strategies are presented below:

- Treatment policy strategy: treatment effect of assigning or initiating a treatment, regardless of the occurrence of the intercurrent event (or including the effects of the intercurrent event, depending on the setup and preference).
- Hypothetical strategy: treatment effect in a scenario where the intercurrent event does not confound the treatment effect desired to be estimated. For example, the effect of a monotherapy treatment might be of interest, where starting other medications for the same disease is an intercurrent event that confounds the effect desired to be estimated. A hypothetical scenario is, therefore, envisaged, in which this intercurrent event would not occur because other medications for the same disease are considered unavailable.
- Composite variable strategy: treatment effect where the intercurrent event is a meaningful outcome, included in the variable definition. For example, starting another medication for the same disease might be considered a treatment failure, and patients with this intercurrent event might be categorized as nonresponders.
- Principal stratum strategy: treatment effect in a stratum (or subpopulation) of patients who would/would not experience the intercurrent event under both investigational and control treatment (or if assigned investigational/control treatment).
- While on treatment strategy: treatment effect while treatment is being taken, prior to the intercurrent event.

For several examples of clinical questions of interest aligned with different intercurrent event strategies, see the estimand examples in the context of MDD from Polverejan et al. (2023).

In confirmatory trials, where a health authority agency is a main trial stakeholder, the clinical question of interest should be of regulatory interest. The trial team should consider whether there is any guidance on what questions are considered relevant in a disease-specific guideline authored by the agency. However, clinical teams may discuss any prior feedback or guidance in case there is a good reason to deviate from it.

The clinical question of interest should be formulated as concisely as possible for easy comprehension. Some attributes of the corresponding estimand might, therefore, not need to be included (e.g., population-level summary) or specified with the same level of detail as in the estimand definition (e.g., treatment and variable).

3.5.1 Case Study Revisited: Formulate Clinical Questions of Interest

In the MDD case study, the clinical question of interest is formulated as follows:

*For patients with MDD for whom acute drug monotherapy would be indicated, what would be the expected effect of being assigned monotherapy Drug X (*versus *placebo) on depression severity at Week 8, had no other antidepressant medications been available?.*

This question is aligned with the trial objective defined in Step 1 of the estimand thinking process (see Sect. 3.3.1). It also addresses how the intercurrent events identified in Step 2 of the estimand thinking process (see Sect. 3.4.1) are handled. We will now explain the individual components of this question.

- The target population includes "*patients with MDD for whom acute drug monotherapy would be indicated.*"
- The variable of interest is "*depression severity at Week 8.*" This variable can be easily understood in the question of interest, but it is not precisely defined. It would need to be further detailed in the variable attribute of the estimand definition included in Section 3.6.
- The treatment regimens that are being compared are "*being assigned monotherapy Drug X (versus placebo).*" Mentioning placebo is considered optional for defining the clinical question of interest and is, therefore, included in parentheses. The reason is that in clinical practice, there is no placebo, and a patient can be assigned or not to a treatment. A prescriber might choose not to treat the patient, or the patient might choose not to start treatment. Sometimes, other phrasings such as "standard of care" can be used (e.g., when a placebo is given on top of standard of care in order to maintain the blinding of the trial).
- The intercurrent event of treatment discontinuation is not directly mentioned in the clinical question of interest. However, the question mentions the effect of "*being assigned monotherapy Drug X (versus placebo).*" This implies that the treatment effect of interest is of treatment assignment, regardless of treatment discontinuation. This clarification can be included in the question, but the question would become longer and more difficult to understand: "… what would be the expected effect of being assigned monotherapy Drug X (versus placebo) on depression severity at Week 8, regardless of treatment discontinuation and had no other antidepressant medications been available?" This question implies that

the treatment policy strategy will be used in the estimand definition for this intercurrent event.

- The intercurrent event of starting other pharmacological treatments for MDD is addressed at the end of the clinical question of interest through the hypothetical scenario "*had no other antidepressant medications been available.*" This implies that the hypothetical strategy will be used in the estimand definition for this intercurrent event.
- The clinical question above does not specifically mention a population-level summary. However, the use of "*expected effect*" can imply that a difference in means will be used in the estimand definition.

3.6 Describe Estimands

The fourth step of implementing the estimand thinking process in a trial is to describe the estimand attributes paired with the clinical questions of interest formulated in the previous step. As described in Chap. 2, an estimand is described by the following attributes: population, variable, treatment, intercurrent events, and population-level summary. Below are some key guiding recommendations on how each attribute of the estimand should be described in the estimand definition.

(a) Population
The target population should refer to patients in a disease setting (e.g., patients with a diagnosis of MDD in a current major depressive episode with at least moderate symptom severity). As the target population for treatment, it needs to be distinguished from the set of participants from the trial and be described in terms of patients rather than participants. It should not be defined based on analysis sets such as "all randomized participants" or "all treated participants." The target population could also be a subset of an overall population, defined either by baseline characteristics or by post–treatment initiation events (e.g., the stratum of patients who would not have an intercurrent event of interest, regardless of treatment assignment, see Chap. 19 for more details).

(b) Variable
The variable attribute should be based on an accepted measure from both clinical and trial stakeholder perspectives. It needs to reflect on the qualitative aspect of the expected treatment effect (e.g., achieving or avoiding a certain discrete variable, such as treatment success or failure, time to event, or change in a continuous score) as well as its temporal aspect (e.g., effect at a fixed time point or over a fixed or variable period). The variable should be measurable for each patient. It can be measured as a continuous (e.g., change from baseline for an outcome), binary (e.g., achieving or not achieving a response), time-to-event, or a count measure. Selection of the appropriate measure will depend on the clinical question of interest. In addition, the variable definition should reflect the intercurrent events that are handled with the composite variable strategy

(e.g., a patient with an intercurrent event being considered a nonresponder) or the patient-dependent treatment duration if the while on treatment strategy is used (e.g., area under curve or average of on-treatment measurements).

(c) Treatment
Treatment can be defined as an individual intervention or a combination of interventions administered concurrently or sequentially, as discussed in Chap. 2 and Sect. 3.3. The treatment attribute should be detailed to include dosage, frequency of administration, route of administration (e.g., oral tablets, intravenous, or subcutaneous), duration of treatment, type of treatment (monotherapy versus add-on therapy), type of background therapy for add-on treatment, allowed rescue medications, and subsequent therapy (if applicable).

(d) Intercurrent Events
Intercurrent events need to be identified before a clinical question of interest can be formulated, as described in Sect. 3.4. The formulation of the clinical question of interest should drive the selection of the strategies for intercurrent events, as described in Chap. 2 and Sect. 3.5. According to the ICH E9(R1) guideline, only the intercurrent events not covered in the other attributes ("remaining") should be specified. Additionally, one might list all intercurrent events and corresponding strategies in a tabular format, as reflected in the MDD example below, see also EMA (2023). There are scenarios under which patients could experience overlapping intercurrent events, which are handled using different strategies. If this is the case, the priority order of applying these strategies should be specified. This will depend on the clinical context. For example, the composite variable strategy will likely have higher priority over strategies such as treatment policy or hypothetical. Further details on identification of intercurrent events and key elements to consider in team discussions are detailed in Sect. 3.4.

(e) Population-Level Summary
Defining the population-level summary needs to take into account both the variable attribute and its clinical relevance in the disease setting. In the case of a continuous variable, the difference in means between treatment regimens is a common summary. For a binary variable, examples of summaries include the difference in rates, risk ratio, and odds ratio. For a time-to-event endpoint, hazard ratio and the difference between event-free rates at a fixed time point are examples of population-level summaries. Given the number of choices, the team should discuss what a clinically meaningful measure is, taking into account established clinical and regulatory precedence. In addition, there is no need to restate the variable when defining the population-level summary, as it is already specified in another attribute. This attribute should not include the estimation method or a statistical test.

In summary, the estimand is about "what" to estimate and not "how" to estimate. The estimand definition should not include any data-handling procedures or analysis specifications. Once the clinical question of interest and the corresponding estimand are defined, the trial team needs to justify their utility to the trial stakeholders.

3.6.1 Case Study Revisited: Describe the Estimand

In the MDD case study, the clinical question of interest was formulated in Sect. 3.5.1 as follows:

For patients with MDD for whom acute drug monotherapy would be indicated, what would be the expected effect of being assigned monotherapy Drug X on depression severity at Week 8, had no other antidepressant medications been available?

Next, we construct the estimand that is paired with this clinical question of interest.

(a) Population: Patients with a diagnosis of MDD in a current major depressive episode with at least moderate symptom severity, for whom acute drug monotherapy would be indicated.
(b) Variable: Change from baseline to Week 8 in the total score of the 17-item version of the Hamilton depression rating scale (HDRS).
(c) Treatments: Monotherapy Drug X and placebo at the selected dose and frequency of administration, regardless of treatment discontinuation and as if other pharmacological treatments for MDD were not available.
(d) Intercurrent events and corresponding strategies:

- Treatment discontinuation is handled with the treatment policy strategy, as reflected in the treatment attribute. This strategy targets the effect of treatment assignment, regardless of treatment discontinuation.
- The start of other pharmacological treatments for MDD is handled with the hypothetical strategy, as reflected in the treatment attribute. Under this strategy, a hypothetical scenario is envisaged in which other pharmacological treatments for MDD are not available so that the estimand can capture the treatment effect as monotherapy.

(e) Population-level summary: Difference in means between Drug X and placebo treatment.

All components of the clinical question of interest discussed in Sect. 3.5 are reflected with additional details in the estimand attributes. The treatment attribute includes the selected dose and frequency of administration and how the intercurrent events are addressed. As intercurrent events are reflected in the treatment attribute, a separate description of the intercurrent events and corresponding strategies is optional. For clarity, we have included it above in (d). The population-level summary defines the treatment effect based on the difference in means between Drug X and placebo treatment for the defined variable.

Once the estimand is defined, it is important to justify its utility to the relevant trial stakeholder(s). The estimand in this case study captures the short-term effect of assignment to treatment, regardless of treatment discontinuation. It is considered of interest to a health authority agency, a main trial stakeholder. This is because treatment discontinuation occurs not only in trials but also in clinical practice, and a treatment effect in an ideal condition, where there is perfect compliance, would be unrealistic. At the same time, this estimand aims to capture the treatment effect as monotherapy so that the effect of other antidepressants that might be used after assignment to either Drug X or placebo is considered to not be of interest.

3.7 Align Trial Design Choices

The fifth step of implementing the estimand thinking process in a trial is to align choices on trial design, including data collection. After defining all trial objectives, clinical questions of interest, and corresponding estimands, the trial team needs to design a trial that can effectively provide all information necessary to estimate all trial estimands and address all objectives. As mentioned earlier in this chapter, the estimand thinking process is initially designed to be sequential, but it allows for adaptation as the trial planning progresses. Ideally, an estimand should correspond to a true question of interest in the target population, and then, a trial should be designed to estimate it. In practice, the feasibility of different aspects of trial design can influence the estimand. For example, the selected patients might have to be restricted to those with moderate disease severity so that the sample size can be manageable and the trial can detect a clinically meaningful treatment effect. While the treatment of interest might be envisioned to be taken with many types of allowed rescue medication, the trial might restrict them to a single type that can be taken across multiple regions. A team should aim to design a trial that is feasible but able to address estimands as close as possible to the true questions of interest.

Members of the team representing various disciplines need to collaborate and provide input to determine all trial design aspects to be documented in the trial protocol, with sections covering the following:

- Type of design and its schema, its rationale, and further design details, including any interim analysis, trial stopping rules, and start/end of trial.
- Description of the trial's inclusion and exclusion criteria.
- Description of and rationale for the investigational trial intervention and any alternative treatment used for comparison, any non-investigational trial interventions, or permitted or prohibited concomitant therapy.
- Description of procedures for permanent or temporary discontinuation of trial interventions and trial withdrawal, including failure to follow-up.
- Trial assessments and procedures, including the schedule of activities, screening or baseline assessments and procedures, efficacy, safety, and other assessments and procedures.
- Statistical considerations, including the main and sensitivity estimators aligned with the selected estimands, as discussed in Sect. 3.8.

The type of design and its schema should be able to address all defined trial objectives. The team might initially consider a parallel, double-blind, randomized design, considered the gold standard design to demonstrate superiority, non-inferiority, or equivalence. However, this type of design may not always be the most appropriate for the selected trial objectives. If a trial objective is to assess the superiority of continuing versus discontinuing the investigational treatment in patients who have shown a stable response to initial treatment with the investigational treatment, then a randomized withdrawal design can be used. In this design, patients can be stabilized on the investigational treatment in a run-in, open-label phase and then randomized into a parallel, double-blind, placebo-controlled phase to either continue treatment or switch to placebo. There are many variations of other types of trial designs, such as a consolidation-followed-by-maintenance trial design, a single-arm design in a rare disease population, or a crossover design. The trial team should have thorough discussions on the considered type of design and its ability to address the trial objectives and estimands.

When defining the trial's inclusion and exclusion criteria, the trial team needs to provide the rationale for the selection of patients and justify that they will provide a good, feasible representation of the target population reflected in the trial objectives and estimands. The treatment regimens included in the treatment attribute of the defined estimands might include the investigational trial interventions, non-investigational trial interventions (e.g., promotion of lifestyle changes), and other concomitant treatments (e.g., using rescue medications as needed). Deviations from the predefined treatment regimens will typically lead to intercurrent events. For example, treatment discontinuation is usually an intercurrent event, and all procedures for permanent or temporary discontinuation of trial intervention need to be documented. While trial withdrawal is not considered an intercurrent event, it is an event that could lead to missing data and loss of information. Consequently, the procedure for trial withdrawal (including failure to follow-up) also needs to be clearly documented in the protocol. All variables included in the estimand definitions are based on efficacy, safety, pharmacokinetics, biomarkers, or other assessments that need to be defined and scheduled at relevant time points.

Data collection is an important aspect of trial design, linked to the defined estimands and the selected strategies for intercurrent events. An estimand using the treatment policy strategy for an intercurrent event requires the values of the variable to be collected before and after the intercurrent event. In contrast, estimands based on other strategies might not require data collection after the intercurrent event. However, that data might be needed for different purposes. Data needed to estimate an estimand but not collected leads to a missing data problem, which has to be addressed through the chosen analysis approach. Missing data is usually linked to untestable assumptions and requires sensitivity analyses to assess the robustness of results. Collecting the reasons for data being missing is helpful to select appropriate analyses that address the missing data. The date of occurrence of each intercurrent event should also be collected.

Multidisciplinary collaboration is essential at the trial design stage. Members of the trial team can start with the ideal design for a particular estimand. After they discuss what is feasible to be implemented in the design, they need to decide whether to modify the trial design or adjust the trial objectives and estimands so that they can be addressed by a realistic design.

3.7.1 Case Study Revisited: Align Trial Design Choices

For the MDD case study, a parallel, double-blind, placebo-controlled, randomized trial design is considered appropriate to address the defined trial objective, clinical question of interest, and corresponding estimand, as described in Sects. 3.3.1, 3.5.1, and 3.6.6. As the treatment policy strategy is used for treatment discontinuation, the HDRS scores after treatment discontinuation are directly relevant to this estimand, and efforts should be made to collect them. A hypothetical strategy is used for the intercurrent event of starting other pharmacological treatments for MDD. Under the selected estimators (see the next section), HDRS scores after this intercurrent event are not relevant. However, the trial protocol should plan to collect this information if the data are relevant for other purposes (e.g., to assess the treatment effect, regardless of starting other pharmacological treatments for MDD).

3.8 Select Suitable Analysis Approaches

The sixth step of implementing the estimand thinking process in a trial is to select the main and sensitivity estimators aligned with each estimand. An aligned analysis method (or estimator) needs to be selected to provide an estimate for each estimand, based on the trial data. Any estimator specifications for an estimand should address the following components, as described in Polverejan et al. (2023):

- Data handling
- Specification of the main estimator with its assumptions
- Specification of the sensitivity estimator(s) with corresponding assumptions

In addition, the analysis used for decision-making (e.g., superiority, non-inferiority, or equivalence) under the corresponding trial objective also needs to be specified. If applicable, specification of any supplementary analyses should also be included. We will describe each of these components.

The data-handling component should include specifications for the analysis set (i.e., the patients used for analysis, such as all randomized patients) and specifications for the selection of data to be used for each patient. It is important to also specify what data points are not used in analysis versus missing versus not existing, if applicable. Data not used are data that may be collected but are not used for the selected estimator due to the strategy selected for an intercurrent event. As an example, data not used could refer to the endpoint values collected after an intercurrent event handled with a hypothetical strategy, if the selected estimator does not use them. According to the ICH E9(R1) guideline, missing data are data that would have been useful but could not be collected (e.g., due to withdrawal from the trial or due to missed visits or data collection). Data not existing could refer to data after terminal events, such as death.

Specifications for the main estimator include the statistical model description, together with the corresponding assumptions for the model and for data not used and missing data. The trial statistician should lead the multidisciplinary discussions around the main estimator selection and should be able to present and discuss the assumptions for the considered estimators using nontechnical language. The assumptions of an estimator should be aligned with the corresponding estimand. For example, if a hypothetical strategy is used for an intercurrent event and data after this event are not used in estimation, the assumptions for the data not used should be based on the potential patient trajectories in the hypothetical scenario that is envisaged.

The sensitivity estimators target the same estimand as the main estimator. According to the ICH E9(R1) guideline, the sensitivity estimators should verify whether or not the estimate derived from the main estimator is robust to departures from its assumptions (ICH 2019, Section A.5.2.1). Their specifications need to clearly state how elements and assumptions differ from those of the main estimator. Ideally, sensitivity estimators should stress-test one assumption at a time. Assumptions could be those related to the statistical model, data not used, or missing data. The ICH E9(R1) guideline mentions that the assumptions for data not used versus missing data could give rise to separate sets of assumptions to be examined in sensitivity analysis (ICH 2019, Section A.5.2.2). A structured approach to sensitivity analysis is preferred, such as a tipping point analysis, as described in Chaps. 15 and 16 of this book, focused on analysis of different types of variables. Clinical feedback is also needed in the context of sensitivity analysis, such as when the assumptions become clinically implausible after the initial main assumptions were stress-tested.

Each estimand is aligned with a trial objective, which states what a trial needs to demonstrate to support the stakeholder's decision-making (e.g., superiority, non-inferiority, or equivalence), as described in Sect. 3.3. When possible, the primary analysis used for decision-making (e.g., the analysis that provides p-values for hypothesis testing) should estimate the population-level summary. However, there are situations when they could be different, for example, when the log-rank test is used to provide p-values, but the hazard ratio derived from Cox regression is used to derive the population-level summary. If that is the case, the analysis used for decision-making should also have clear specifications, including the statistical model description and its assumptions, and be accompanied by sensitivity analyses that stress-test its assumptions.

The multidisciplinary trial team should also discuss the need for supplementary estimands and analyses, as described in Chap. 2. Supplementary estimands to a main estimand could be defined to investigate other types of treatment effects than those defined in the main estimand. They might be different but related to the main estimand (see also Chap. 2). For example, a supplementary estimand could keep the same attributes except for the strategy used for an intercurrent event. Different but relevant and related questions of interest could help the trial stakeholders better understand treatment benefits from different angles. If a trial has multiple stakeholders, a main estimand for a stakeholder could be considered supplementary for another stakeholder. The estimators of supplementary estimands are called supplementary analyses. Other types of supplementary analyses are those investigating different estimators for the same main estimand. They are different than sensitivity analyses, which stress-test the main estimator assumptions.

Different strategies for intercurrent events generally lead to different estimators. For the treatment policy strategy, all data points collected after the intercurrent event are included in the estimation. Missing data due to study withdrawal are usually still present, and assumptions for missing data would need to be made. Estimators aligned with this strategy need to account for the intercurrent event, which is expected to change the patient outcome trajectory.

For the hypothetical strategy, the data points after the intercurrent event might not be of interest, depending on the specific analysis approach being used. For an aligned analysis approach, the underlying assumptions highly depend on the specific situation in hypothetical scenarios. It is necessary to consider what would have happened or what might be allowed to happen, instead of just assuming that the intercurrent event would not have happened. As the amount of data not used and missing data could be large under the hypothetical strategy, performing sensitivity analyses under different assumptions is particularly important. There are also methods that apply adjustments to post-intercurrent event data to model the patient trajectory under the envisaged hypothetical scenario (see, for example, Sect. 15.2.2 in Chap. 15 of this book).

Applying the composite variable strategy is straightforward for a binary or time-to-event endpoint. For a binary endpoint, a patient with an intercurrent event is usually considered a nonresponder or treatment failure. For a time-to-event endpoint, the intercurrent event could be considered an event. There are different ways of applying this strategy for a continuous variable, leading to different estimators (see Sect. 15.2.3). Incorporating different intercurrent events in the variable might make results difficult to interpret. Supplementary analyses could help by exploring the treatment effect on separate composite variable components.

The while on treatment strategy is mostly captured in the definition of the variable. Estimators aligned with this strategy might have lesser degrees of complexity, as the amount of missing data is reduced under this strategy. As discussed in Sect. 2.5.2 of Chap. 2, however, care is required if the occurrence of the intercurrent event differs between the treatments being compared, leading to the need for rigorous sensitivity analysis.

Under the principal stratum strategy, membership in a stratum cannot be observed for all patients. Estimators use various modeling techniques, requiring different assumptions (see Chap. 19).

3.8.1 Case Study Revisited: Select Suitable Analysis Approaches

In the MDD case study, we will now briefly describe the main and sensitivity estimators selected for the estimand defined in Sect. 3.6.6. This description includes all necessary components: data handling, specification of the main estimator with its assumptions, and specification of the sensitivity estimator with its assumptions. We will also clarify the analysis used for decision-making and describe how the superiority claim from the trial objective can be assessed. It is important to emphasize that the estimators from this case study are presented as an example and are not to be taken as guidance for MDD or for a similar estimand in another disease area.

3.8.1.1 Data Handling

The analysis set is based on all randomized patients. Data points used for analysis include outcome values collected from baseline to Week 8, including the values collected after treatment discontinuation. Outcome values collected after the intercurrent event of starting other pharmacological treatments for MDD, addressed by a hypothetical strategy, are not used in the analysis. Missing data occurs after study withdrawal or due to missed visits.

3.8.1.2 Main Estimator/Analysis Assumptions

For intermittent missing data: Missing at random assumption is used, implying that intermittent missing measurements are assumed to be similar to those from the other patients from the same treatment group, who do not have intermittent missing measurements. For data not used and monotone missing data: Conditional on observed baseline attributes and post-baseline values, outcomes are assumed similar to those in the placebo arm, as if patients from the investigational arm would always have been members of the placebo arm. This assumption is considered aligned with the assumed hypothetical scenario of other pharmacological treatments for MDD not being available and appropriate for missing data due to study withdrawal. If no other MDD treatments are available, patients could be considered similar to those receiving no treatment, i.e., the placebo arm. Similarly, missing values could also be considered similar to those from patients receiving no treatment.

3.8.1.3 Main Estimator/Analysis Description

The main estimator is based on the copy-reference multiple imputation method. This method imputes data under the assumption that patients from the investigational arm would always have been assigned to the placebo arm. For additional details on control-based multiple imputation methods, see Chap. 15. After multiple imputation, an analysis of covariance (ANCOVA) model is applied to each multiply imputed dataset, and the results are then combined across multiple imputations. The decision rule used to assess superiority can be based on the one-sided p-value of the contrast test at the Week-8 visit.

3.8.1.4 Sensitivity Analysis

The sensitivity analysis is based on the same steps as in the main estimator, except that in the second step, a jump-to-reference multiple imputation method is used instead. The jump-to-reference method assumes that if a patient is doing worse at a visit than the mean of the patient's own treatment arm, then the patient is imputed to do worse than the mean of the control arm. For additional details on this method, see Chap. 15.

3.8.1.5 Supplementary Analysis

A supplementary estimand is defined, where both intercurrent events are handled with the composite variable strategy and reflected in the variable definition. The variable is defined as achieving response at Week 8, which means reaching at least 50% reduction from baseline at Week 8 in the HDRS total score, without discontinuing treatment or starting other pharmacological treatment for MDD by Week 8. The population-level summary is the difference in proportions of patients achieving response between Drug X and placebo, which will be estimated from the trial data.

3.9 Document Chosen Estimands

The final step of implementing the estimand thinking process in a trial is to document the chosen estimands. The ICH E9(R1) guideline recommends that the primary estimand along with estimands for secondary trial objectives (e.g., related to secondary variables) that are likely to support regulatory decisions should be documented in the trial protocol. The trial protocol should detail all clinical questions of interest aligned with defined trial objectives, with justification on how answering the proposed questions would support stakeholder decision-making. Each estimand should be aligned with a trial objective and have a corresponding clinical question of interest. Estimand attributes, such as intercurrent events and corresponding strategies, should be detailed in the estimand definitions. Main and sensitivity estimators also need to be specified in the protocol, and it is critical that they are aligned with the defined estimands. The statistical analysis plan includes further details on statistical analysis, including assumptions for estimators and details on how to handle missing data. Supplementary estimands should also be detailed to ensure that there is alignment on the supportive analyses that will facilitate regulatory assessment and different stakeholder requirements. Study report and regulatory submission documents should detail the results, addressing all the defined estimands. Chap. 4 provides further information on the documentation of estimands and reporting of results.

3.10 Multidisciplinary Collaborations

The estimand framework implementation can prevent misalignment across trial objectives, design, data collection, and statistical analyses. An effective implementation requires collaborative efforts from multidisciplinary teams, including statisticians, clinicians, and professionals from other groups such as regulatory affairs and clinical operations. Their involvement is critical, from the planning phase to the conduct and reporting of the trial.

The statisticians and clinicians on the trial team are critical for driving the implementation of the estimand thinking process. While the clinicians should assist in identifying clinical questions of interest, the statisticians should clearly introduce the estimand terminology to lay a foundation for efficient discussions, aid in translating the estimand concepts, and elicit the necessary information throughout the various steps of the estimand thinking process. The use of statistical terminology related to estimands in multidisciplinary team discussions (e.g., using hypothetical or treatment policy terms when discussing the clinical question of interest) should be avoided. Statistical terminology is not likely to facilitate effective collaboration, as it can affect the level of understanding and involvement of the clinicians and other functions. Cross-functional discussions should be in simple terms and can be broken down into multiple parts, such as identification of trial stakeholders and what decisions they need to make, taking into account the therapeutic context and the intended application of the treatment when discussing the target population, treatment regimen, variable of interest, potential intercurrent events and how they can be addressed, and clinically meaningful summaries that can be considered when quantifying the treatment effect of interest. Formulation of the trial objectives and questions of interest is based on the clinical setting, so they are mainly based on the clinician's decision. The statistician can facilitate the discussions and also highlight when an estimand is difficult or impossible to estimate. The statistician also needs to provide clear and unambiguous estimand definitions in the trial protocol and other trial documents, where precise estimand terminology can be used.

Implementation of some steps of the estimand thinking process can be straightforward, for example, when there is extensive prior regulatory precedence in the disease setting that is highlighted in a health authority guideline. However, there can also be settings where the implementation can turn out to be lengthy and complex due to multiple aspects, such as different trial stakeholder requirements, complex disease settings, or complex potential patient journeys in the disease setting. Hence, the need for cross-functional collaboration to construct a clinically relevant estimand is crucial.

It is important that estimands for a trial are discussed early with the key trial stakeholders (e.g., health authority agencies and payers) to ensure alignment on the selected estimands and the corresponding estimation approaches. Ideally, this discussion should occur before or at the trial design stage. If there is no agreement among trial stakeholders on the selection of the estimands supporting primary or key secondary objectives, a main estimand for a stakeholder could be considered supplementary for another stakeholder.

3.11 Concluding Remarks

The estimand framework introduced in Chaps. 1 and 2, along with the thinking process described in this chapter, provides clear steps that a trial team needs to take when implementing the ICH E9(R1) guideline in trial planning. This process can be effectively carried out only through multidisciplinary collaborations. The examples presented in later parts of this book essentially follow the estimand thinking process and can be used together with the case study presented in this chapter for a deeper understanding of implementing the estimand framework in clinical trials across various disease areas.

The ICH E9(R1) guideline states in Section A.2 that trial planning should proceed in sequence. As mentioned throughout this chapter, we have described the estimand thinking process as initially designed to be sequential, following steps 1–7 introduced in Sect. 3.2 and detailed in Sects. 3.3 through 3.9. However, this process can be adapted and made fit-for-purpose for each trial setup. It can accommodate iterations, refinements, and adaptations, allowing feedback loops from one step to a previous one, as the trial planning progresses and new insights emerge.

References

Bell, J., Hamilton, A., Sailer, O., & Voss, F. (2021). The detailed clinical objectives approach to designing clinical trials and choosing estimands. *Pharmaceutical Statistics, 20*(6), 1112–1124. https://doi.org/10.1002/pst.2129

EMA. Day 80 assessment report - Clinical template with guidance - Rev.10.23 Revamp. European Medicines Agency Committee for Medicinal Products for Human Use. Updated Oct 12, 2023. Accessed Mar 20, 2024, https://www.ema.europa.eu/en/assessment-templates-guidance#ema-inpage-item-8164

ICH. (2019). *E9(R1) addendum on estimands and sensitivity analysis in clinical trials to the guideline on statistical principles for clinical trials*. Step 4 document available at www.ich.org

ICH. (2021). *E9(R1) training material*. Available at https://ich.org/

Polverejan, E., O'Kelly, M., Hefting, N., Norton, J. D., Lim, P., & Walton, M. K. (2023). Defining clinical trial estimands: A practical guide for study teams with examples based on a psychiatric disorder. *Therapeutic Innovation & Regulatory Science, 57*(5), 911–939. https://doi.org/10.1007/s43441-023-00524-2

WHO. Target product profiles. Accessed Mar 20, 2024. https://www.who.int/observatories/global-observatory-on-health-research-and-development/analyses-and-syntheses/target-product-profile/who-target-product-profiles

Chapter 4
Documentation of Estimands and Reporting of Results

Hongying Li, Melanie Wright, and Christine Fletcher

Abstract This chapter focuses on the impact of the ICH E9(R1) guideline on the documentation of estimands in clinical trial documents and on the planning and reporting of clinical trial results. Throughout the chapter, these aspects are illustrated through a generic example. Points to consider regarding the documentation of the estimand and analysis methods in the trial protocol are described. The impact of the estimand on the statistical analysis plan is also discussed, and considerations are described that will facilitate clinical study report writing. Recommendations are given for reporting the frequency of intercurrent events and the way to a clear presentation of the link between the estimands, the analysis sets, and the statistical analysis methods, and key assumptions underpinning the methods in the clinical study report are discussed. Emerging practices regarding the description of results in the prescribing information and publications are also mentioned.

4.1 Introduction

The adoption of the estimand framework has gained significant momentum globally since the official release of the ICH E9(R1) guideline in November 2019 (ICH, 2019). The release has sparked extensive discussions and growing expertise in understanding and incorporating estimands in clinical studies.

H. Li (✉)
China Statistical Sciences, Eli Lilly and Company, Shanghai, China
e-mail: li_hong_ying@lilly.com

M. Wright
Advanced Quantitative Sciences, Novartis, Basel, Switzerland
e-mail: melanie.wright@novartis.com

C. Fletcher
Biostatistics, GSK, Stevenange, UK
e-mail: chrissie.a.fletcher@gsk.com

J. Wei et al. (eds.), *Estimands in Clinical Trials*, Springer Series in Pharmaceutical Statistics, https://doi.org/10.1007/978-3-032-02192-2_4

The incorporation of estimands into trial protocols will inevitably impact the trial objectives, trial design, trial conduct, and statistical considerations sections. This chapter discusses key considerations arising from this change, focusing on the trial objectives and statistical considerations sections and the downstream implications for the statistical analysis plan (SAP). While there has been significant focus on integrating estimands into trial protocol and the SAP, lesser attention has been given to the best way to report their results in the clinical study report (CSR) and in publication(s). This chapter will also discuss considerations on these aspects.

4.2 Generic Example

For the purposes of illustration throughout this chapter, a generic example in the indication of type 2 diabetes will be used, as described in the European Medicines Agency's (EMA) guideline on clinical investigation of medicinal products in the treatment or prevention of diabetes mellitus (EMA, 2023a). Please refer to Sect. 12.2 in Chap. 12 for more discussion on the disease and the EMA guideline.

The EMA guideline describes the treatment goal as improving blood glucose concentrations and puts forward a change in glycated hemoglobin A1c (HbA1c) from baseline as an appropriate primary endpoint. The document continues to discuss the target of estimation (estimand), as follows:

> The primary target should be the estimation of a treatment effect based on the difference in HbA1c from baseline to the end of trial...between the test compound and a control treatment... The main expected intercurrent events to be considered include treatment discontinuation, additional medications, and rescue medication.

The document then provides some guidance on the appropriate strategies for intercurrent events, as described below:

> Treatment discontinuation: Since patients are not expected to benefit once treatment is discontinued (e.g., due to adverse events) the treatment effect should be estimated based on observed or modelled data reflecting adherence to treatment as observed in the clinical trial (treatment policy strategy).
>
> Additional/rescue medication: Considering introduction of other medication that will influence HbA1c values, the impact of additional medication complicates the evaluation of the effect of the test product compared to placebo or active control. Therefore, the treatment effect can be estimated under the assumption that rescue medication, or use of other medications that will influence HbA1c values, was not introduced (hypothetical scenario).

4.3 Documentation of Estimands

As described in Chap. 3, the estimand is defined through the estimand thinking process, which promotes an interdisciplinary collaboration within the clinical trial team and ensures that the defined trial objectives, the corresponding clinical question(s) of interest, and associated estimands are meaningful to stakeholders and will support decision-making. Often, there is no clear guidance on which estimand is appropriate to be the primary estimand, and different estimands may be relevant to different stakeholders, so each situation should be considered carefully.

Once the primary estimand(s) and estimands aligned to key secondary objectives have been agreed upon, it will be important to provide documentation in the clinical trial protocol. The following recommendations are provided in the ICH E9(R1) guideline:

> A trial protocol should define and specify explicitly a primary estimand that corresponds to the primary trial objective. The protocol and the analysis plan should prespecify the main estimator that is aligned with the primary estimand and leads to the primary analysis, together with a suitable sensitivity analysis to explore the robustness under deviations from its assumptions. Estimands for secondary trial objectives (e.g., related to secondary variables) that are likely to support regulatory decisions should also be defined and specified explicitly in the protocol and analysis plan, each with a corresponding main estimator and a suitable sensitivity analysis.

4.3.1 Documenting Estimands in the Protocol

Although there is no standardized way to document estimand(s) in the protocol, we can gain insights from the currently available public protocol templates that incorporate the estimand framework or literature that addresses this question.

In the 2024 release from TransCelerate, the common protocol template (CPT) provides guidance relating to the documentation of estimands (TransCelerate, 2024). Estimands impact many sections of the protocol; however, the explicit documentation of the chosen estimands for the trial is reflected in protocol Sect. 4.3 (Objectives, Endpoints, and Estimands) and protocol section 9 (Statistical Considerations). The estimand(s) aligned to each objective are defined under the objectives and endpoints table in protocol Sect. 4.3, whereas the analysis methods aligned to each estimand are described under separate subsections in protocol section 9. For other protocol sections, the guidance suggests ensuring that the contents are aligned with the estimand(s).

In November 2018, the ICH endorsed the task of developing the ICH M11 guideline, which includes a clinical electronic structured harmonized protocol template. To date, a draft version has been released for public comments, which has incorporated the estimand framework (ICH, 2022). It is expected that the final template will incorporate estimand-related language, with detailed instructions provided in all the relevant sections to ensure alignment with the estimand framework introduced in the ICH E9(R1) guideline. Please see Sect. 11.3 in Chap. 11 of this book for more discussions about the template. When the final ICH protocol template becomes available, it is anticipated that it will become the standard protocol template to be used in all clinical trials.

Considerations for incorporating estimands into the protocol template were discussed by Lynggaard et al. (2022). They proposed to describe the estimand early in the protocol before the trial design or statistical analysis sections since the choice of estimand will have consequences on the trial design, conduct, and analysis. The authors recommend having either a single section dedicated to objectives and estimands or two adjacent sections, given that the trial objectives and estimands are closely related. Lynggaard et al. (2022) also point out that sufficient details of estimands should be provided so that different stakeholders can have a clear understanding of the targeted treatment effects that will be estimated. But providing excessive technical details such that the clinical principle is obscured should be avoided. Such details can be described elsewhere in the protocol (e.g., in a dedicated intercurrent events section). The goal is to ensure that all required information on the intercurrent events and their strategies is available in the protocol, regardless of whether the description is in the protocol objectives and estimands section or in a later dedicated section. They also recommend providing a rationale for the choice of the key estimands, including a justification of the choice of intercurrent event strategies from a clinical/scientific perspective.

The implementation of the estimand framework also has an impact on the trial design, conduct, and schedule of assessments/data collection. All these design aspects need to be aligned with the chosen estimands by the clinical trial team and clearly documented in the protocol. Please refer to Chap. 3 for more considerations on these aspects.

Sections 4.3.1.1 and 4.3.1.2 below focus on the aspects of documentation that are new or require changes since the implementation of the ICH E9(R1) guideline.

4.3.1.1 Describing an Estimand

Considerations about the process of defining clinical objectives and formulating clinical questions of interest, which lead to defining estimands, are discussed in Chaps. 1, 2, and 3 of this book. Very detailed examples are given to help understand the process in the literature (Bell et al., 2021; Polverejan et al., 2023). Essentially, an estimand is a more detailed expression of a clinical question of interest, with its five associated attributes clearly stated (ICH, 2019, Section A.3.3).

Two forms for describing an estimand are proposed: prose and a structured form using bullet points (Lynggaard et al., 2022). In the first one, the estimand, including the five attributes, is written in one or two sentences. Using the generic example as illustration, the primary estimand could be described as:

The primary estimand is the difference in mean change from baseline to week 24 in HbA1c of Drug X vs. *placebo in adult patients with type 2 diabetes managed by diet and exercise alone, including the effects of treatment discontinuation due to any reason and as though no other additional/rescue medication is available.*

While this is a valid method and may be more appealing to non-statisticians compared to a list of bullet points, it will become increasingly difficult to write and read such prose when there are more intercurrent events to describe. A structured format is a good complementary approach. The proposed structured format is similar to the format used for describing an estimand in the CPT proposed by TransCelerate (2024).

The recommendation is to first describe the clinical question of interest aligned to the clinical objective. Second, define the five attributes of the estimand, namely the target population, target variable (or endpoint), treatment conditions, intercurrent events (and strategies to address them), and population-level summary. Finally, explain the rationale for choosing this estimand. This ensures that the attributes are clearly stated and that intercurrent event strategies are explained; also, see Sects. 3.5 and 3.6 in Chap. 3 of this book for a related discussion. Following this format, we can write the estimand for the generic example in Sect. 4.2 as below:

The clinical question of interest is: For adult patients with type 2 diabetes managed by diet and exercise alone, what would be the expected effect of prescribing Drug X on glycemic control as measured by a change in HbA1C from baseline to week 24, had no other additional/rescue medications been available and regardless of treatment discontinuation?

The estimand is described by the following attributes:

(a) *Population: Adults with type 2 diabetes managed by diet and exercise alone.*
(b) *Variable (or endpoint): Change from baseline to week 24 in HbA1c.*
(c) *Treatment: Drug X and placebo, regardless of treatment discontinuation and as if other rescue medication were not available.*
(d) *Intercurrent events and strategies to address them:*
    - *Initiation of rescue medication (hypothetical strategy, as captured in the treatment attribute above).*
    - *Treatment discontinuation due to any reason (treatment policy strategy, as captured in the treatment attribute above).*
(e) *Population-level summary: Difference between means.*

Rationale for estimand: This aligns with regulatory guidance and addresses the clinical question of interest. Of note, the EMA guideline (CPMP/EWP/1090/00 Rev.2) states:

> *Since patients are not expected to benefit once treatment is discontinued (e.g., due to adverse events) the treatment effect should be estimated based on observed or modelled data reflecting adherence to treatment as observed in the clinical trial (treatment policy strategy).*
>
> *Considering introduction of other medication that will influence HbA1c values, the impact of additional medication complicates the evaluation of the effect of the test product compared to placebo or active control. Therefore, the treatment effect can be estimated under the assumption that rescue medication, or use of other medications that will influence HbA1c values, was not introduced (hypothetical scenario).*

4.3.1.2 Implications for Planning and Documenting Statistical Analyses

A clear description of the analysis methods targeting the primary estimand(s) and secondary estimands (or any other supplementary estimands) that are important for regulatory decision-making should be provided in the protocol, while the full details of all the planned analysis methods targeting all estimands can be specified in the SAP.

The estimand has implications for the specification of the analysis set (ICH, 2021). It is no longer sufficient to define the population of trial participants to be used in the analyses, but the data points to be used in relation to intercurrent events must also be specified. Different approaches to defining analysis sets may be taken. A conventional approach to defining the analysis population can still be used to specify the selection of participants, provided that the data points to be included in the analysis are specified when describing the estimator. Alternatively, we can also define the analysis dataset directly corresponding to a specific estimand. In this case, the analysis set definition will consider two dimensions, i.e., the selection of participants and the selection of data points (visits). A third approach is to define the analysis set on the participant level (i.e., analysis population) and data point level (i.e., data point sets) separately. Then, the two sets are combined to provide the full specification of the data points to be included in an analysis. In the TransCelerate CPT, three examples are given, which reflect the three approaches described (TransCelerate, 2024). Another approach described by Lynggaard et al. (2022) is to include a dedicated intercurrent events section (in the statistical section of the protocol).

This is an evolving area, and standard conventions, such as the specification of the "Full Analysis Set" when presenting a summary table of the analysis results, are still being utilized. Provided the data points to be utilized for an analysis are carefully specified as part of the planned statistical analysis, clarity can be achieved. As dataset standards are also evolving (e.g., Clinical Data Interchange Standards Consortium (CDISC) Analysis Data Model (ADaM) standards relating to intercurrent events), the approach to define the analysis set may be revised to align with those in the future.

A key aspect of the ICH E9(R1) guideline is the clarification of the role of sensitivity analysis in regulatory decision-making. Sensitivity analyses are defined as those with the intent to explore the robustness of inferences from the main estimator to deviations from underlying statistical assumptions and limitations in the data. A recommendation is provided such that (ICH, 2019, Section A.5.2.1)

> sensitivity analysis should be planned for the main estimators of all estimands that will be important for regulatory decision making and labeling in the product information.

Hence, it is important to prespecify in the protocol, not only the main analysis method(s) (e.g., to target the primary estimand(s)) but also one or more sensitivity analyses, which will be applied to assess the robustness of results to underlying assumptions inherent to the chosen methods and to any limitations of the data. Depending on the importance of other (secondary) estimands in the study (for example, for those associated with potential label claims), it is also prudent to consider prespecification of the associated main and sensitivity analyses in the same way.

The ICH E9(R1) guideline also points out that supplementary analyses can be conducted to provide additional insights to deepen the understanding of the treatment effect, but these are considered of lower importance compared to the main and sensitivity analyses. Please refer to Lynggaard et al. (2022) for more discussions on the role of supplementary analyses. The need for prespecification of supplementary analysis in the protocol will depend on the situation; Sect. 4.4.1.3 provides more information on this topic.

Note that for a given estimand, there is no need to repeat the description of the estimand attributes in the statistical analysis section if these are already clearly described in the protocol section for objectives, endpoints, and estimands. Rather, additional details that are not covered when defining estimands can be provided when describing the statistical analysis method, for example, the impact of the intercurrent event strategies on the selection of the data to be included in an analysis and which data will be used in the analysis.

In consideration of the full specification of the main analysis required for the protocol, it will be important to document the following:

1. The selection of data to be included in the analysis, i.e., the impact of intercurrent event strategies on the selection (or exclusion) of data.
2. The main analysis methodology, including any assumptions underpinning the statistical model. If applicable, specify methods (e.g., multiple imputation) to be applied to target the hypothetical scenario in the case of an estimand specifying a hypothetical strategy for an intercurrent event.
3. How missing data will be handled, including any assumptions inherent in the chosen methods.
4. One or more sensitivity analyses to understand the robustness of results to underlying assumptions of the main analysis

Following these recommendations, the text in the protocol for the generic example could be written as follows. Note that the content is expected to adopt the structure in the ICH M11 template (ICH, 2022), which would become best practice once released in its final form (see also Sect. 11.3 in Chap. 11 of this book):

Main Analysis Approach *The main analysis targeting the primary estimand will include post-baseline HbA1c values collected until the start of intake of rescue medication (if applicable) or until the week-24 visit* (i.e., *HbA1c values collected after rescue medication intake will be discarded from the analysis).*	Selection of data to be included in the analysis
Data for visits following the intake of rescue medications will be predicted to reflect that the participant would have had a worsening in response, had the participant not received such medications. This will be achieved through multiple imputation and by applying a copy reference approach for participants randomized to drug X and by assuming missing at random (MAR) for participants randomized to placebo.	Methods relating to targeting a hypothetical scenario

Statistical analysis will be carried out using a mixed model of repeated measures (MMRM) (for each imputed dataset) for the change from baseline in HbA1c at each visit through week 24. This model will include treatment, visit, treatment by visit, and visit by baseline as fixed effects and baseline HbA1c as a covariate. The correlations between visits within patients will be modeled using an unstructured covariance matrix The difference between adjusted means for drug X vs. *placebo (and 95% confidence interval) will be estimated for the 24-week time point (and the results will be combined according to Rubin's rules).*	Main analysis methodology
Handling of missing data *In cases where participants who previously discontinued treatment have missing data due to early study withdrawal, missing data will be imputed to indicate a worsening in condition* (i.e., *a copy reference approach for participants randomized to drug X will be applied). MMRM implicitly imputes missing data under a MAR assumption; hence, missing data occurring on the placebo arm or intermittent missing measurements caused due to administrative reasons will be implicitly handled through the analysis model.*	Handling of missing data, which would have been useful in the analysis had it been collected
Sensitivity analyses *The following sensitivity analysis will be conducted to assess the robustness of results to underlying assumptions made in the main analysis targeting the primary estimand.* • *Multiple imputation using a jump-to-reference approach, following the occurrence of missing data following treatment discontinuation.* • *Multiple imputation using a copy reference approach will be applied for all missing data (regardless of the reason for missingness).*	Specification of sensitivity analyses, testing robustness of results to underlying assumptions

4.3.2 Impacts of Estimands on the SAP

As mentioned in Sect. 4.3.1, the important estimand(s) supporting primary and secondary objectives(s) likely to support regulatory decisions and associated analysis methods should be specified in the protocol. The details of other estimands, such as those aligned to the exploratory objectives, may be omitted from the protocol and described in the SAP. The SAP will provide full details of the main, sensitivity, and supplementary analyses for all estimands.

At the time of SAP writing, it is important to look ahead to what may be needed to ensure clarity in the CSR. There are four main points to consider for the SAP, which will facilitate writing of the CSR at the end:

1. Plan displays of the number and timing of intercurrent events by treatment arm.
2. Ensure that there is clarity in the description of the main and sensitivity analyses for each estimand (the assumptions made and tested) (see Sect. 4.3.1.2).
3. Consider planning additional displays to illustrate the data included and discarded from an analysis and/or the degree of missing data.
4. Consider the approach used to identify the estimands addressed in the shell tables/figures, as appropriate (see Sect. 4.4.1.3)

As stated in the ICH E9(R1) guideline, summaries of the number and timings of each intercurrent event in each treatment arm should be reported in the CSR; hence, the SAP will need to provide details of planned summary analyses for this new requirement. The method to summarize the intercurrent events may depend on the strategy specified for each estimand, as illustrated in Table 4.1 below. Another point to consider is the type of endpoint adopted. For example, for a time-to-event endpoint, the timing of the intercurrent events becomes very important, and separate displays may be required to understand the impact of the occurrence of an intercurrent event, for example, in consideration of censoring. A display of the frequency of participants with intercurrent events occurring prior to the outcomes of interest would be helpful for this purpose (for example, prior to the first heart failure hospitalization or death).

Consider planning figures to illustrate (i) how much of the observed data is included in an analysis, (ii) the observed data impacted by intercurrent events and discarded, and (iii) the amount of data that would be useful but was not observed and, hence, is truly missing. Such displays are extremely valuable to aid the interpretation of sensitivity analyses. An interesting example is Fig. 3 presented in the publication by Aroda et al. (2019b). The authors illustrated the proportion of participants over time with data impacted by the occurrence of the intercurrent events and also the proportion of missing data.

4.3.3 Impact of Estimands on Analysis Datasets

The introduction of estimands has shifted the focus toward the careful derivation of the set of data that forms the basis for the planned analysis targeting each estimand. As described in Sect. 4.3.1.2, it is no longer sufficient to specify only the participants to be included in each analysis. It is now necessary to identify for each estimand, which combination of participants and data collected will be used as the basis of the planned statistical analysis in an ADaM dataset. This can be achieved in various ways, for example, by creating a new ADaM dataset for intercurrent events and using this in conjunction with analysis population flags to determine which data from each participant will form the basis for estimation (as currently proposed by the Pharmaceutical User Software Exchange (PhUSE) and a new CDISC draft white paper; also, see Sect. 6.6 in Chap. 6), having a separate analysis set for each estimand defined in an ADaM dataset that defines the participants and data to be used for estimation, or a combination of these.

It is important that there is complete documentation that accompanies these datasets so that users can understand the structure and content and are able to determine the set of data that forms the basis of each analysis aligned to each estimand.

Table 4.1 Link between intercurrent event strategy and display of intercurrent events

Strategy	Interpretation for reporting	Example of displays
Treatment policy	Occurrence of intercurrent event is part of the treatment strategy; hence, provide displays providing information about the intercurrent event considered to be part of the treatment strategy. The timing of the intercurrent event may also be important	Display the frequency of participants with the intercurrent event (at a minimum). Additionally, display the frequency of intercurrent events per participant (e.g., swimmer plot), or consider the time to an intercurrent event
Composite variable	The intercurrent event becomes a component of the endpoint and, hence, is considered to be meaningful for the assessment of the outcome for a participant. For reporting, it would be important to assess the influence of the intercurrent event on the endpoint (e.g., if used as part of a response definition, how many times has an intercurrent event led to a participant being classified as a "nonresponder")	Display the number (%) of participants, with at least one intercurrent event, as part of a breakdown of the components of the endpoint
Hypothetical	When a hypothetical strategy has been applied, it is considered desirable to evaluate the treatment effect as though the intercurrent event had not occurred. The methods applied to evaluate such an estimand often lead to the exclusion of observed data following the intercurrent event. As such, it is helpful to include in the report the degree of data impacted by intercurrent events and, hence, excluded from an analysis	Use of graphical approaches to display the proportion of data impacted by intercurrent events and the timing at which the event occurred
While on treatment	The response prior to the occurrence of an intercurrent event is of interest, and as such, the intercurrent event defines the end of a period of time over which an outcome is to be assessed. Hence, for reporting purposes, it may be important to assess the timing of the intercurrent events and the time periods over which the endpoint has been derived	Graphical approaches to display the period of time of evaluation of the endpoint for each participant until the intercurrent event (e.g., a swimmer plot). Summaries of the time period over which an endpoint has been evaluated by treatment, for example, exposure time
Principal stratum	The occurrence (or nonoccurrence) of the intercurrent event defines the target population of interest	If an active run-in design is applied, a consort style diagram may be helpful. Otherwise, a simple display of the frequency of participants by treatment in each stratum of interest (as defined by the intercurrent event) may be sufficient

4.4 Impact of Estimands on the Transparency of Reporting of Results

As described in Chap. 1, the estimand framework facilitates alignment between the trial objectives, clinical questions of interest, estimands, trial design, trial conduct, and planned statistical analyses. The estimand framework ensures that the best trial design and analysis methods are in place to answer the key clinical questions and that sensitivity analyses are aligned to demonstrate the robustness of estimates derived from the main analysis. Upon trial readout, it is important to consider how to present and communicate the results in order to ensure that the clarity achieved through the documentation of estimands in the protocol leads to clarity in the report and, ultimately, leads to facilitating regulatory decision-making and an assessment of benefits and risks.

Consider the setting of a phase III confirmatory trial and the range of documents presenting the results (see Table 4.2). There are a variety of stakeholders who need to be involved in making decisions based on the trial results. It is thus important to ensure that treatment effects are consistently described and documented clearly in all clinical trial–related documents and can be understood by these different stakeholders.

At the time of writing this chapter, examples are emerging where estimands and results are being reported across different communication channels, including press releases, journal articles, and drug labeling. However, given that phase III trials often take several years to readout, there are relatively few published cases to date. Hence, this is an evolving area, whereby best practices will continue to unfold over time. Interestingly, there has been more movement in this direction for specific therapy areas, such as type 2 diabetes and obesity. The two manuscripts published on the PIONEER 1 trial (Aroda et al., 2019a, b) led the way in terms of how clear reporting of results with relation to estimands can be achieved. The results

Table 4.2 Example of documents presenting trial results and associated stakeholders

Timing	During trial	Trial readout	Registration	Final product	Pricing
Document	Interim analysis, DMC safety review	Topline results, CSR, press release, publication, clinical trial registries, IB	SCS, SCE, clinical overview, briefing materials	Prescribing information, patient information leaflet, layman summary	HTA dossier
To whom	DMC, internal decision-makers	Sponsor, investigators, external clinical experts, clinical trialists, investors	Health authorities, advisory committee, patient advocacy groups	Prescribers, patients	HTA bodies

Abbreviations: *DMC* = Data Monitoring Committee, *CSR* = clinical study report, *IB* = investigator brochure, *SCS* = summary of clinical safety, *SCE* = summary of clinical efficacy, and *HTA* = health technology assessment

manuscripts for the AWARD-1 diabetes trial (Frias et al., 2021) and a trial in the obesity indication (Wilding et al., 2021) are also good examples of reporting estimands and results and are referred to in the next few sections.

4.4.1 Reporting Results in the CSR

Section A.6 in the ICH E9(R1) guideline recommends that results from the main, sensitivity, and supplementary analyses should be reported systematically in the clinical trial report, specifying whether each analysis was prespecified, introduced while the trial was still blinded, or performed post hoc. It also recommends that summaries of the number and timing of each intercurrent event in each treatment arm should be reported.

In Module 3 of the training material provided by the ICH E9(R1) expert working group (ICH, 2021), it further says that the results from the main, sensitivity, and supplementary analyses should be systematically presented and discussed with reference to the estimand. It also recommends that the robustness of inferences should be discussed based on the results from the sensitivity analysis. The information in this section is based on these recommendations. Emerging best practices with regard to the impact of estimands on report writing are also discussed.

4.4.1.1 Reporting the Frequency (and Timing) of Intercurrent Events

As discussed in Sect. 4.3.2, following trial readout, it will be important to understand the frequency (and potentially timing) of intercurrent events occurring during the trial by treatment arm. This will be a key output to include up front in the study report, whereby a reviewer can assess which of the intercurrent events have occurred with high or low frequency, thus allowing an appreciation of the difference (or similarity) between results associated with estimands applying different intercurrent event strategies. Where additional or supplementary estimands have been defined for a specific objective, this information may also help the trial team and the medical writer focus on the interpretation of each treatment effect relative to each clinical question of interest that the estimand is addressing.

4.4.1.2 Ensuring a Clear Link between Estimands, Statistical Analysis Methods, and Reporting of Sensitivity Analyses in the Report

In the analysis methods section of the CSR, a clear presentation of the link between the estimands, the analysis sets, and the statistical analysis methods will help the reviewer assess the different treatment effects being estimated and how key assumptions underpinning the methods have been assessed in sensitivity analyses.

To facilitate this, a tabular layout may be helpful. To ensure clarity, it is recommended to separate the assumptions made relating to the impact of intercurrent event strategies (and whether any observed data will be ignored/excluded) from the assumptions made in the case of truly missing data. Such descriptions should include the appropriate level of details suitable for a statistician to understand the methodology.

A similar approach can then be applied to describe the main analysis results, together with the results from the planned sensitivity analyses. However, in this display, it is recommended to use descriptions of the sensitivity analyses, such that a clinical reviewer can understand what has changed compared to the main analysis. Please see Tables 4.3 and 4.4 below as illustrations using the diabetes case study example in Sect. 4.4.2.

As indicated in Sect. 4.3.1.2, a key area for consideration is to document any data points that were collected but have been discarded from the statistical analysis. If this information does not fit within the main body of the study report, consider whether the statistical appendix could be utilized for this purpose.

4.4.1.3 Emerging Concepts: Use of Labeling Conventions

When reporting the trial results, an important consideration is that there may be more than one estimand employing the same endpoint attribute. In the past, trial results have often been reported according to the endpoint, and all additional analyses relating to the primary endpoint may have been labeled "sensitivity analyses." However, it is likely that many of such analyses would have been addressing an alternative estimand. As a motivating example, see the publication of the results in the PIONEER 1 trial (Aroda et al., 2019a) in which two sets of results are described, targeting two different estimands but utilizing the same endpoint.

Hence, it may be necessary to report the results from several supplementary estimands, whereby the intercurrent events are reflected in different ways (keeping other estimand attributes the same), thus answering different questions. Such a scenario, requiring more than one estimand, may occur in case different stakeholders have alternative opinions about the estimand of most interest. In this case, it is conceivable that the analyses targeting each estimand may need their own suite of sensitivity analyses (see Fig. 4.1 for illustration). Note that it is important to clarify which estimand will be the primary estimand to address the objective.

To address this situation, a method of communicating results, such that the estimand can be identified in the output, needs to be developed. Several options are available, such as (i) writing the full estimand out in the table or figure titles, (ii) developing a catalogue of estimands and using a numbering approach for each estimand, or (iii) developing a set of labels with clinical meaning and definitions to allow us to distinguish between estimands in a shorthand way (for example, in the table or figure title). Such an approach could capture the spirit of the estimand framework, providing the information that can inform a reviewer how intercurrent events have been addressed in the output. This method was applied in the

Table 4.3 Example table separating assumptions related to the estimation of hypothetical scenario from assumptions related to handling of missing data

	Estimand			Estimation assumptions		
				Hypothetical scenario	Missing data handling	
Endpoint	Intercurrent events	Impact of intercurrent events on data selection	Analysis	Rescue medication	Following treatment discontinuation	Missing due to administrative reasons
Change from baseline in HbA1c at week 24	Rescue medication: Hypothetical Treatment discontinuation: Treatment policy	Discard HbA1c data after rescue medication intake Use all available data observed after treatment discontinuation	Main	CR for investigational, MAR for placebo	CR for investigational under MNAR assumption, MAR for placebo	MAR for investigational and placebo
			Sensitivity 1	Same as main analysis	JR for investigational under the MNAR assumption, MAR for placebo	Same as main analysis
			Sensitivity 2	Same as main analysis	Same as main analysis	CR for investigational under MNAR assumption, MAR for placebo

Abbreviations: *CR* = copy reference (pattern mixture model), *JR* = jump to reference, *MAR* = missing at random, and *MNAR* = missing not at random

Table 4.4 Example table of results from the main analysis and sensitivity analyses

Endpoint	Analysis	Assumptions following rescue medication use	Assumptions for missing data	Difference between means (Drug X vs. placebo)	95% confidence interval	p-value
Change from baseline in HbA1c at week 24	Main	Assume that the HbA1c trajectory for participants in the drug X arm moves toward the trajectory in the placebo arm	If missing data follows treatment discontinuation, assume that the HbA1c trajectory for participants in the drug X arm moves toward the trajectory in the placebo arm. Assume that the HbA1c trajectory for participants in the placebo arm follows the HbA1c collected for others in the placebo arm	xx.x	(xx.x, xx.x)	x.xxxxx
	Sensitivity 1	Same as main analysis	If missing data follows treatment discontinuation, assume that the HbA1c trajectory for participants in the drug X arm jumps quickly toward the trajectory in the placebo arm. Assume that the HbA1c trajectory for participants in the placebo arm follows the HbA1c collected for others in the placebo arm	xx.x	(xx.x, xx.x)	x.xxxxx

(continued)

Table 4.4 (continued)

Endpoint	Analysis	Assumptions following rescue medication use	Assumptions for missing data	Difference between means (Drug X vs. placebo)	95% confidence interval	p-value
	Sensitivity 2	Same as main analysis	Assume that the HbA1c trajectory for participants in the drug X arm moves toward the trajectory in the placebo arm, regardless of the reason for missing data. Assume that the HbA1c trajectory for participants in the placebo arm follows the HbA1c collected for others in the placebo arm	xx.x	(xx.x, xx.x)	x.xxxxx

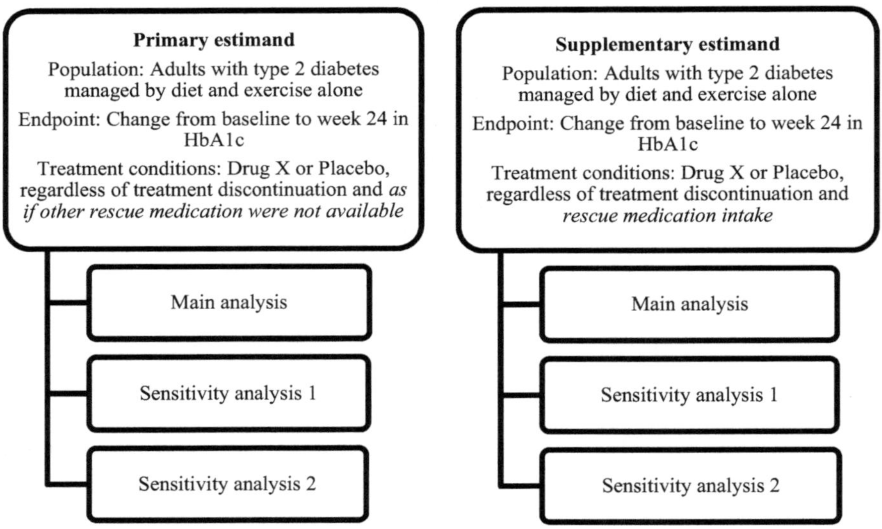

Fig. 4.1 Structure of estimands and analyses

publication of the results in the PIONEER 1 trial (Aroda et al., 2019a, b), the AWARD-1 diabetes trial (Frias et al., 2021), and a trial to assess once-weekly semaglutide in adults with overweight or obesity (Wilding et al., 2021). In these three published examples, shorthand labels were defined clearly in the manuscripts and were used to reflect the clinical question of interest of the estimand when presenting two sets of results (both based on the same primary endpoint).

A key point to note is that it is of utmost importance to ensure that labeling conventions associated with estimands are clearly documented and described together with the results. Labeling conventions can be helpful to assist the team in communicating results within a drug development program and use consistent labels, where appropriate, across trials. At the time of writing this chapter, no standard labeling conventions are available, and caution is warranted since similar-sounding labels created by different authors may have different meanings.

4.4.2 Implications in the Submission Dossier

If the recommendations laid out in Sect. 4.4.1 have been followed for the CSR, for example, in the case of a phase III confirmatory trial, it is natural that a similar approach to communication of the results can be brought through to the summary of clinical efficacy (SCE), the summary of clinical safety (SCS), and the clinical overview (CO). In particular, the labels for the different estimand philosophies can be used throughout these documents.

For certain cases, it may become very beneficial to consider the specification of estimands to clarify the evaluation of key safety risks as well as to frame the efficacy benefits; for more details about estimands for safety assessment, please see Sect. 21.3 in Chap. 21. The recommendations in terms of communication of safety results would be similar to those for efficacy. If such an approach were applied, then clarity may be provided to the SCS safety summaries, and in addition, estimands for safety may also be considered for the assessment of benefit/risk in the clinical overview section. For example, when considering the diabetes case study, a scenario could be envisaged, whereby the study team may like to characterize a safety risk emerging from Drug X alone and without any safety effects from rescue medication intake (i.e., to evaluate the safety of the new treatment purely vs. placebo). In this case, it would be helpful to specify such a safety estimand and have clarity with regard to weighing up the relative benefits and risks of the new product. Alternatively, characterizing safety risks for the new treatment in conjunction with rescue medication may also be of interest. As for efficacy evaluation, specification of estimands for important safety risks can also provide clarity to decision-makers and help inform benefit–risk considerations.

4.4.2.1 Impact on Prescribing Information

Ultimately, the goal is to provide clarity about the clinical meaning of the observed treatment effects (i.e., the quantified benefits and risks) of a new product and ensure that these are clearly described in prescribing information. If estimands have enabled a clearer communication of results throughout the dossier and language has been used that a general audience can understand, then a natural flow of the communication of results into the drug labeling will be facilitated. Labeling specialists can also help provide guidance with regard to clearly describing treatment effects and can assist with finding nontechnical terms that reflect the essential aspects of the estimands, without necessarily using estimand terminology.

Examples in the public domain where labeling language has been overtly influenced by estimands remain rare. However, one example is in the Rybelsus label for a type 2 diabetes indication, where Rybelsus is the brand name for oral semaglutide that was investigated in the PIONEER 1 trial (Aroda et al., 2019a). In this case, a treatment policy strategy was applied for rescue medication usage during the trial. The footnote of the key results table explains the percentage of participants who received rescue medication during the trial to provide clarity that, in fact, many more participants on placebo required rescue medication usage than those on active treatment.

Health authorities have also started thinking more about these aspects. For example, the EMA has recently released a draft guidance on the assessment of the summary of product characteristics, in which the impact of estimands has been mentioned (EMA, 2023b).

4.4.3 Implications for Publications and Downstream Communication

As mentioned in previous sections, a small selection of examples now exists, whereby results have been published with clear reference to the estimands that they address; for example, see Aroda et al. (2019a), Frias et al. (2021), and Wilding et al. (2021). Further, in the PIONEER 1 example (Aroda et al., 2019a), the labeling conventions used to distinguish between results from different estimands were consistently carried through to all secondary manuscripts, hence providing further clarity when comparing results across publications.

4.5 Concluding Remarks

Implementation of the ICH E9(R1) guideline helps improve transparency to different stakeholders throughout the trial process, from the design to the result reporting. The benefit from the efforts of incorporating the estimand framework can only be realized by good documentation practice. This chapter has focused on new requirements regarding the documentation of estimands in the trial protocol and SAP, impact on the analysis datasets, and new expectations on reporting results in the CSR, submission dossiers, and publications. Practices on these aspects are still evolving, and it is expected that more examples will emerge soon.

References

Aroda, V. R., Rosenstock, J., Terauchi, Y., Altuntas, Y., Lalic, N. M., Morales Villegas, E. C., Jeppesen, O. K., Christiansen, E., Hertz, C. L., & Haluzík, M. (2019a). PIONEER 1: Randomized clinical trial of the efficacy and safety of oral semaglutide monotherapy in comparison with placebo in patients with type 2 diabetes. *Diabetes Care, 42*(9), 1724–1732.

Aroda, V. R., Saugstrup, T., Buse, J., Donsmark, M., Zacho, J., & Davies, M. (2019b). Incorporating and interpreting regulatory guidance on estimands in diabetes clinical trials: The PIONEER 1 randomized clinical trial as an example. *Diabetes, Obesity & Metabolism, 21*, 2203–2010.

Bell, J., Hamilton, A., Sailer, O., & Voss, F. (2021). The detailed clinical objectives approach to designing clinical trials and choosing estimands. *Pharmaceutical Statistics, 20*(6), 1112–1124.

EMA. (2023a). *Guideline on clinical investigation of medicinal products in the treatment or prevention of diabetes mellitus—Revision 2. CPMP/EWP/1080/00 Rev 2*. Available at www.ema.europa.eu

EMA. (2023b). *Assessment of SmPC section 5.1 (draft). EMA/CHMP/566497/2023*. Available at www.ema.europa.eu

Frias, J. P., Bonora, E., Nevarez Ruiz, L., Li, Y. G., Yu, Z., Milicevic, Z., Malik, R., Bethel, M. A., & Cox, D. A. (2021). Efficacy and safety of dulaglutide 3.0 mg and 4.5 mg versus dulaglutide 1.5 mg in metformin-treated patients with type 2 diabetes in a randomized controlled trial (AWARD-11). *Diabetes Care, 44*(3), 765–773.

ICH. (2019). *E9(R1) addendum on estimands and sensitivity analysis in clinical trials to the guideline on statistical principles for clinical trials*. Step 4 document available at www.ich.org

ICH. (2021). *E9(R1) training material*. Available at https://ich.org/

ICH. (2022). *M11 Clinical electronic structured harmonized protocol*. (Draft) Step 2 document available at www.ich.org

Lynggaard, H., Bell, J., Lösch, C., Besseghir, A., Rantell, K., Schoder, V., & Lanius, V. (2022). Principles and recommendations for incorporating estimands into clinical study protocol templates. *Trials, 23*(1), 685.

Polverejan, E., O'Kelly, M., Hefting, N., Norton, J. D., Lim, P., & Walton, M. K. (2023). Defining clinical trial Estimands: A practical guide for study teams with examples based on a psychiatric disorder. *Therapeutic Innovation & Regulatory Science, 57*, 1–29.

TransCelerate BioPharma INC. (2024). *Clinical Content & Reuse Solutions; Common Protocol Template (CPT)*. Available at www.transceleratebiopharmainc.com

Wilding, J. P., Batterham, R. L., Calanna, S., Davies, M., Van Gaal, L. F., Lingvay, I., McGowan, B. M., Rosenstock, J., Tran, M. T., Wadden, T. A., & Wharton, S. (2021). Once-weekly semaglutide in adults with overweight or obesity. *New England Journal of Medicine, 384*(11), 989–1002.

Chapter 5
Estimands and Causal Inference

Mouna Akacha, Jonathan Bartlett, Bjorn Bomkamp, Tianmeng Lyu, Hege Michiels, and Kaspar Rufibach

Abstract Although the ICH E9(R1) guideline introduces the estimand framework for clinical trials without explicitly using the term "causal," it refers to treatment effects as how the outcome of treatment compares to what would have happened to the same subjects under an alternative treatment. This definition of estimands is aligned with the potential outcomes framework utilized in causal inference. Randomized controlled trials (RCTs) are the gold standard for estimating the average causal treatment effect in drug development. More broadly, causal inference plays a crucial role whenever care and assumptions are needed to account for confounding factors and selection biases, such as in observational studies or RCTs subject to intercurrent events. In this chapter, we will review causal inference and its assumptions, discuss the role it can have in drug development (in randomized trials and observational data analyses), and discuss the interplay between causal inference and the ICH E9(R1) guideline. In this context, we will stress the importance of well-defined interventions and estimands, proper trial designs, and transparent assumptions to ensure valid and reliable conclusions.

M. Akacha (✉) · B. Bomkamp
Advanced Methodology and Data Science, Novartis Pharma AG, Basel, Switzerland
e-mail: mouna.akacha@novartis.com; bjoern.bornkamp@novartis.com

J. Bartlett
Department of Medical Statistics and Faculty of Epidemiology and Population Health, London School of Hygiene & Tropical Medicine, London, UK
e-mail: Jonathan.Bartlett1@lshtm.ac.uk

T. Lyu
Advanced Methodology and Data Science, Novartis Pharmaceuticals Corporation, East Hanover, NJ, USA
e-mail: tianmeng.lyu@novartis.com

H. Michiels
Quantitative Sciences, Argenx, Ghent, Belgium

K. Rufibach
Advanced Biostatistical Sciences, Clinical Measurement Sciences, Merck KGaA, Darmstadt, Germany
e-mail: kaspar.rufibach@merckgroup.com

J. Wei et al. (eds.), *Estimands in Clinical Trials*, Springer Series in Pharmaceutical Statistics, https://doi.org/10.1007/978-3-032-02192-2_5

5.1 What is Causal Inference?

Causal inference can be defined as the scientific discipline that considers the assumptions, trial designs, and estimation strategies that allow researchers to draw causal conclusions from experiments and data (Hill & Stuart, 2015). Here, "causal conclusion" refers to a conclusion regarding the effect of a particular variable (e.g., treatment) on some outcome(s) of interest. Importantly, observed association does not necessarily imply causation. This was also famously discussed in the 1950s when the first studies showing a correlation between smoking and lung cancer were published (Doll & Hill, 1950). While nowadays there is no doubt that smoking causes lung cancer, in the 1950s, it remained unclear, and, for example, Fisher (1958) argued:

> The curious associations with lung cancer found in relation to smoking habits do not, in the minds of some of us, lend themselves easily to the simple conclusions that the products of combustion reaching the surface of the bronchus induce, though after a long interval, the development of cancer.

An alternative explanation for the observed association was the possible existence of a common cause for both smoking and lung cancer. If this were true, then the association would be observed even if there was no causation between smoking and lung cancer (Doll & Hill, 1950; Fisher, 1958).

5.1.1 Potential Outcomes Framework

The potential outcomes framework (Neyman, 1923; Rubin, 1978) allows us to formally define causal effects. The first to formalize this was Neyman, who, in his master's thesis (Neyman, 1923), introduced what we know today as the potential outcomes framework. This framework postulates that at inclusion in a trial (be it randomized or not), each patient has two potential outcomes. With Y the outcome and Z the intervention, $Y(Z = 1)$ represents the potential outcome if the patient were on treatment and $Y(Z = 0)$ the potential outcome if the patient were on control.

While Neyman considered randomization-based inference where only the treatment assignment is random (see Chapter 6 in Imbens and Rubin (2015) for an introduction), Rubin later extended the idea of potential outcomes beyond randomization-based inference and situations where the treatment assignment is randomized (Rubin, 1978).

5.1.2 Causal Effects

The potential or counterfactual outcomes require a thought experiment on what the outcome would be if the same patient were assigned to different treatment options. In the aforementioned example, $Y(1)$ represents whether a subject would have lung cancer or not if (s)he smoked and $Y(0)$ whether the same subject would have lung cancer or not if (s)he did not smoke. Smoking has a causal effect on patient i if $Y_i(1) \neq Y_i(0)$. In practice, however, we can only observe one of the two potential outcomes $Y(1)$ and $Y(0)$ but not both.

The population-level causal effect is defined as a contrast of functionals of potential outcomes. For example, the average causal effect of treatment Z on outcome Y can be defined as $E[Y(1) - Y(0)]$. Note that the causal effects are all defined based on potential outcomes, while the contrasts in the outcomes conditional on the received treatment, $E(Y|Z = 1)$ vs. $E(Y|Z = 0)$, are referred to as an association effect. In other words, causation answers questions like "What is the treatment effect if all patients were on treatment compared to if all of them were on control?" whereas association answers questions like "What is the outcome in patients who are on treatment compared to the outcome in patients who are on control?" For a graphical representation of association vs. causation, we refer to Fig. 1.1 of Hernán and Robins (2020).

The definition of causation and association is, hence, different, and the average causal effect may not equal the association contrast. This is especially true in observational studies, as treatment and control patients are not necessarily comparable due to potential treatment–outcome confounding.

5.1.3 Commonly Used Identification Assumptions

The main challenge with causal inference is that we will never observe the two potential outcomes for the same patient simultaneously and, therefore, need to rely on assumptions about the missing potential outcomes. In the following, the three most commonly used identification assumptions will be introduced, along with a discussion on their relevance in randomized controlled trials (RCTs) and observational studies.

First, the stable unit treatment value assumption (Little & Rubin, 2000) is needed to infer the population causal effects from randomized and observational data.

Assumption 5.1 Stable unit treatment value assumption (SUTVA). This assumption includes two parts:

1. Consistency: For every patient i, if $Z_i = z$, then $Y_i = Y_i(z)$.
2. No interference: Patient i's outcome does not depend on patient j's treatment $(i \neq j)$.

The consistency assumption states that the observed outcome is equal to the potential outcome under the received treatment. This assumption requires the treatment to be well-defined. If there are potentially different versions of treatment, for example, for the same treatment, "heart transplant," different doctors may use different surgical techniques (Hernán & Robins, 2020); then, the consistency assumption can be violated, see also Sect. 5.3 for further discussion. Potential violation of the no-interference assumption may occur, for example, in vaccine studies, where the infection outcome of a patient may depend on whether others are vaccinated or not.

Relying on Assumption 5.1 and randomization, the causal effect $E[Y(1) - Y(0)]$ is identifiable, which means that it can be expressed as an expectation of a function of the observed data, see Sect. 5.2 for a derivation. Without randomization, such as in observational studies, it may still be possible to estimate causal effects, albeit only by introducing additional assumptions. In fact, causal inference methods (e.g., Rubin, 1978; Robins, 1986; Greenland et al., 1999; Pearl 2001a, b) were initially developed for observational studies, where the primary issue involves treatment–outcome confounding (Lipkovich et al., 2020). These methods rely on the assumption of no unmeasured confounders or exchangeability.

Assumption 5.2 Exchangeability. The potential outcomes are independent of treatment assignment, conditional on confounders X; i.e., $Y(z) \perp Z \mid X$, for all z.

If X impacts both treatment assignment Z and potential outcomes $Y(z)$, then X is called a confounder of Z and $Y(z)$. The exchangeability assumption holds if all confounders impacting Z and $Y(z)$ are identified and observed; i.e., there are no unmeasured confounders. This assumption is expected to hold in randomized controlled trials where the treatment assignment is either completely random or depends on known covariates (e.g., in a stratified randomization). In observational studies, the confounders to condition upon to achieve exchangeability are unknown, and care needs to be taken to identify the confounders. In fact, the exchangeability assumption cannot be verified from the observed data in an observational study.

Finally, the positivity assumption is (implicitly) assumed to ensure that there is a probability greater than zero of being assigned to each of the treatment levels.

Assumption 5.3 Positivity. Here, we assume that conditional on the selected covariates X, the probability of receiving each treatment is positive; i.e., for all z and x, $0 < P(Z = z|X = x) < 1$.

This assumption is expected to hold by randomization but is not guaranteed in observational studies. For example, in the smoking example (see Sect. 5.1.2), the positivity assumption may be violated as health-conscious patients are usually nonsmokers.

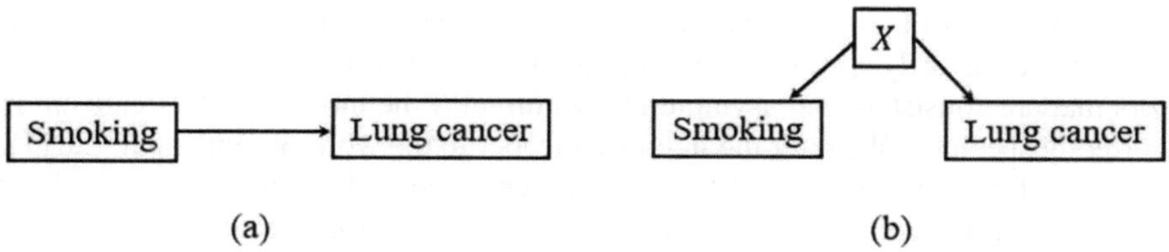

Fig. 5.1 Causal directed acyclic graphs to illustrate two possible underlying mechanisms to explain the observed association between smoking and lung cancer

5.1.4 Causal Directed Acyclic Graphs

To evaluate the plausibility of the above assumptions, causal directed acyclic graphs (Greenland et al., 1999; Pearl, 1995) can be used as they provide graphical representations of the assumed data-generating mechanism. These graphical models are nonparametric, in the sense that they do not impose assumptions on the functional relationships between variables or on the distributions of the variables. Moreover, they enable us to incorporate expert knowledge in the form of causal assumptions. More information can be found in the work by Hernán and Robins (2020). For example, we can use causal directed acyclic graphs to illustrate the different possible underlying data mechanisms to explain the observed association between smoking and lung cancer (Doll & Hill, 1950; Fisher, 1958). Figure 5.1a illustrates the option that smoking causes lung cancer, whereas Fig. 5.1b illustrates the alternative explanation where there are common causes to both smoking and lung cancer, which induce the observed association. Note that important assumptions are made by the arrows that are left out. For example, in Fig. 5.1(a), we assume that there are no common causes of smoking and lung cancer.

5.1.5 Estimation Techniques

Over the years, different estimation techniques have been developed to draw conclusions from observational data, based on the aforementioned identification and additional model assumptions. For example, inverse probability weighting (Horvitz & Thompson, 1952) creates a pseudo-population in which every patient appears as a treated and as a control patient. Every observed outcome is inversely weighted by the probability of the observed treatment, given the covariates. In doing so, population causal effects can be estimated, as a situation is mimicked where treatment assignment is random. Standardization (Robins, 1986), also called g-computation, is an alternative method that relies on modeling the outcome, given treatment and confounders, rather than modeling the treatment, given confounders. In addition, doubly robust estimation (Scharfstein et al., 1999; Robins, 2000) relies on a model for the treatment and a model for the outcome but is guaranteed to be consistent, even when one of these models, but not both, is misspecified. Moreover, when both models are correctly specified, it has the smallest asymptotic variance of all estimators that are consistent and asymptotically normal if the model for the treatment is correctly specified. We refer the interested reader to the work of Funk et al. (2011).

In randomized clinical trials, causal inference methods were initially used for settings with noncompliance (Robins, 1998; Rubin, 1998). Recently, the focus on causal inference techniques within clinical trials has expanded to settings involving intercurrent events beyond noncompliance, such as competing event settings (Schmidli et al., 2023; Young et al., 2020). We will discuss additional examples in the next section.

5.2 What is the Role of Causal Inference in Drug Development?

In this section, we will illustrate the value of causal inference in drug development by focusing on different drug development settings. Before doing so, we discuss the interplay of randomization, the cornerstone of drug development, and causal inference.

5.2.1 Randomized Controlled Trials

Regulatory agencies stress the importance of randomization in drug development through various guidelines. For example, the European Medicines Agency (EMA) discusses the role of randomization in its rare disease guideline (EMA, 2007) by emphasizing that most orphan drugs and pediatric indications submitted for regulatory approval are based on randomized controlled trials and that deviation from such standards should only be considered when completely unavoidable. Even more prominently, EMA's reflection paper on single-arm trials (EMA, 2023) states in its opening that randomized controlled trials (RCTs) are the standard for providing confirmatory evidence on the efficacy of a new treatment. Similarly, the US Food and Drug Administration (FDA) generally considers randomized superiority trials with a placebo- or active-control design to be the strongest provider of evidence of effectiveness (FDA, 2019).

This emphasis in the guidelines of two major regions invites the question as to why randomization is so crucial for drug approval. One explanation is that randomization allows trialists to make a causal statement about drug efficacy with few assumptions (Chapters 5 and 6 in Imbens & Rubin, 2015; Rosenberger et al., 2019). To formally show that randomization allows us to estimate a causal effect, suppose we are interested in estimating the average treatment effect, ATE $=E(Y(1) - Y(0))$ in a sampling-based inference framework. To do so, we make the three assumptions laid out in Sect. 5.1, and together with the linearity of the expectation, we get:

$$\begin{aligned}
\text{ATE} &= E\big(Y(1)-Y(0)\big)=E\big(Y(1)\big)-E\big(Y(0)\big) && \text{linearity of } E(.)\\
&= E_x\big(E\big(Y(1)|X\big)\big)-E_x\big(E\big(Y(0)|X\big)\big) && \text{law of total expectation}\\
&= E_x\big(E\big(Y(1)|Z=1,X\big)\big)-E_x\big(E\big(Y(0)|,Z=0|,X\big)\big) && \text{exchangeability}\\
&= E_x\big(E\big(Y|Z=1,X\big)\big)-E_x\big(E\big(Y|Z=0,X\big)\big) && \text{consistency.}
\end{aligned}$$

In randomized controlled trials, the benefit of randomly assigning well-defined interventions to two groups of patients is that the consistency, positivity, and exchangeability assumptions generally hold, even without conditioning on further baseline covariates. Consequently, estimation of the average treatment effect becomes straightforward. So one crucial role that causal inference plays in drug development is that it provides a rigorous justification for randomized clinical trials, notably the cornerstone of pharmaceutical drug development, as discussed above.

However, there is more to the usefulness of causal inference for drug development. As exemplified above, causal inference surfaces the assumptions that are needed to make a causal claim. These assumptions can then be transparently discussed within a trial team, between sponsor and regulator, and among any other stakeholders. Many of these assumptions are trivially met when randomizing and running a tightly controlled trial.

In the following sections, we will consider the value of causal inference in settings beyond randomized controlled trials and the average treatment effect.

5.2.2 *Non-randomized Trials*

In the last section, we discussed the interplay of randomization and causal inference. However, there are situations in drug development where we still want to make a causal claim but where randomization is not feasible or ethical, such as in situations where standard treatments are not effective at all (e.g., in terminally ill oncology patients), or we want to draw a causal conclusion from data that has already been collected outside of a randomized controlled trial, such as observational or real-world data studies. That was the setup where the target trial framework was first proposed (Hernán & Robins, 2016; Hernán et al., 2022), and it is broadly applied today. The first step in the target trial framework is a proper formulation and documentation of the causal question of interest in the protocol of a hypothetical randomized controlled trial that would allow the estimation of this effect. The protocol must specify certain key elements that define the causal estimand: eligibility criteria, treatment strategies, treatment assignment, the start and end of follow-up, outcomes, and causal contrasts. Estimation of the targeted estimand is specified either in this protocol or in a separate data analysis plan. Typically, a randomized trial that would allow estimation of the causal estimand of interest is then described in such a protocol, and this trial then becomes the target trial for the causal estimand of interest. The second step is to emulate the components of that protocol using the observational (or real-world) data: finding eligible individuals, assigning them to a treatment strategy compatible with their data, following them up from assignment (time zero) until outcome or the end of follow-up, and conducting the analysis as specified for the corresponding target trial. To emulate random treatment assignment, typically, adjustment for baseline confounders is performed.

5.2.3 Single-Arm Trials

If randomization is considered to not be feasible or ethical, single-arm trials are oftentimes considered, and causal inference offers a framework to display the assumptions needed to be able to make causal claims, see Rippin et al. (2022) for a comprehensive discussion. Hampson et al. (2023) provide an example of contextualizing a single-arm trial with real-world data in relapsed–refractory follicular lymphoma. Starting from the clinical question of interest, "To evaluate the efficacy of tisagenlecleucel as compared to the current standard-of-care as measured by complete response, overall survival, and progression free survival," the authors combine the target trial with the ICH E9(R1) estimand framework (ICH, 2019), where the latter primarily contributes the concept of intercurrent events. The causal effect that is then formulated by combining the two frameworks is "What is the causal effect of prescribing tisagenlecleucel vs. standard -of-care in patients meeting the inclusion/exclusion criteria of the single arm trial?" This causal effect corresponds to the average treatment effect on the treated (ATT), which is different from the ATE defined above. Emulating the causal question of a target randomized controlled trial complemented by considerations about intercurrent events offers, at least, the following advantages: (i) clarity on the causal effect one is estimating, which, here, is the average treatment effect on the treated; (ii) understanding of the differences between the inclusion and exclusion criteria; (iii) listing of intercurrent events (here, new anticancer treatment) and defining strategies on how to deal with them; and (iv) decision on what to take as the index date (i.e., the date of inclusion of the patient in the emulated trial).

5.2.4 Causal Effects of Interest in Drug Development

In drug development, we are often interested in the effect of the initially randomized treatment on an outcome while accounting for intercurrent events, such as discontinuation of treatment, initiation of rescue therapy, or treatment switching. Hernán et al. (2013) argued that randomized trials are only expected to be free from baseline confounding but not from post-randomization confounding and selection bias. Here, selection bias refers to potentially different follow-up patterns between treatment arms.

The original ICH E9 guideline (ICH, 1998) suggested utilizing the intention-to-treat (ITT) principle, which, in that guideline, implies that (i) all randomized patients should be included in the analysis and (ii) that

> the effect of a treatment policy can be best assessed by evaluating on the basis of the intention to treat a subject (i.e., the planned treatment regimen) rather than the actual treatment given.

An argument for this principle given in the ICH E9 guideline was that the preservation of the initial randomization in analysis is important in preventing bias and in providing a secure foundation for statistical tests. It is important to note that the ITT principle, as introduced in the ICH E9 guideline, is not an estimand but rather a principle that refers to what the ICH E9(R1) guideline now calls analysis sets. These refer to the patients recruited in the clinical trial (the sample drawn from the population), which should be included in the analysis and pertains entirely to estimation. The ICH E9(R1) guideline refers to this as the full analysis set, which is defined to be as close as possible to including all randomized patients.

The ICH E9 guideline mentions that implementing the ITT principle necessitates complete follow-up of all randomized patients for trial outcomes. In case some data are not available for certain patients, the ICH E9 guideline suggests the use of imputation methods. Over the years, it has become clear that this guidance is not sufficiently clear, in the sense that imputations are driven by assumptions, but to assess the validity of those assumptions, one needs to clarify what estimand one is targeting. In addition, clinical events, such as discontinuation of treatment, initiation of rescue therapy, or treatment switching, are informative by themselves. How to address such events in an efficacy analysis goes beyond just a missing data-handling problem. Hernán et al. (2013) argued that

> what started as an RCT may effectively become an observational study that requires analyses that complement, but go beyond, intention-to-treat analyses,

and these analyses are often rooted in causal inference. In the ICH E9(R1) guideline, such post-baseline events are called intercurrent events, and five strategies are proposed to account for the interplay of the intercurrent events and other estimand attributes like outcome variable or population, see Chap. 2 in this book for a detailed introduction. All these strategies can be embedded in a causal frame using potential outcomes, as discussed by Lipkovich et al. (2020). This again emphasizes the relevance of causal inference for drug development. Of the proposed five strategies, the treatment policy strategy can arguably be considered the closest in spirit to the ITT principle. The subtle differences between the ITT principle and applying a treatment policy strategy for an intercurrent event have been discussed by Fletcher et al. (2022).

The ICH E9(R1) guideline acknowledges that treatment effect measures other than treatment policy effects may be of interest in certain settings. In these situations, causal inference plays an even more crucial role in (i) enabling a precise definition of the estimands through the potential outcome framework and (ii) providing tailored estimation techniques.

One such example can be found in the context of per-protocol set (PPS) analyses. Protocol violations are often documented when conducting clinical trials, and according to the original ICH E9 guideline, it is often of interest to estimate a treatment effect that most closely reflects the scientific model underlying the protocol. The traditional analysis in these situations compares the outcomes across treatment arms on the subgroups of patients that adhere to the protocol on treatment and on control arms. From the potential outcome perspective, protocol adherence is a post-baseline variable, and each patient thus possesses possibly different potential outcomes for protocol adherence on the treatment and on the control arm. This analysis thus does not estimate a causal effect, unless a strong assumption is made that the potential outcome of protocol adherence is independent of the assigned treatment. This is also reflected in the ICH E9(R1) guideline, which states that it may not be possible to construct a relevant estimand with which the analysis of the PPS is aligned and that, later,

> estimands might be constructed, with aligned method of analysis, that better address the objective usually associated with the analysis of the PPS. If so, analysis of the PPS might not add additional insights.

The role of PPS analyses in the context of vaccine trials and their interplay with causal inference techniques are also considered by Michiels et al. (2022).

An additional illustration of the value of the ICH E9(R1) guideline and causal inference considerations can be drawn in the context of clinical trial disruptions. For example, the coronavirus disease (COVID-19) pandemic and associated measures like lockdowns led to various intercurrent events, such as treatment discontinuation due to drug supply issues. The estimand framework and causal inference thinking proved very valuable when considering the interplay of such intercurrent events and the original research question (Akacha et al., 2020; Meyer et al., 2020; Van Lancker et al., 2023). It may, for example, be relevant to estimate the treatment effect in the absence of logistical challenges caused by the COVID-19 pandemic. This hypothetical estimand may require assumptions or analysis techniques introduced in the causal inference literature (Van Lancker et al., 2023). We refer to Chap. 23 in this book for further details on how the estimand framework can be leveraged for clinical trial disruptions like the COVID-19 pandemic.

Finally, another causal effect, which has found its way into drug development, is based on principal stratification, corresponding to one of the five intercurrent event strategies laid out in the ICH E9(R1) guideline. There are many questions in randomized clinical trials that involve a comparison of subpopulations defined by post-baseline variables. Such post-baseline variables can be the occurrence of an adverse event or dose reductions, the value of a biomarker above some threshold, or exposure below a threshold. All these can be considered intercurrent events, following the framework laid out in the ICH E9(R1) guideline, which defines intercurrent events as events occurring after treatment initiation that affect either the interpretation or the existence of the measurements associated with the clinical question of interest.

One way to deal with such intercurrent events is by principal stratification, where strata are defined based on the potential outcomes of the intercurrent event. Treatment effects of interest are then defined in one or a combination of these strata. In the context of antidrug antibodies for targeted oncology trials, one may, for example, be interested in the question "Do patients that develop anti-drug antibodies on the treatment arm still benefit from the treatment?" See Kong et al. (2023) for more details on this example. Various estimation methods making different assumptions have been proposed (e.g., Lipkovich et al., 2022), and we will provide additional considerations in Sect. 5.3. Bornkamp et al. (2021) provide a discussion of the potential role of principal stratification in drug development and offer many examples and some considerations on estimation methods. Bornkamp and Bermann (2020) discuss an illustrative example for an intercurrent event of a biomarker over a certain threshold. Other authors have looked at the effects on adherers, see, for example, Qu et al. (2020). We refer to Chap. 19 in this book for further details on principal stratification.

5.3 What is the Interplay of Causal Inference and the ICH E9(R1) Guideline?

In this section, we discuss the interplay between causal inference concepts and methods and the ICH E9(R1) guideline. Ostensibly, the ICH E9(R1) guideline does not refer to or make use of concepts of methods from the causal inference literature, and indeed, the word "causal" never appears. Nevertheless, as noted by others (Scharfstein, 2019), concepts from causal inference clearly run throughout the guideline. As discussed earlier, the estimands following from the five intercurrent event strategies can all be written using potential outcomes notation (Lipkovich et al., 2020). Likewise, Drury et al. (2024) emphasize that the estimand framework and causal inference are complementary, not competing, paradigms. In the remainder of this chapter, we consider commonalities of the addendum and causal inference literature and discuss topics where concepts in the ICH E9(R1) guideline have been discussed potentially under different names or notation in the causal inference literature.

5.3.1 Definition of Treatment Effect

The ICH E9(R1) guideline adopts a counterfactual viewpoint to define treatment effects. In Section A.3, the guideline states:

> Central questions for drug development and licensing are to establish the existence, and to estimate the magnitude, of treatment effects: how the outcome of treatment compares to what would have happened to the same subjects under alternative treatment.

This is very close to the definition of causal effect in parts of the causal inference literature: In their Technical Point 1.1, Hernán and Robins (2020) state:

> The average causal effect, defined by a contrast of means of counterfactual outcomes, is the most commonly used population causal effect. [...] In general, a population causal effect can be defined as a contrast of any functional of the marginal distributions of counterfactual outcomes under different actions or treatment values.

This definition implies that treatment effect model parameters in some regression models may not necessarily be causal effects (or only under certain additional assumptions). This has caused some discussion. For a summary, see, for example, Daniel et al. (2021), who discuss marginal and conditional treatment effect measures, as well as the closely related concept of collapsibility of effect measures. Despite the similarity in definition of the treatment effect, the ICH E9(R1) guideline does not go into these technical details or even use the word causal effect. So even if the definition in the ICH E9(R1) guideline could be read to imply a certain restriction of the treatment effects to be used, this conclusion does not seem to be implied.

5.3.2 The Separation of Estimand Definition from Statistical Assumptions

The ICH E9(R1) guideline advocates a framework where the definition of the trial estimand comes first, followed by the specification of statistical estimation methods and their assumptions, see Chap. 1 in this book for details. This separation of estimand definition from statistical assumptions is in line with the causal inference literature, in particular van der Laan and Rose's targeted learning roadmap (van der Laan & Rose, 2011) and more recent developments in so-called assumption-lean inference (Vansteelandt & Dukes, 2022). Within this literature, the motivation for this separation is principally the idea that we should define the scientific question or quantity of interest without reference to statistical assumptions, not least because, often, the latter cannot be known to hold with certainty.

5.3.3 *Intercurrent Events and the Hypothetical Strategy*

A fundamental concept in the ICH E9(R1) guideline is the introduction of the term and notion of intercurrent events. Looking at the literature of modern causal inference, one does not see a concept clearly corresponding to intercurrent events. A link can, however, be made if one views the intercurrent event as a time-varying treatment, noting that this "treatment" is distinct from the initially randomized treatment (Lipkovich et al., 2020; Olarte Parra et al., 2023). For example, consider a trial in patients with diabetes where, if during follow-up, a patient's glycemic control becomes sufficiently poor, they receive rescue treatment with insulin. Here, we could contemplate the use of a hypothetical estimand that asks what would have happened had the insulin rescue treatment not been available. In this case, the receipt of rescue during the follow-up can be viewed as a time-varying treatment, and the hypothetical estimand of interest can be cast as the effect of A vs. B, had this time-varying treatment been set to zero at all follow-up time points (i.e., intervening on rescue so that it would not be available in the trial). From a causal mediation perspective, such a hypothetical estimand corresponds to a controlled direct effect (Pearl, 2001a, b), with the receipt of rescue medication taking the role of a mediator of the effect of randomized treatment on the final outcome.

Having made the connection between adopting a hypothetical strategy for addressing an intercurrent event and viewing it as a time-varying treatment, we are then able to leverage the developments from the causal inference literature on the identification and estimation of such effects (Olarte Parra et al., 2023). In particular, this raises the possibility of using data after the occurrence of such an intercurrent event in the estimation process, which is generally not done, with the potential for increased efficiency (Lasch et al., 2023).

5.3.4 *The Importance of Well-Defined Interventions*

A long-running debate among causal inference researchers concerns whether the notion of causal effects can only be attributed to interventions. This goes back to the motto "no causation without manipulation," which was coined in the paper by Holland (1986), arguing that causal effects should be reserved for interventions. Holland uses race and sex as examples of attributes that cannot be manipulated and, therefore, cannot be causes. This notion is also reflected in the SUTVA/consistency assumption (see Sect. 5.1.3) for the potential outcome to be well-defined. On the other hand, Bollen and Pearl (2013) disagree with the motto "no causation without manipulation." They consider it restrictive as it is reserved only to human interventions and excludes causal questions such as whether the moon causes the tides.

Hernán (2005), however, goes further and argues that in order to be well-defined, the effect of an exposure or treatment requires one to clearly define how exactly the exposure or treatment would be manipulated. For example, we might use data from an observational study to try and estimate the effects of body composition, measured by the ratio of lean body mass to fat mass, on functional outcomes in the elderly. Such an analysis, with suitable adjustment for confounding, contrasts outcomes between those with high and those with low lean-to-fat ratio. Arguably, the resulting estimate does not correspond to a well-defined causal effect because we have not considered possible interventions that would manipulate the lean-to-fat ratio. Various interventions could be possible (even if obviously unethical), such as vigorous exercise, starvation, and surgery (Hernán, 2005). Each may well alter the lean-to-fat ratio, but they would presumably have quite different effects on the functional outcome endpoint. As such, there really is a collection of possible causal effects of varying lean-to-fat ratio, and it is not clear which, if any, the estimate from the observational study corresponds to.

This issue would seem at first sight to be of little relevance to the topic of estimands in designed randomized studies. Here, we have two (or more) treatments to be compared, and the protocol contains the exact details on how the treatments are defined and should be administered. However, if we contemplate addressing an intercurrent event, the preceding discussion becomes relevant.

Consider, for example, the hypothetical strategy—how would we hypothetically prevent the intercurrent event from occurring, such that the effect of the intercurrent event is well-defined? In the earlier described case of insulin rescue in a diabetes trial, we could conceive of running the trial and not allowing patients to have access to insulin rescue treatment. Such a trial would not be ethical, and we would not run such a trial, but in principle, we could. Consider in the same trial that some patients may need to discontinue their randomized treatment due to adverse event occurrence. We may again contemplate adopting the hypothetical strategy to address this intercurrent event, asking what would have happened had we somehow forced patients to continue their randomized treatment despite the adverse event. Now, apart from the important point of whether the resulting estimand would be relevant to stakeholders, it is less clear that such an effect is well-defined—how would we force patients to continue taking treatment and convince physicians to be a part of this if it was contraindicated medically? Again, one could imagine various unethical ways of achieving this, but, analogous to the lean-to-fat ratio example, different approaches to forcing patients to remain on their randomized treatment may lead to material differences in outcomes. As such, one can argue that the estimand comparing treatment A to B in the hypothetical scenario where patients remain on randomized treatment throughout follow-up is ill-defined.

Also, for the treatment policy strategy, the notion of the exact definition of the "treatment" becomes relevant. Hernán and Scharfstein (2018), in a constructive criticism of the draft ICH E9(R1) guideline from 2017, note that treatment strategies should also be precisely defined in terms of prescribing how investigators and patients should react to intercurrent events. For example, the treatment condition "take treatment A" could mean "begin and continue taking treatment A until the end of follow-up (irrespective of, for example, adverse events)" or "begin treatment A and take it until the end of follow-up unless adverse events occur, in which case, take treatment C," or something else. Thus, Hernán and Scharfstein advocated incorporating the possible occurrence of intercurrent events into the treatment regimen's definition if its occurrence would or may alter the treatment(s) the patient receives. The final version of the ICH E9(R1) guideline from 2019 introduced "treatment" as a new estimand attribute, and the idea underlying the treatment policy strategy is that a subsequent treatment discontinuation and potential intake of alternative medication afterward can become part of this treatment attribute (as they reflect the actual experience of patients with the drug). However, it may not always be feasible to prespecify precisely how investigators or patients should react to events like treatment discontinuations or which follow-up medication will be prescribed. Medical practice may be different across regions for certain diseases; in a certain region, for example, a highly effective rescue medication may be prescribed, while in other regions, it may not be prescribed. This would then constitute a violation of the SUTVA/consistency assumption. In other situations, however, the specific difference in rescue medication will not have an important impact on the outcome. The SUTVA/consistency assumptions are an important reminder that the treatment estimand attribute should be carefully specified.

5.3.5 Principal Stratum Strategy

The one area in which the ICH E9(R1) guideline most obviously connects with the literature from causal inference is the discussion of using the principal stratum strategy to address intercurrent events, see also Sect. 5.2. Here, the estimand is defined in a subset of the population defined by the values of the potential outcomes of the intercurrent event under the different randomized treatments, although the ICH E9(R1) guideline describes this without formally using the terminology or notation of potential outcomes. From a drug development perspective, it has been argued that several relevant (often post hoc) questions can be identified to be of principal-stratum type (Bornkamp et al., 2021). Akacha et al. (2017) argue that a particular tripartite estimand approach is of most interest from the perspective of patients, physicians, regulators, and payers, in which one of three estimands is of principal-stratum type. At the same time, the causal inference community seems split about the usefulness of the principal stratum estimands. The use of the estimand has, for example, been criticized by Scharfstein (2019) and Stensrud and Dukes (2022) since, for a given patient, it is not definitively known at baseline whether they will belong to the principal stratum of patients to which the effect pertains. In addition, the authors criticize that the estimation of principal stratum effects relies on the use of assumptions that are not verifiable from the observed data, in particular, when across-worlds assumptions are required, which are controversially discussed in the causal inference community, see also Richardson and Robins (2013).

These are important caveats, even after taking into account that one can sometimes model principal stratum membership in terms of baseline covariates (which would allow us to predict the likelihood at baseline of whether or not certain intercurrent events will occur for an individual patient) or that sensitivity analyses are performed with respect to the assumptions.

Despite these considerations, there is interest in principal stratum estimands. While in many situations, for such questions, naive post hoc analyses are performed, the utilization of a principal stratum and potential outcomes perspective may lead to more reasonable analyses. One example, mentioned already earlier, is the development of antidrug antibodies for biological treatments. Antidrug antibodies may bind to the drug, and it is, thus, an important question whether the occurrence of such antibodies affects the efficacy or safety of the drug. The existence of antidrug antibodies is a post-baseline event, which, sometimes, may only occur in the investigational treatment arm. Naively comparing the outcomes of patients on the treatment arm with antidrug antibodies' occurrence vs. the outcomes of all patients on the control arm (or patients without antidrug antibodies' occurrence on treatment with all patients on the control arm) will, in general, not have a causal interpretation. This can be seen from noting that on the treatment arm, one conditions (subsets) on the post-baseline event, while no such conditioning or sub-setting is performed on the control arm. The baseline characteristics of the group developing or not developing antidrug antibodies on treatment may be different, so a causal conclusion of treatment effect cannot be given, see Kong et al. (2023) for more details or Peters et al. (2022) for an example.

5.3.6 The Importance of Assumptions and Sensitivity Analysis

The ICH E9(R1) guideline says little about specific statistical methods and assumptions, but in Section A.2, it defines a framework in which, in addition to a main estimator, a series of sensitivity estimators are also considered, see Chaps. 1 and 2 in this book for details. The latter targets the same estimand but explores the sensitivity of the main estimator to one or more of its statistical assumptions. This approach aligns with the strong emphasis made within the causal inference literature to explicate assumptions required to identify estimands from the observed data and develop methods that permit the assessment of the sensitivity of inferences to key assumptions. For example, the use of causal diagrams and assumptions relating to potential outcomes may help those involved in trials understand whether assumptions being made are plausible and, hence, whether the resulting treatment effect estimate can be relied upon (Olarte Parra et al., 2023). In regard to sensitivity analyses, while within pharmaceutical trials, sensitivity analyses for not-at-random missingness are now commonly conducted, thus far, sensitivity analysis methods from causal inference (e.g., Brumback et al., 2004) are, to the best of our knowledge, less used. We anticipate in the future greater uptake of such methods from those analyzing trials.

5.4 Concluding Remarks

In this chapter, we discussed the interplay of estimands and causal inference in global drug development. Not surprisingly, we conclude that causal thinking and inference play an important role. We believe that the ultimate goal of drug development is to answer causal questions about the desired and undesired effects of treatments. Patients and health care providers want to know whether taking a specific treatment vs. not taking it will have an effect on the patient's health status. In addition, they want to know the magnitude of such effects. It seems natural and intuitive to frame such questions using the potential outcome framework.

In global drug development, we refer to the ICH E9(R1) guideline when defining treatment effects of interest. Section 5.3.1 discusses in detail how similar the definitions of treatment effects in the ICH E9(R1) guideline and the causal effects in the causal inference literature are. The FDA guideline on covariate adjustment (FDA, 2023) also mentions causal inference approaches, highlighting the relevance of causal inference methodology in the regulatory setting.

More broadly, causal inference provides the following:

- A language to define scientific questions precisely.
- Clarity on the assumptions needed.
- Statistical methods to estimate the effects.

Throughout this chapter, we discussed that causal inference concepts and methods can:

- Add clarity for the validity of established approaches.
- Raise questions for the validity of established approaches.
- Help address intercurrent events.
- Allow targeting estimands other than treatment policy effects.
- Provide clarity on how to estimate treatment policy effects.
- Guide appropriate approaches to leverage trial external data.
- Support principled analysis of observational data.

While all these aspects are very valuable and promising, it is also fair to say that we are just at the beginning of understanding and evaluating the potential impact of causal inference in drug development. The examples mentioned in this chapter showcase the importance of causal thinking in the context of randomized trials, single-arm trials, and observational studies. However, more experience is needed, and it is unlikely that we will see general recommendations on relevant causal estimands, plausible identification assumptions, or appropriate estimation approaches in the near future. Indeed, for example, identification assumptions have not been explicitly mentioned in the ICH E9(R1) guideline. While the guideline distinguishes broadly between two tasks (defining the estimand and specifying appropriate statistical analyses), in causal inference, three tasks are often distinguished. Stensrud and Dukes (2022) state that they

> find it helpful to distinguish between the following three tasks of data analyses: (i) translation of the research question into a formal causal estimand, (ii) assessing conditions for identification of the causal estimand, and (iii) estimation of the causal estimand from observed data.

One potential contributing factor to the gradual adoption of causal inference in drug development is the existence of different schools of thought within the causal inference community. Prominent researchers in the field seem to disagree on some foundational aspects, for example, "What is the definition of a causal effect?" and "What type of assumptions are acceptable?" Some examples of these differences were discussed in Sect. 5.3. Furthermore, there is a lack of a single overarching causal inference framework. As discussed in Sect. 5.2.2., Hernán and Robins (2016) introduced the target trial framework for drawing causal conclusions from observational data. Petersen and van der Laan (2014) provide an alternative formal framework for causal inference from observational data. They focus on integrating causal modeling and statistical estimation rather than mimicking a randomized clinical trial. The alignment between these two frameworks and their interplay with the ICH E9(R1) guideline are not entirely clear. Hampson et al. (2023) provide a view on combining the target trial framework with the ICH E9(R1) estimand framework.

Another contributing factor to the gradual adoption of causal inference in drug development is the hesitance toward untestable assumptions in the analysis of clinical trials. Hernán et al. (2013) write:

> A key obstacle in the adoption of these complementary methods is a widespread reluctance to accept that overcoming the limitations of intention-to-treat analyses necessitates untestable assumptions. Embracing these more sophisticated analyses will require a new framework for both the design and conduct of randomized trials.

While the ICH E9(R1) guideline can be considered such a framework, a widespread reluctance toward relying on untestable assumptions still holds true.

The examples discussed in this chapter only give a small snapshot of application areas where causal thinking can contribute significantly. Additional areas include not only drug discovery (Cai et al., 2022) and pharmacometrics (Rogers et al., 2023) but also considerations around diversity in clinical trials, where causal inference concepts around generalizability and transportability (Dahabreh et al., 2020) may play an important role.

We believe that the clinical trialist and causal inference communities will need to collaborate more closely and understand each other's perspectives, terminologies, and constraints. In this context, the role of trial designs and regulatory requirements needs careful consideration. We owe it to patients and health care providers to answer causal questions about the treatments at hand and communicate the answers clearly through the label. While experience is still limited, we believe that causal thinking and inference have an important role to play.

References

Akacha, M., Bretz, F. And Ruberg, S. (2017). Estimands in clinical trials–broadening the perspective. Statistics in Medicine 36, 5–19.

Akacha, M., Branson, J., Bretz, F., Dharan, B., Gallo, P., Gathmann, I., Hemmings, R., Jones, J., Xi, D., & Zuber, E. (2020). Challenges in assessing the impact of the COVID-19 pandemic on the integrity and interpretability of clinical trials. *Statistics in Biopharmaceutical Research, 12*(4), 419–426.

Bollen, K. A., & Pearl, J. (2013). Eight myths about causality and structural equation models. In *Handbook of causal analysis for social research* (pp. 301–328). Springer.

Bornkamp, B., & Bermann, G. (2020). Estimating the treatment effect in a subgroup defined by an early post-baseline biomarker measurement in randomized clinical trials with time-to-event endpoint. *Statistics in Biopharmaceutical Research, 12*, 19–28.

Bornkamp, B., Rufibach, K., Lin, J., Liu, Y., Mehrotra, D. V., Roychoudhury, S., et al. (2021). Principal stratum strategy: potential role in drug development. *Pharmaceutical Statistics, 20*(4), 737–751.

Brumback, B. A., Hernán, M. A., Haneuse, S. J., & Robins, J. M. (2004). Sensitivity analyses for unmeasured confounding assuming a marginal structural model for repeated measures. *Statistics in Medicine, 23*(5), 749–767.

Cai, Z., Xi, D., Zhu, X., & Li, R. (2022). Causal discoveries for high dimensional mixed data. *Statistics in Medicine, 41*(24), 4924–4940.

Daniel, R., Zhang, J., & Farewell, D. (2021). Making apples from oranges: Comparing noncollapsible effect estimators and their standard errors after adjustment for different covariate sets. *Biometrical Journal, 63*(3), 528–557.

Dahabreh, I. J., Robertson, S. E., Steingrimsson, J. A., Stuart, E. A., & Hernán, M. A. (2020). Extending inferences from a randomized trial to a new target population. *Statistics in Medicine, 39*(14), 1999–2014.

Doll, R., & Hill, A. B. (1950). Smoking and carcinoma of the lung. *British Medical Journal, 2*(4682), 739.

Drury, T., Bartlett, J. W., Wright, D., and Keene, O. N. (2024). The estimand framework and causal inference: Complementary not competing paradigms. arXiv preprint arXiv:2412.12380.

EMA. (2007). Guideline on Clinical Trials in Small Populations. Available at https://www.ema.europa.eu.

EMA. (2023). Reflection paper on establishing efficacy based on single-arm trials submitted as pivotal evidence in a marketing authorization. Available at https://www.ema.europa.eu.

FDA. (2019). Demonstrating substantial evidence of effectiveness for human drug and biological products. Available at https://www.fda.gov

FDA. (2023). Adjusting for Covariates in Randomized Clinical Trials for Drugs and Biological Product. Available at https://www.fda.gov

Fisher, R. A. (1958). Cancer and smoking. *Nature, 182*(4635), 596.

Fletcher, C., Hefting, N., Wright, M., Bell, J., Anzures-Cabrera, J., Wright, D., Lynggaard, H., & Schueler, A. (2022). Marking 2-years of new thinking in clinical trials: The Estimand Journey. *Therapeutic Innovation & Regulatory Science, 56*(4), 637–650.

Funk, M. J., Westreich, D., Wiesen, C., Stürmer, T., Brookhart, M. A., & Davidian, M. (2011). Doubly robust estimation of causal effects. *American Journal of Epidemiology, 173*(7), 761–767.

Greenland, S., Pearl, J., & Robins, J. M. (1999). Causal diagrams for epidemiologic research. *Epidemiology, 10*, 37–48.

Hampson, L. V., Chu, J., Zia, A., Zhang, J., Hsu, W.-C., Parzynski, C. S., Hao, Y., & Degtyarev, E. (2023). Combining the target trial and estimand frameworks to define the causal estimand: An application using real-world data to contextualize a single-arm trial. *Statistics in Biopharmaceutical Research*. to appear.

Hernán, M. A. (2005). Invited commentary: Hypothetical interventions to define causal effects—Afterthought or prerequisite? *American Journal of Epidemiology, 162*(7), 618–620.

Hernán, M. A., Hernández-Díaz, S., & Robins, J. M. (2013). Randomized trials analyzed as observational studies. *Annals of Internal Medicine, 159*(8), 560–562.

Hernán, M. A., & Robins, J. M. (2016). Using big data to emulate a target trial when a randomized trial is not available. *American Journal of Epidemiology, 183*, 758–764.

Hernán, M. A., & Scharfstein, D. (2018). Cautions as regulators move to end exclusive reliance on intention to treat. *Annals of Internal Medicine, 168*(7), 515–516.

Hernán, M. A., & Robins, J. M. (2020). *Causal inference: What if.* Chapman & Hall/CRC.

Hernán, M. A., Wang, W., & Leaf, D. E. (2022). Target trial emulation: A framework for causal inference from observational data. *JAMA, 328*(24), 2446–2447.

Hill, J., & Stuart, E. A. (2015). *Causal inference: overview. International Encyclopedia of the Social & Behavioral Sciences* (2nd ed., pp. 255–260).

Holland, P. W. (1986). Statistics and causal inference. *Journal of the American Statistical Association, 81*(396), 945–960.

Horvitz, D. G., & Thompson, D. J. (1952). A generalization of sampling without replacement from a finite universe. *Journal of the American Statistical Association, 47*(260), 663–685.

ICH (1998). E9 guideline on statistical principles for clinical trials. Step 4 document available at www.ich.org

ICH (2019). E9(R1) addendum on estimands and sensitivity analysis in clinical trials to the guideline on statistical principles for clinical trials. Step 4 document available at www.ich.org

Imbens, G. W., & Rubin, D. B. (2015). *Causal inference in statistics, social, and biomedical sciences*. Cambridge University Press.

Kong, S., Heinzmann, D., Lauer, S., & Tian, L. (2023). Weighted approach for estimating effects in principal strata with missing data for a categorical post-baseline variable in randomized controlled trials. *Statistics in Biopharmaceutical Research, 15*(1), 187–197.

Lasch, F., Guizzaro, L., Petavy, F., & Gallo, C. (2023). A simulation study on the estimation of the effect in the hypothetical scenario of no use of symptomatic treatment in trials for disease-modifying agents for Alzheimer's disease. *Statistics in Biopharmaceutical Research, 15*(2), 386–399.

Little, R. J., & Rubin, D. B. (2000). Causal effects in clinical and epidemiological studies via potential outcomes: Concepts and analytical approaches. *Annual Review of Public Health, 21*(1), 121–145.

Lipkovich, I., Ratitch, B., & Mallinckrodt, C. H. (2020). Causal inference and estimands in clinical trials. *Statistics in Biopharmaceutical Research, 12*(1), 54–67.

Lipkovich, I., Ratitch, B., Qu, Y., Zhang, X., Shan, M., & Mallinckrodt, C. (2022). Using principal stratification in analysis of clinical trials. *Statistics in Medicine, 41*(19), 3837–3877.

Meyer, R. D., Ratitch, B., Wolbers, M., Marchenko, O., Quan, H., Li, D., Fletcher, C., Li, X., Wright, D., Shentu, Y., et al. (2020). Statistical issues and recommendations for clinical trials conducted during the COVID-19 pandemic. *Statistics in Biopharmaceutical Research, 12*(4), 399–411.

Michiels, H., Vandebosch, A., & Vansteelandt, S. (2022). Estimation and interpretation of vaccine efficacy in COVID-19 randomized clinical trials. *Statistical Communications in Infectious Diseases, 14*(1).

Neyman, J. Sur les applications de la theorie des probabilites aux experiences agricoles: Essai des principes. Master's Thesis (1923). Excerpts reprinted in English, Statistical Science, Vol. 5, pp. 463–472. (D. M. Dabrowska, and T. P. Speed, Translators). Available at https://www.ics.uci.edu/~sternh/courses/265/neyman_statsci1990.pdf

Olarte Parra, C., Daniel, R. M., & Bartlett, J. W. (2023). Hypothetical estimands in clinical trials: A unification of causal inference and missing data methods. *Statistics in Biopharmaceutical Research, 15*(2), 421–432.

Pearl, J. (1995). Causal diagrams for empirical research. *Biometrika, 82*(4), 669–688.

Pearl, J. (2001a). Direct and indirect effects. In *Proceedings of the seventeenth conference on uncertainty and artificial intelligence* (pp. 411–420). Morgan Kaufmann, San Francisco.
Pearl, J. (2001b). Causal inference in the health sciences: A conceptual introduction. *Health Services and Outcomes Research Methodology, 2*, 189–220.
Peters, S., Galle, P. R., Bernaards, C. A., Ballinger, M., Bruno, R., Quarmby, V., et al. (2022). Evaluation of atezolizumab immunogenicity: Efficacy and safety (part 2). *Clinical and Translational Science, 15*, 141–157.
Petersen, M. L., & van der Laan, M. J. (2014). Causal models and learning from data: Integrating causal modeling and statistical estimation. *Epidemiology (Cambridge, Mass.), 25*(3), 418.
Qu, Y., Fu, H., Luo, J., & Ruberg, S. J. (2020). A general framework for treatment effect estimators considering patient adherence. *Statistics in Biopharmaceutical Research, 12*(1), 1–18.
Richardson, T. S., & Robins, J. M. (2013). Single world intervention graphs (SWIGs): A unification of the counterfactual and graphical approaches to causality. *Center for the Statistics and the Social Sciences, University of Washington Series. Working Paper, 128*(30).
Rippin, G., Ballarini, N., Sanz, H., Largent, J., Quinten, C., & Pignatti, F. (2022). A review of causal inference for external comparator arm studies. *Drug Safety, 45*, 815–837.
Robins, J. (1986). A new approach to causal inference in mortality studies with a sustained exposure period—Application to control of the healthy worker survivor effect. *Mathematical Modelling, 7*(9–12), 1393–1512.
Robins, J. M. (1998). Correction for non-compliance in equivalence trials. *Statistics in Medicine, 17*(3), 269–302.
Robins, J. M. (2000). Robust estimation in sequentially ignorable missing data and causal inference models. *Proceedings of the American Statistical Association, 1999*, 6–10.
Rogers, J. A., Maas, H., & Pitarch, A. P. (2023). An introduction to causal inference for pharmacometricians. *CPT: Pharmacometrics & Systems Pharmacology, 12*, 27–40.
Rosenberger, W. F., Uschner, D., & Wang, Y. (2019). Randomization: The forgotten component of the randomized clinical trial. *Statistics in Medicine, 38*, 1–12.
Rubin, D. B. (1978). Bayesian inference for causal effects: The role of randomization. *The Annals of Statistics, 6*, 34–58.
Rubin, D. B. (1998). More powerful randomization-based p-values in double-blind trials with noncompliance. *Statistics in Medicine, 17*(3), 371–385.
Scharfstein, D. O., Rotnitzky, A., & Robins, J. M. (1999). Adjusting for nonignorable drop-out using semiparametric nonresponse models. *Journal of the American Statistical Association, 94*(448), 1096–1120.
Scharfstein, D. O. (2019). A constructive critique of the draft ICH E9 addendum. *Clinical Trials, 16*(4), 375–380.
Schmidli, H., Roger, J. H., & Akacha, M. (2023). Estimands for recurrent event endpoints in the presence of a terminal event. *Statistics in Biopharmaceutical Research, 15*(2), 238–248.
Stensrud, M. J., & Dukes, O. (2022). Translating questions to estimands in randomized clinical trials with intercurrent events. *Statistics in Medicine, 41*(16), 3211–3228.
Van der Laan, M. J., & Rose, S. (2011). *Targeted learning* (Springer Series in Statistics). Springer.
Van Lancker, K., Tarima, S., Bartlett, J., Bauer, M., Bharani-Dharan, B., Bretz, F., Flournoy, N., Michiels, H., Olarte Parra, C., Rosenberger, J. L., & Cro, S. (2023). Estimands and their estimators for clinical trials impacted by the Covid-19 pandemic: A report from the NISS Ingram Olkin forum series on unplanned clinical trial disruptions. *Statistics in Biopharmaceutical Research, 15*(1), 94–111.
Vansteelandt, S., & Dukes, O. (2022). Assumption-lean inference for generalized linear model parameters. *Journal of the Royal Statistical Society Series B: Statistical Methodology, 84*(3), 657–685.
Young, J. G., Stensrud, M. J., Tchetgen Tchetgen, E. J., & Hernán, M. A. (2020). A causal framework for classical statistical estimands in failure-time settings with competing events. *Statistics in Medicine, 39*(8), 1199–1236.

Chapter 6
Global Initiatives Since the Release of ICH E9(R1)

Jingjun Qiu, Hans Ulrich Burger, Paul Delmar, Evgeny Degtyarev, Christine Fletcher, Elena Polverejan, Chris Price, Stephen J. Ruberg, Kaspar Rufibach, Nikolaos Sfikas, Lori Van Meter, and Siyue Wang

J. Qiu (✉)
Biometrics and Data Science, FosunPharma, Beijing, China
e-mail: qiujingjun@fosunpharma.com

H. U. Burger
Roche, Basel, Switzerland
e-mail: hans_ulrich.burger@roche.com

P. Delmar
Data Science, Basel, Switzerland
e-mail: paul.delmar@roche.com

E. Degtyarev
Advanced Quantitative Sciences, Basel, Switzerland
e-mail: evgeny.degtyarev@novartis.com

C. Fletcher
Biostatistics, Stevenage, UK
e-mail: chrissie.a.fletcher@gsk.com

E. Polverejan
Quantitative Sciences and Clinical Pharmacology, Johnson & Johnson, Titusville, NJ, USA
e-mail: epolvere@its.jnj.com

C. Price
Data Sciences, Roche, Welwyn, UK
e-mail: chris.price.cp1@roche.com

S. J. Ruberg
Analytix Thinking / Purdue University, Indianapolis, USA

K. Rufibach
Methods, Collaboration, and Outreach Group (MCO), Product Development Data Sciences, Basel, Switzerland

J. Wei et al. (eds.), *Estimands in Clinical Trials*, Springer Series in Pharmaceutical Statistics, https://doi.org/10.1007/978-3-032-02192-2_6

N. Sfikas
AQS, Biostatistics, Basel, Switzerland
e-mail: nikolaos.sfikas@novartis.com

L. Van Meter
Integrated Data and Analytics, Johnson & Johnson, Titusville, NJ, USA
e-mail: lvanmet@its.jnj.com

S. Wang
Harvard T.H Chan School of Public Health, Boston, MA, USA
e-mail: siyuewang@hsph.harvard.edu

Abstract This chapter provides a comprehensive overview of global initiatives to implement the International Council for Harmonisation of Technical Requirements for Pharmaceuticals for Human Use (ICH) E9(R1) guideline and its estimand framework across diverse therapeutic areas and statistical disciplines. It highlights the work of seven international working groups, each contributing to the refinement and practical application of the estimand framework in clinical trials. This chapter summarizes the background, objectives, and main activities of each working group. Key initiatives such as the publication of white papers, development of best practices, and engagement with regulatory bodies are discussed, emphasizing the importance of interdisciplinary collaboration. This chapter also highlights how these working groups have fostered global communication through seminars, workshops, and collaborative publications, including the development of the Drug Information Association's (DIA) Estimand Bluebook in Chinese, which forms the basis of this book. This chapter underscores the ongoing efforts to ensure accurate interpretation and implementation of the estimand framework to enhance the quality and efficiency of clinical trials worldwide as new concepts, methodologies, and guidelines continue to emerge.

6.1 Introduction

This chapter provides an overview of global initiatives that were created in response to the release of the International Council for Harmonisation of Technical Requirements for Pharmaceuticals for Human Use (ICH) E9(R1) guideline (ICH, 2019), aimed at developing and implementing the estimand framework. It recognizes the simultaneous contributions of various working groups and peers from different regions. This chapter summarizes the objectives and scope of the following seven working groups:

- European Federation of Pharmaceutical Industries and Associations (EFPIA)/ European Federation of Statisticians in the Pharmaceutical Industry (EFSPI) Estimand Implementation Working Group.
  (https://www.efspi.org/EFSPI/Working_Groups/EFSPI_EFPIA_EIWG.aspx)
- Neuroscience Estimand Working Group.

(https://www.psiweb.org/sigs-special-interest-groups/neuroscience-estimands)
- Oncology Estimand Working Group. (https://oncoestimand.github.io/oncowg_webpage/docs/)
- Tripartite Working Team (TWT).
- Pharmaceutical Users Software Exchange (PHUSE) Estimand Working Group (https://advance.hub.phuse.global/wiki/spaces/WEL/pages/26804662/Implementation+of+Estimands+ICH+E9+R1+using+Data+Standards)
- International Society for Central Nervous System (CNS) Clinical Trials and Methodology (ISCTM) Estimands and Missing Data Working Group (https://isctm.org/missing-data-working-group-activity-deliverables/)
- China Drug Information Association (DIA)-China Clinical Trial Statistics (CCTS) Estimand Working Group (DC-EWG).

Each section describes the background, objectives, main activities, forms of collaboration, and deliverables. We extend our gratitude for the significant contributions made by all working group members and promote the continued exchange of knowledge and innovative ideas.

6.2 EFPIA/EFSPI Estimand Implementation Working Group

6.2.1 Background and Objectives

The Estimand Implementation Working Group (EIWG) was established in October 2019, around the time of the release of the ICH E9(R1) guideline in December 2019. Sponsored by the European Federation of Statisticians in the Pharmaceutical Industry (EFSPI) and the European Federation of Pharmaceutical Industries and Associations (EFPIA), the EIWG includes clinical and statistical representatives from various sectors, including sponsor companies, contract research organizations, independent consultants, academia, and regulatory agencies.

The EIWG aims to bring together statisticians and clinicians to facilitate the implementation of estimands. It provides a cross-industry forum to:

- Share experiences from industry, academia, and regulatory agencies in implementing the estimand framework introduced by the ICH E9(R1) guideline.
- Discuss practical issues emerging from the implementation of the estimand framework.
- Engage in scientific discussions about the benefits and applications of the framework.

The goal is to provide feedback and recommendations for best practices, promote a broad understanding and awareness of the framework within the field of statistics and across other scientific disciplines, and compile relevant issues and topics arising from the implementation of the ICH E9(R1) guideline.

6.2.2 Main Activities

The EIWG engages in a range of activities aimed at supporting and promoting the ICH E9(R1) guideline. A key focus of the group is on raising awareness of the guideline's significance and implications across the industry. In addition, the EIWG develops and shares recommendations on best practices to ensure effective and consistent adoption. The group actively supports the broad implementation of the guideline across various types of clinical trials, ensuring that its principles are understood and applied correctly. Alongside these efforts, the EIWG conducts methodological research to address challenges and refine approaches associated with the guideline's implementation. Finally, the group collaborates with a diverse set of stakeholders (including regulatory agencies, sponsors, and academics) who are impacted by the guideline, fostering dialogue and partnerships that facilitate smooth integration and application.

6.2.3 Forms of Collaboration

To raise awareness and demonstrate the value of the estimand framework, the EIWG established an Estimand Training Academy. This initiative offers training and illustrates the application of the estimand framework through case studies.

The EIWG provides recommendations on best practices, based on experiences from implementing the estimand framework. EIWG members actively support the broader implementation of the estimand framework across various clinical settings beyond confirmatory clinical trials. For example, one group of statisticians and pharmacokinetic experts is investigating the application of estimands in early phases, such as dose finding, clinical pharmacology, bioequivalence, and bioavailability studies. Another group, including both estimand experts and health outcome researchers, is exploring the use of estimands in late-phase studies, such as those supporting health technology assessments (HTAs). This is particularly relevant, as the Regulation (EU) 2021/2282 on health technology assessment entered into force on 11 January 2022 and applies from 12 January 2025 (European Parliament and Council, 2021).

EIWG members are discussing the relevance of various estimands in non-inferiority settings and how these estimands align with existing guidelines. They share recent regulatory feedback on non-inferiority trials and are exploring questions such as the following:

- What is the underlying clinical question in a non-inferiority trial?
- Are two estimands with different strategies for intercurrent events required to reflect the spirit in the European Medicines Agency's (EMA) guideline on switching between superiority and non-inferiority?
- Can protocol violations be addressed as intercurrent events?
- Is there any remaining role for a per-protocol analysis set?

- Can different estimands be used to show non-inferiority and superiority in the same trial (hierarchical setup)?
- How does the estimand framework impact the choice of the non-inferiority margin?

EIWG members are engaged in methodological research. For instance, an estimation sub-team is assessing the performance of various methods for estimating treatment effects, specifically when treatment policy strategies are applied to address intercurrent events.

EIWG members are also developing guidance for reporting estimands in clinical trial reports, scientific publications, and press releases. They are engaged in discussions with representatives from Cochrane to review the inclusion of estimands in the Consolidated Standards of Reporting Trials (CONSORT) Handbook for Systematic Reviews. Additionally, they are collaborating with representatives from CONSORT regarding their reporting guidelines. There have also been connections with the National Institutes of Health (NIH) in the United States (U.S.) on incorporating estimands into clinical trial registration and reporting on ClinicalTrials.gov.

The EIWG collaborates with other groups on estimand-related activities, such as sharing implementation experiences with TransCelerate BioPharma to update its Common Protocol Template and working with Pharmaceutical Users Software Exchange (PHUSE, see Sect. 6.6) on incorporating estimands into analysis datasets.

6.2.4 Deliverables and Further Information

EIWG members have presented their research at scientific meetings and conferences and published key findings on central topics related to estimands and their application. A complete list of publications and conference materials is available from the working group's webpage. The training academy has also hosted a series of webinars. These webinars provide key insights into the practical applications of the estimand framework across different clinical research areas.

All training sessions are available as video-on-demand. These materials can be accessed through EFPIA's YouTube channel, accessible from the working group's webpage, which features the latest updates on research and innovation activities of the EFPIA. Further information on ongoing activities and access to materials generated by the EIWG can be found on its official webpage, provided in Sect. 6.6.1.

6.3 Neuroscience Estimand Working Group

6.3.1 Background and Objectives

In 2015, statistical leaders working in neuroscience founded a community to exchange and discuss common statistical challenges and offer mutual support. In 2017, this community was formally established as a Special Interest Group (SIG) governed by EFSPI and Statisticians in the Pharmaceutical Industry (PSI). When the draft ICH E9(R1) guideline was released in August 2017, this group began discussing the application of the estimand framework for various neuroscience indications. The SIG recognized the complexity of applying the estimand framework in neuroscience due to the heterogeneity of indications, which is often associated with high missing data rates. Due to the heterogeneity in clinical features, trial designs, and endpoints, neurological diseases require a tailored approach to effectively applying the estimand framework.

6.3.2 *Main Activities*

The application of the estimand framework in neuroscience proved to be particularly challenging due to the complexity of neurological diseases and the high rates of missing data caused by intercurrent events. The neuroscience community recognized that addressing these challenges with a single working group focused on one specific indication would not suffice. As a result, three separate working groups were established, each focusing on a different area: Parkinson's disease, multiple sclerosis, and pain/migraine. Additionally, the group aligned its efforts with an existing working group for Alzheimer's disease under the American Statistical Association (ASA).

These four working groups collectively covered a broad range of endpoints in neuroscience, including longitudinal endpoints with long-term follow-up, those with short- to mid-term follow-up, and time-to-event endpoints. The primary research questions addressed by these groups focused on integrating clinical trials and their analyses within the estimand framework. This included identifying the key intercurrent events, developing strategies to address them, and exploring their implications for estimation, testing strategies, and the handling of missing data in clinical trials.

In addition, the SIG created a working group dedicated to decentralized trials, with a particular focus on neuroscience. This group examined various aspects of decentralized trials, including the application of the estimand framework in these settings. With the establishment of these working groups, the SIG expanded to include over 40 statisticians from a wide range of companies and regulatory agencies in both Europe and the U.S.

6.3.3 *Forms of Collaboration*

Collaboration within the SIG involved statisticians from a wide range of global pharmaceutical companies, including AbbVie, AstraZeneca, Biogen, Denali, Janssen, Lilly, Lundbeck, Novartis, PPD, and Roche, as well as regulatory agencies, such as the Medicines and Healthcare products Regulatory Agency (MHRA) in the

United Kingdom. These collaborations encompassed various activities, including joint research and publications, organizing seminars, and maintaining ongoing communication and support among participating companies and regulatory agencies.

The group held regular virtual meetings, typically on a monthly basis, with sessions for all working group members and separate meetings for the individual working groups. A designated colleague was responsible for coordinating the regular meetings for both the overall community and each working group. The consistent scheduling of these meetings was essential to ensuring progress, both for the entire group and the individual working groups. Occasionally, the group also arranged face-to-face meetings at conferences, when enough members were present. While these in-person meetings were valuable for fostering group cohesion and social interaction, they were less critical for advancing the group's objectives.

6.3.4 Deliverables and Further Information

The SIG initially planned four publications. To date, two papers have been published (Donohue et al., 2020; Noci et al., 2022), with two more in the final stages of preparation. Additionally, the working group on decentralized clinical trials in neuroscience has successfully published its first paper (Burger et al., 2023), which utilizes the estimand framework to clarify and discuss the unique aspects of decentralized trials.

Beyond publications, the working groups have actively contributed to numerous conferences, presenting both oral presentations and posters. A particularly noteworthy event was a seminar organized by the British and Belgian Sections of the EFSPI, which was entirely led by the SIG and focused solely on the application of the estimand framework in neuroscience.

Perhaps, the most significant accomplishment has been the ongoing collaboration between various companies and regulatory agencies engaged in neuroscience. This collaboration has not only facilitated knowledge sharing but also deepened the understanding and practical application of the estimand framework in neurosciences, see Chap. 9 for various case studies in this field.

6.4 Oncology Estimand Working Group

6.4.1 Background and Objectives

Although the estimand framework was developed for various clinical trial settings and endpoints, early examples predominantly focused on symptomatic studies and continuous, longitudinal endpoints. In oncology, however, primary endpoints are typically time-to-event outcomes, such as overall survival, progression-free survival, or event-free survival. Many questions remained regarding estimand definition, analysis methods, data collection, trial interpretation, and the use of oncology endpoints in drug development. It quickly became evident that collaboration between industry and regulators was essential to operationalize the estimand framework for sponsors of oncology clinical trials and beyond.

The Oncology Estimand Working Group was formally established in February 2018, following informal discussions among statisticians in Basel. Initial research questions for the working group included the following:

- How can time-to-event endpoints be embedded in the estimand framework?
- What are the most relevant estimands and intercurrent events in oncology clinical trials?
- How do the five strategies for addressing intercurrent events outlined in the ICH E9(R1) guideline apply to time-to-event endpoints?
- How can analysis methods traditionally used in oncology, such as treatment switching or missing data schemes, be embedded in the estimand framework? Can the estimands implicitly targeted by these analyses be made more explicit and transparent?
- Although the ICH E9(R1) guideline does not (explicitly) require a causal interpretation of a proposed estimand, are there parts of the drug development life cycle that necessitate a causal interpretation of an estimand? Given that the hazard ratio from a Cox regression does not (immediately) admit a causal interpretation, what effect measures for time-to-event endpoints are more suitable for causal interpretation?

6.4.2 Main Activities

These topics were highly relevant and generated significant interest, both within the working group and among external stakeholders. In November 2018, the working group was officially recognized as an SIG in oncology by the EFSPI and PSI. In June 2019, the ASA Biopharmaceutical Section granted the group the official status as an ASA Scientific Working Group. As of June 2023, the group included 99 members (37 from Europe, 52 from the U.S., and 10 from Asia), representing 48 pharmaceutical companies or academic institutions.

6.4.3 Forms of Collaboration

The scientific objectives were initially addressed by five sub-teams (solid tumors, hematology, causal inference, censoring, and treatment switching), which have so far resulted in seven scientific publications: Lawrance et al. (2020), Degtyarev et al. (2020), Casey et al. (2021), Sun et al. (2021), Bornkamp et al. (2021), Manitz et al.

(2022), and Siegel et al. (2024), in addition to numerous presentations at global scientific conferences and webinars. In a second wave, task forces were established to address emerging topics, such as estimand engagement, principal stratification, patient-reported outcomes, and duration of responses. Additional topics included quantification of follow-up, real-world data and estimands, conditional and marginal effects, time-to-event endpoints with prognostic or predictive biomarker subgroups, early development estimand nexus, and estimands for safety analyses.

Since its inception, the working group has organized hybrid seminars and webinars featuring speakers from clinical, regulatory, and payer perspectives, sessions at conferences, and has given numerous talks sharing the results of its work. These events were often organized in collaboration with other statistical groups, including the ASA Biopharmaceutical Section, EFSPI, PSI, Basel Biometric Society, ASA New Jersey Chapter, EIWG (see Sect. 6.6.2), and ASA Lifetime Data Science Section.

The working group maintains a flat organizational structure, with task forces operating independently and holding regular meetings among the task force leaders. In addition, teleconferences of the full working group are held periodically. Key communication tools include periodic newsletters and the working group's webpage, provided in Sect. 6.6.1. To keep things simple, the working group opted for a simple markdown webpage hosted on GitHub.

With the support of ICH E9(R1) working group members (Frank Bretz and Devan Mehrotra), the working group established early connections with statisticians from eight regulatory agencies: EMA, MHRA, US Food and Drug Administration (FDA), Pharmaceuticals and Medical Devices Agency (PMDA, Japan), Health Canada, Swissmedic, National Medical Products Administration (NMPA, China), and Center for Drug Evaluation (CDE, Taiwan). The working group regularly organizes teleconferences with these regulatory colleagues to share the working group's progress within the task forces and invite regulatory colleagues to share their experiences and open questions that the working group might take as an inspiration for further research. These regular teleconferences offered a good opportunity for both sides to have a constructive dialogue on scientific problems related to estimands and regularly update each other on ongoing developments.

The large number of dedicated statisticians and the collaborative spirit were key factors in the working group's productivity over the past five years. Additional recommendations to future working groups from our experience include the following:

- Co-leadership: Combining two networks, leadership styles, and perspectives proved beneficial for the working group's success, allowing co-leads to support each other and enhance the group's cohesion.
- Flat organization: The two co-leads facilitated the group's initial communication and administrative tasks, but the task forces quickly became self-sufficient, with members proactively forming teams and setting their own pace.
- Communication strategy: Early planning for conference submissions, seminars, and publications helped ensure timely presentations of working group results.

The working group webpage played an instrumental role in maintaining communication.

- Representing the industry: While an affiliation with a larger society was not needed at the initiation of the working group, receiving the status of an EFSPI SIG and an ASA Biopharmaceutical Section Scientific Working Group later made it easier to collaborate with other groups on the organization of webinars and conference sessions and to interact with regulators, even if the working group did not directly use any resources from these umbrella societies.

6.4.4 Deliverables and Further Information

As of April 2025, the working group has published 16 scientific publications. In addition to the seven publications mentioned above, this includes Sridhara et al. (2022), Rufibach et al. (2023), Liu et al. (2023), Englert et al. (2023), Weber et al. (2024), Lawrance et al. (2023), Mercier et al. (2024), Wei et al. (2024), and Mozumder et al. (2025).

Notable achievements include publications addressing the impact of the coronavirus disease (COVID-19) pandemic on clinical trials (also, see Chap. 23 in this book), widely cited papers in *Pharmaceutical Statistics*, and significant contributions to understanding the principal stratum in the pharmaceutical industry (also, see Chap. 19). Several of these papers have had a direct influence on guidelines from the European Network for Health Technology Assessment (EuNetHTA), highlighting the practical impact of the group's research.

The Oncology Estimand Working Group has established a global network of about 100 statisticians who collaborate across industry, academia, and regulatory agencies. Regular teleconferences with regulatory agencies facilitate dialogue on scientific challenges and advancements related to estimands. All resources produced by the working group (including talks, papers, and software) are available on its webpage, provided in Sect. 6.6.1. We refer to Chap. 7 in this book for various case studies in oncology and hematology.

The working group was founded on the understanding that while internal workstreams within companies are useful and necessary, collaboration across companies and stakeholders is essential to addressing shared challenges and leading the implementation of the estimand framework. The journey of this working group exemplifies how an informally started group can become a global and productive network of statisticians, and we hope that it can serve as an example for future groups. We are confident that the network of statisticians from this working group will continue collaborating on estimands and potentially other topics, even if formal working group activities eventually come to a close.

6.5 Tripartite Working Team

6.5.1 Background and Objectives

The Tripartite Working Team (TWT) is composed of volunteers from various pharmaceutical companies and is named after the Tripartite Estimand Approach (TEA), initially published by Akacha et al. (2017), as well as Ruberg and Akacha (2017). Funded by selected pharmaceutical companies and Purdue University, the TEA follows the ICH E9(R1) guideline's definition of a treatment effect, focusing on three key treatment effects derived from discussions with physicians and patients regarding their understanding of treatment. The objective is to address critical questions for drug development and licensing, particularly in understanding the probability of treatment discontinuation due to adverse events or a lack of efficacy, and the effect of the treatment for patients who adhere to it.

6.5.2 Main Activities

The TWT primarily focuses on investigating estimands and estimators related to the direct effect of treatment, particularly for patients who adhere to the prescribed treatment (Estimand 3 in Akacha et al. (2017)). This approach contrasts with the traditional intent-to-treat principle, which estimates the effect of initiating a treatment regardless of adherence. The TWT has been active in delivering short courses and conference presentations to communicate causal inference concepts for pharmaceutical clinical trials, with a focus on the Adherer Average Causal Effect (AdACE). Additionally, the TWT has developed the Clinical Trials with Intercurrent Events Simulator (CITIES), a data-generating model that mimics published trials and explores statistical methodologies under various clinical trial scenarios (Wahab et al., 2024).

Ongoing research efforts within the TWT include comprehensive simulation studies evaluating the performance of different strategies described in the ICH E9(R1) guideline, further development of the CITIES model to incorporate additional outcomes and features, and continued research on AdACE methodologies. The TWT also studies the baseline characteristics of adherers versus non-adherers across different disease states.

6.5.3 Forms of Collaboration

The TWT meets monthly and is open to all individuals interested in exploring the TEA or AdACE approaches. The current leader of the TWT is Stephen Ruberg, with members from various organizations, including Analytix Thinking, Gilead, Janssen,

Lilly, Merck, Moderna, Novartis, and Unlearn AI. Financial support has been provided by Janssen, Lilly, and Purdue University, with in-kind contributions from all participating parties, including time, computational resources, and video conferencing. The TWT represents a collaborative effort among statisticians, supported by both pharmaceutical companies and academic institutions, to advance research on the TEA and AdACE methodologies.

6.5.4 Deliverables and Further Information

The TWT has made significant contributions to the field through the development and publication of the CITIES model, which is available with the `cities` package in `R` (Wahab et al., 2023). This CITIES model allows researchers to assess treatment effects and explore the impact of intercurrent events in clinical trials. The TWT continues to refine the model and extend its applicability to a broader range of clinical outcomes. Additionally, the TWT's research has led to the development of short courses, presentations at statistical conferences, and ongoing research into the AdACE methodology. The TWT is committed to providing clear and clinically relevant treatment effect estimates that inform decision-making by physicians and patients, following the principles laid out in the ICH E9(R1) guideline.

6.6 PHUSE Estimand Working Group

6.6.1 Background and Objectives

The ICH E9(R1) guideline addresses important statistical and clinical considerations for implementation, including aspects of trial design and conduct, but it does not cover the technical implementation in the dataflow. Many regulatory agencies mandate adherence to the Clinical Data Standards Interchange Consortium (CDISC) data standards, which must be evaluated to ensure that they sufficiently support the ICH E9(R1) guideline.

Informal discussions between clinical data scientists and data standards experts identified the potential benefits of a joint effort between PHUSE and CDISC. Such a collaboration could provide guidance on how to use existing data standards and identify where extensions to these standards may be necessary. PHUSE and CDISC regularly partner on projects that address both standards development and implementation.

As the project was established, its research topics quickly attracted numerous volunteers. The project's success relied on the integration of a broad range of expertise. Volunteers, including statisticians from PSI, EFSPI, and ASA, as well as experts from CDISC for their Clinical Data Acquisition Standards Harmonization

(CDASH) model and Analysis Data Model (ADaM), were invited to contribute. By the project's launch in March 2022, more than 70 participants from over 30 organizations, with expertise in biostatistics, statistical programming, data management, and standards development, had joined the initiative.

The initial scope of the project was to evaluate existing CDISC standards, identify and recommend necessary updates to CDISC standards, and share best practices. Specifically, the project team will address the collection of precise data to describe intercurrent events, in particular, relating to study drug discontinuation and concomitant medications; the storing of intercurrent event data in analysis datasets; and the identification of observations for analyses based on different intercurrent event strategies.

6.6.2 *Main Activities*

The project team's final deliverable is a white paper published by PHUSE, outlining a framework for implementing estimands using CDISC data standards, accompanied by examples. This framework is intended to be light, flexible, and consistent to accommodate the diverse situations encountered in estimand definitions and implementation. Note that the design of an individual estimand within a protocol and statistical analysis plan is beyond the scope of the project.

In addition to the white paper, the project has also investigated the current implementation of estimands using data standards. A survey conducted in spring 2023 within the PHUSE community aimed to assess the adoption of estimands in internal data standards. The survey results have informed the project's efforts to address the identified challenges with best practices and examples.

6.6.3 *Forms of Collaboration*

To address the identified challenges, volunteers were organized into two sub-teams focused on data collection and data analysis. The sub-team's co-leads held regular meetings with the project leads and other key stakeholders to maintain alignment and ensure progress. The team conducted a comprehensive review of existing standards, identified areas requiring further development, and examined studies on implementations of the estimand framework. They also assessed the current practices of the participating organizations. Based on these steps, they proposed a technical implementation framework for the estimand.

An important objective of the project was to upskill participants with limited prior knowledge of estimands, enabling them to effectively contribute their expertise. The project included numerous informational and working sessions to enhance the understanding of estimands and data standards. Knowledge sharing highlighted the need for end-to-end examples illustrating the impact of estimands on case report forms, as well as on CDISC Study Data Tabulation Model (SDTM) and ADaM datasets. The team was also fortunate to be able to build on the work published by Qu et al. (2023) and Polverejan et al. (2023), as well as the authors' contributions to this project.

The project's success has been significantly supported by representatives from the CDISC foundational standards teams and the backing of PHUSE and CDISC leadership, who have provided ongoing oversight and support.

The project team maintains regular communication through PHUSE forums, presenting their work at various events across the globe. Additionally, the adoption survey and the project have been presented at the Drug Information Association (DIA) Global Annual Meeting to raise awareness.

6.6.4 Deliverables and Further Information

In December 2023, the project team released a draft version of the white paper and accompanying examples for public comments. During this public comment period, feedback was received from regulatory agencies, industry groups, pharmaceutical companies, and individuals. The project team reviewed these comments and held collaborative sessions with EIWG and CDISC to address and incorporate their feedback.

The project team planned to release the final version of the white paper and examples by the end of 2024 on the PHUSE webpage, serving as an aid for estimands implementers in the data standards community. Further proposed extensions to data standards will be submitted to CDISC for consideration in future versions of the foundational data standards.

6.7 ISCTM Estimands and Missing Data Working Group

6.7.1 Background and Objectives

The International Society for Central Nervous System (CNS) Clinical Trials and Methodology (ISCTM) is a multidisciplinary organization focused on advancing and disseminating clinical research methods related to CNS therapeutics. ISCTM brings together international stakeholders from academia, industry, government, payers, policymakers, and the public to address strategic clinical, regulatory, methodological, and policy challenges in clinical research.

The Estimands and Missing Data Working Group of the ISCTM ("ISCTM Estimand Working Group") was formed in February 2017, following a session on missing data presented at the 2016 ISCTM Autumn Conference. The draft ICH E9(R1) guideline was released shortly after, in August 2017. The ISCTM community recognized the need for multidisciplinary collaboration in the implementation of the estimand framework. This working group began by holding broad meetings with ISCTM members interested in estimands, discussing topics ranging from intercurrent events to interpretations of the ICH E9(R1) guideline recommendations. The need emerged to develop an interdisciplinary process for implementing the estimand framework at the clinical trial planning stage. This became the main objective of this working group.

6.7.2 Main Activities

In 2020, a core group from this working group, comprising representatives from clinical and statistical functions with trial and regulatory experience, was formed to develop a scientific paper. This paper was published in 2023 as an open-access resource, sponsored by ISCTM (Polverejan et al., 2023). It describes an interdisciplinary process for implementing the estimand framework, illustrated by specific examples using hypothetical trials evaluating a treatment for major depressive disorder (MDD).

The paper uses MDD to demonstrate the process of selecting and constructing an estimand because it is highly prevalent and extensively studied, with widely accepted endpoints. However, MDD is a complex indication, with challenges such as high treatment dropout rates. Several issues encountered in defining estimands in clinical trials of the treatment for MDD can be generalized and applied to clinical trials in other disease areas. These issues, including a relatively high number of discontinuations from treatment, (partial) compliance, and starting other pharmacological treatments for the same disease, are ones that could influence the trial outcomes.

While all examples are applicable to MDD, based on the authors' experience, the main objective of the paper was not to recommend best estimands for MDD but to describe a practical guide for study teams to define clinical trial estimands. This guide can then be applied to clinical trials across many disease areas.

A consistent template is used for each estimand example. This template ensures that all steps in the proposed estimand implementation process are considered and addressed, including identifying the trial stakeholder(s), the decisions they need to make about the investigated treatment in their specific role, and the questions that would support their decision-making. Each of the five strategies for addressing intercurrent events is covered by at least one example, with diverse endpoints including continuous, binary, and time-to-event outcomes. Several examples were presented with specifications for a potential trial design, key trial implementation elements needed to address the estimand, and main and sensitivity estimators. This template could be used in a variety of settings for a clinical trial, such as for protocols and statistical analysis plans.

Both clinical and statistical representation in the ISCTM Estimand Working Group ensured deep discussions on many aspects of the estimand process, including how to formulate trial objectives and clinical questions of interest. Particular focus was placed on formulating the clinical questions of interest in natural, nontechnical language for easier comprehension, as reflected in the paper's examples. While the target treatment effect is formalized in the estimand definition, formulating the clinical question of interest is an important step, as it allows a cross-disciplinary discussion in the study team. It has also been emphasized that different question formulations would imply different intercurrent event strategies, and team discussions should be guided to follow this order instead of the other way around.

The clinical and statistical collaboration also influenced other aspects. For example, it shaped the definition of the target population in the context of a maintenance monotherapy treatment for MDD: patients with a diagnosis of MDD, who have shown a stable response to initial treatment with a new investigational treatment and for whom continuing monotherapy would be clinically acceptable. A randomized withdrawal trial was considered appropriate in the context of the defined estimand. However, the potential occurrence of withdrawal-syndrome-induced relapse after discontinuing the experimental drug was one of the concerns of the proposed estimand and corresponding design. As a result, a supplementary estimand was defined to mitigate this concern.

The work of Polverejan et al. (2023) contains multiple estimand examples from MDD, see Chap. 9 in this book for other estimand examples from neurosciences.

6.7.3 Forms of Collaboration

The ISCTM Estimand Working Group collaborates through regular meetings and continuous communication on interesting topics. This working group has an open meeting during every ISCTM Annual Scientific Meeting, welcoming any attendees with interest in this topic. Sessions on estimands were organized by this working group in the 2020 and 2024 ISCTM Annual Scientific Meetings.

Any ISCTM working group benefits from continuous support from ISCTM, including open-access sponsorship for the resulting publications and organization of regular meetings and sessions during ISCTM meetings. Engagement within the ISCTM community is also facilitated through an ISCTM communication channel.

6.7.4 Deliverables and Further Information

A half-day session on estimands was held during the 2020 ISCTM Annual Scientific Meeting, featuring clinical and statistical speakers from the pharmaceutical industry, EMA, and FDA. Another session in 2024 addressed deeper estimand-related topics by presenting many examples and pairing clinicians and statisticians in each presentation. Slides and recordings from all previous ISCTM meetings are available for open access at the ISCTM webpage, provided in Sect. 6.6.1, under the Meetings/

Activities tab, and all ISCTM-sponsored publications are available under the Publications tab.

The initial main objective of the ISCTM Estimand Working Group has been accomplished by Polverejan et al.'s (2023) publication. Future directions include outreach to nonstatistical communities, improving communication between different functions in implementing the estimand framework and discussing estimands in specific CNS-related research areas.

6.8 China DIA-CCTS Estimand Working Group

6.8.1 Background and Objectives

In the fall of 2017, pharmaceutical statistics experts in China became aware of the ICH E9(R1) guideline. A working group was quickly formed to review and discuss the implications of the ICH E9(R1) guideline, with a focus on clinical trials in China. In collaboration with industry experts from the DIA Statistics Community, the China Clinical Trial Statistics (CCTS) established the DIA-CCTS Estimand Working Group (DC-EWG). The group's primary goals are to reach consensus on the interpretation of the ICH E9(R1) guideline, better understand the estimand framework, address outstanding questions, and provide reference guidance for implementation.

6.8.2 Main Activities

The working group conducted an extensive literature review and held multiple teleconferences to discuss their findings. Their first DC-EWG seminar, held at Nanjing Medical University, was highly productive, covering a range of important topics related to the ICH E9(R1) guideline. Discussions began with an overview of the guideline, along with its associated training materials and sharing insights on estimand-related topics from international pharmaceutical working groups and experts. The seminar also explored applied case studies from therapeutic areas such as oncology, diabetes, and cardiovascular diseases, providing a practical context for understanding the estimand framework.

A significant portion of the seminar was dedicated to intercurrent events and missing data, with detailed discussions on how these issues are addressed differently within the estimand framework. The group also reviewed how estimand frameworks are applied in clinical trial protocols and statistical analysis plans across different companies, highlighting significant variations in approaches. Regulatory feedback was discussed, particularly focusing on justifications for chosen estimands, estimators, and the handling of missing data. This led to the recognition of a need for protocol and statistical analysis plan templates that incorporate the estimand framework.

Another key topic was the translation of key terms and sentences from the ICH E9(R1) guideline. The group worked to reach consensus on accurate translations to ensure consistency in implementation. Additionally, the seminar raised several challenges for further discussion, including the potential impact of the estimand framework on trial design, conduct, statistical analysis, and registration reviews, as well as the influence of estimand implementation on trial sample sizes. The group also considered how to address differing estimand requirements among drug approval agencies in multiregional clinical trials.

Finally, the working group emphasized the importance of activities in China, such as hosting seminars and workshops to facilitate communication with national and international experts, aiming to reach a deeper consensus within the professional community in China.

6.8.3 Forms of Collaboration

DC-EWG organizes training and discussions on the ICH E9(R1) guideline at various seminars and conferences each year, such as the DIA China Annual Meeting, the Quantitative Science Forum, and the China Biostatistics Summit Forum.

Following China's accession to the ICH, the NMPA and its Center for Drug Evaluation have actively collaborated with the DC-EWG. These collaborations focus on providing training and discussions about the implementation of the ICH E9(R1) guideline in China, encouraging sponsors to proactively consider potential intercurrent events and strategies to address them, and integrating the estimand framework into protocols. This approach enables earlier data collection and more effective answers to scientific questions.

6.8.4 Deliverables and Further Information

In 2021, the DC-EWG organized the writing of an estimand book in Chinese ("Bluebook") to support the implementation of the ICH E9(R1) guideline in China. The authoring team comprises statisticians from pharmaceutical companies and academia who collaborate to collect and interpret case studies across various therapeutic areas. The two Chinese editions of the estimand book (DC-EWG, 2021, 2022) form the basis for this book. The DC-EWG, along with other statistical working groups, will continue to foster communication among experts from different regions and functions worldwide. Through case studies, roundtable discussions, training workshops, and other initiatives, the working group aims to improve clinical trial design, conduct, analysis, and interpretation.

6.9 Concluding Remarks

The implementation of the ICH E9(R1) guideline and the estimand framework represents a significant advancement in the design, conduct, and analysis of clinical trials. The collaborative efforts of numerous global working groups, spanning diverse therapeutic areas and statistical disciplines, have played a pivotal role in refining and operationalizing these concepts. Through detailed case studies, interdisciplinary discussions, and practical guidance, these groups have demonstrated the importance of integrating the estimand framework into clinical trial protocols to better align trial planning, design, conduct, and analysis.

This chapter highlights the value of global collaboration, knowledge sharing, and continuous engagement with regulatory agencies to ensure consistency in the application of the estimand framework. Ongoing challenges, such as the need for standardized documentation practices and addressing differing regulatory requirements, remain important areas for future focus. However, the collective progress made thus far is a testament to the framework's potential to strengthen the dialogue between disciplines involved in the formulation of clinical trial objectives, design, conduct, analysis, and interpretation, as well as between sponsor and regulator regarding the treatment effect(s) of interest that a clinical trial should address.

As the field continues to evolve, the contributions of these working groups will remain crucial in shaping future guidelines, improving clinical trial efficiency, and fostering a deeper understanding of estimands across the global scientific and regulatory communities.

References

Akacha, M., Bretz, F., & Ruberg, S. (2017). Estimands in clinical trials—broadening the perspective. *Statistics in Medicine, 36*(1), 5–19. https://doi.org/10.1002/sim.7033

Bornkamp, B., Rufibach, K., Lin, J., Liu, Y., Mehrotra, D. V., Roychoudhury, S., Schmidli, H., Shentu, Y., & Wolbers, M. (2021). Principal stratum strategy: Potential role in drug development. *Pharmaceutical Statistics, 20*(4), 737–751. https://doi.org/10.1002/pst.2104

Burger, H. U., Van de Casteele, T., Rantell, K. R., Corey-Lisle, P., Sfikas, N., Abt, M., & Working group on Decentralized Trials as part of the European Scientific Interest Group (ESIG) in Neuroscience. (2023). Opportunities and challenges with decentralized trials in neuroscience. *Biometrical Journal. Biometrische Zeitschrift, 65*(8), e2200370. https://doi.org/10.1002/bimj.202200370

Casey, M., Degtyarev, E., Lechuga, M. J., Aimone, P., Ravaud, A., Motzer, R. J., Liu, F., Stalbovskaya, V., Tang, R., Butler, E., Sailer, O., Halabi, S., & George, D. (2021). Estimand framework: Are we asking the right questions? A case study in the solid tumor setting. *Pharmaceutical Statistics, 20*(2), 324–334. https://doi.org/10.1002/pst.2079

China Clinical Trial Statistics (CCTS)—Drug Information Association (DIA) ICH E9(R1)/Estimand Working Group (CD-EWG). (2021). ICH E9(R1) estimands and sensitivity analysis (1st ed.). Retrieved September 2, 2024, from https://www.diaglobal.org.cn/ichxskc

China Clinical Trial Statistics (CCTS)—Drug Information Association (DIA) ICH E9(R1)/Estimand Working Group (CD-EWG). (2022). ICH E9(R1) estimands and sensitivity analysis (2nd ed.). Retrieved September 2, 2024, from http://www.diachampion.com/index.php?c=show&id=12

Degtyarev, E., Rufibach, K., Shentu, Y., Yung, G., Casey, M., Englert, S., Liu, F., Liu, Y., Sailer, O., Siegel, J., Sun, S., Tang, R., Zhou, J., & Industry Working Group on Estimands in Oncology. (2020). Assessing the impact of COVID-19 on the clinical trial objective and analysis of oncology clinical trials-application of the estimand framework. *Statistics in Biopharmaceutical Research, 12*(4), 427–437. https://doi.org/10.1080/19466315.2020.1785543

Delmar, P., Voyle, N., Caputo, A., Donohue, M. C., Li, D. J., Mackey, H., Quarg, P., Zhu, Y., Bell, J., Model, F., & Liu-Seifert, H. (2018). Estimand in early Alzheimer's disease: Progress update from the International Alzheimer's Disease Scientific Working Group (AD SWG) substream. *Alzheimer's & Dementia, 14*(7S_Part_27), P1437. https://doi.org/10.1016/j.jalz.2018.06.2416

Donohue, M. C., Model, F., Delmar, P., Volye, N., Liu-Seifert, H., Rafii, M. S., Aisen, P. S., & Alzheimer's Disease Neuroimaging Initiative. (2020). Initiation of symptomatic medication in Alzheimer's disease clinical trials: Hypothetical versus treatment policy approach. *Alzheimer's & Dementia: The Journal of the Alzheimer's Association, 16*(5), 797–803. https://doi.org/10.1002/alz.12058

EMA. (2020). *Points to consider on switching between superiority and non-inferiority. CPMP/EWP/482/99*. Available at https://www.ema.europa.eu/

Englert, S., Mercier, F., Pilling, E. A., Homer, V., Habermehl, C., Zimmermann, S., & Kan-Dobrosky, N. (2023). Defining estimands for efficacy assessment in single arm phase 1b or phase 2 clinical trials in oncology early development. *Pharmaceutical Statistics, 22*(5), 921–937. https://doi.org/10.1002/pst.2319

European Parliament and Council. (2021). Regulation (EU) 2021/2282 on health technology assessment and amending Directive 2011/24/EU. *Official Journal of the European Union, L458*, 1–37.

ICH. (2019). E9(R1) addendum on estimands and sensitivity analysis in clinical trials to the guideline on statistical principles for clinical trials. Step 4 document available at www.ich.org

Lawrance, R., Degtyarev, E., Griffiths, P., Trask, P., Lau, H., D'Alessio, D., Griebsch, I., Wallenstein, G., Cocks, K., & Rufibach, K. (2020). What is an estimand & how does it relate to quantifying the effect of treatment on patient-reported quality of life outcomes in clinical trials? *Journal of Patient-Reported Outcomes, 4*(1), 68. https://doi.org/10.1186/s41687-020-00218-5

Lawrance, R., Skaltsa, K., Regnault, A., & Floden, L. (2023). Reflections on estimands for patient-reported outcomes in cancer clinical trials. *Journal of Biopharmaceutical Statistics*, 1–11. Advance online publication. https://doi.org/10.1080/10543406.2023.2280628

Liu, Y., Yang, M., Kil, S., Li, J., Mondal, S., Shentu, Y., et al. (2023). From logic-respecting efficacy estimands to logic-ensuring analysis principle for time-to-event endpoint in randomized clinical trials with subgroups. *Statistics in Biopharmaceutical Research, 15*(3), 560–573. https://doi.org/10.1080/19466315.2023.2186945

Manitz, J., Kan-Dobrosky, N., Buchner, H., Casadebaig, M. L., Degtyarev, E., Dey, J., Haddad, V., Jie, F., Martin, E., Mo, M., Rufibach, K., Shentu, Y., Stalbovskaya, V., Sammi Tang, R., Yung, G., & Zhou, J. (2022). Estimands for overall survival in clinical trials with treatment switching in oncology. *Pharmaceutical Statistics, 21*(1), 150–162. https://doi.org/10.1002/pst.2158

Mercier, F., Homer, V., Geng, J., Zhang, H., Englert, S., Kan-Dobrosky, N., & Victor, A. (2024). Estimands in oncology early clinical development: Assessing the impact of intercurrent events on the dose-toxicity relationship. *Statistics in Biopharmaceutical Research, 1–9*. https://doi.org/10.1080/19466315.2023.2296648

Mozumder, S. I., Grinsted, L., Siegel, J. M., Liu, F., Weber, H. J., & Englert, S. (2025). Time-to-event estimands in oncology trials: What's censoring got to do, got to do with it? *Statistics in Biopharmaceutical Research, 1–14*. https://doi.org/10.1080/19466315.2025.2487127

Noci, A., Wolbers, M., Abt, M., Baayen, C., Burger, H. U., Jin, M., & Robieson, W. Z. (2022). A comparison of estimand and estimation strategies for clinical trials in early Parkinson's disease. *Statistics in Biopharmaceutical Research, 15*(3), 491–501. https://doi.org/10.1080/19466315.2022.2116476

Polverejan, E., O'Kelly, M., Hefting, N., Norton, J. D., Lim, P., & Walton, M. K. (2023). Defining clinical trial Estimands: A practical guide for study teams with examples based on a psychiatric disorder. *Therapeutic Innovation & Regulatory Science, 57*(5), 911–939. https://doi.org/10.1007/s43441-023-00524-2

Qu, Y., Fu, H., Luo, J., & Ruberg, S. J. (2020). A general framework for treatment effect estimators considering patient adherence. *Statistics in Biopharmaceutical Research, 12*(1), 1–18. https://doi.org/10.1080/19466315.2019.1700157

Qu, Y., Luo, J., & Ruberg, S. J. (2021). Implementation of tripartite estimands using adherence causal estimators under the causal inference framework. *Pharmaceutical Statistics, 20*(1), 55–67. https://doi.org/10.1002/pst.2054

Qu, Y., White, R. D., & Ruberg, S. J. (2023). Accurate collection of reasons for treatment discontinuation to better define estimands in clinical trials. *Therapeutic Innovation & Regulatory Science, 57*(3), 521–528. https://doi.org/10.1007/s43441-022-00491-0

Ruberg, S. J., & Akacha, M. (2017). Considerations for evaluating treatment effects from randomized clinical trials. *Clinical Pharmacology and Therapeutics, 102*(6), 917–923. https://doi.org/10.1002/cpt.869

Rufibach, K., Grinsted, L., Li, J., Weber, H. J., Zheng, C., & Zhou, J. (2023). Quantification of follow-up time in oncology clinical trials with a time-to-event endpoint: Asking the right questions. *Pharmaceutical Statistics, 22*(4), 671–691. https://doi.org/10.1002/pst.2300

Siegel, J. M., Weber, H. J., Englert, S., Liu, F., Casey, M., & Pharmaceutical Industry Working Group on Estimands in Oncology. (2024). Time-to-event estimands and loss to follow-up in oncology in light of the estimands guidance. *Pharmaceutical Statistics, 23*. https://doi.org/10.1002/pst.2386. Advance online publication.

Sridhara, R., Barksdale, E., Marchenko, O., Jiang, Q., Ando, Y., Bloomquist, E., Coory, M., Crouse, M., Degtyarev, E., Framke, T., Freidlin, B., Gerber, D. E., Gwise, T., Josephson, F., Hess, L., Kluetz, P., Li, D., Mandrekar, S., Posch, M., Rantell, K., Ratitch, B., Raven, A., Roes, K., Rufibach, K., Sarac, S. B., Simon, R., Singh, H., Theoret, M., Thomson, A., Zuber, E., Shen, Y. L., & Pazdur, R. (2022). Cancer clinical trials beyond pandemic: Report of an American Statistical Association biopharmaceutical section open forum discussion. *Statistics in Biopharmaceutical Research, 15*(2), 444–449. https://doi.org/10.1080/19466315.2022.2103181

Sun, S., Weber, H. J., Butler, E., Rufibach, K., & Roychoudhury, S. (2021). Estimands in hematologic oncology trials. *Pharmaceutical Statistics, 20*(4), 793–805. https://doi.org/10.1002/pst.2108

Wahab, A. H. A., Yongming, Q., Michiels, H., Luo, J., Zhuang, R., McDaniel, D., Xi, D., Polverejan, E., Gilbert, S., Ruberg, S., & Sabbagh, A. (2023). Cities: Clinical trials with intercurrent events simulator. *R package version 0.1.3*. https://CRAN.R-project.org/package=cities

Wahab, A. H. A., Qu, Y., Michiels, H., Luo, J., Zhuang, R., D, M. D., Xi, D., Polverejan, E., Gilbert, S., Ruberg, S., & Sabbaghi, A. (2024). CITIES: Clinical trials with intercurrent events simulator. *Biometrical Journal*. (in press), *66*, e2200103.

Weber, H. J., Corson, S., Li, J., Mercier, F., Roychoudhury, S., Sailer, M. O., Sun, S., Todd, A., Yung, G., & Industry Working Group on Estimands in Oncology. (2024). Duration of and time to response in oncology clinical trials from the perspective of the estimand framework. *Pharmaceutical Statistics, 23*(1), 91–106. https://doi.org/10.1002/pst.2340

Wei, J., Xu, J., Bornkamp, B., Lin, R., Tian, H., Xi, D., Zhang, X., Zhao, Z., & Roychoudhury, S. (2024). Conditional and unconditional treatment effects in randomized clinical trials: Estimands, estimation, and interpretation. *Statistics in Biopharmaceutical Research, 16*(3), 371–381. https://doi.org/10.1080/19466315.2023.2292774

Part II
Case Studies Under the Estimand Framework

This part of the book presents applications of the estimand framework through a series of case studies drawn from a wide range of therapeutic areas. Across all examples, the case studies demonstrate how the estimand framework can be practically applied to address diverse clinical questions. This part begins with examples from oncology and hematology, illustrating the implementation of estimands in trials involving renal cell carcinoma, Chimeric Antigen Receptor T-cell therapy (CAR-T), and non-Hodgkin lymphoma, along with considerations of patient-reported outcome studies. The focus then shifts to immunology and inflammation, with applications in non-radiographic axial spondylarthritis, generalized pustular psoriasis, and atopic dermatitis. Next, the use of the estimand framework is explored in neuroscience, including its application in trials targeting multiple sclerosis, pain and migraines, Parkinson's disease, and Alzheimer's disease. This part concludes with additional case studies from selected therapeutic areas not covered in previous chapters, such as chronic heart failure, asthma, COVID-19, and preventive vaccine trials.

Chapter 7
Applying the Estimand Framework: Case Studies in Oncology and Hematology

Xue Yang, Steven Sun, Jiawei Wei, Evgeny Degtyarev, Zhiyue Huang, and Dongmei Lu

Abstract This chapter reviews the applications of the estimand framework in oncology and hematology, focusing on the unique challenges presented by complex diseases and a variety of treatment options. It stresses the necessity of defining clear trial objectives and establishing reliable estimands to ensure the accurate evaluation of treatment outcomes. Several case studies are included to illustrate the complexities involved in implementing the estimand framework. This chapter highlights how the selection of strategies for the intercurrent events can significantly affect the interpretation of treatment effects and the overall conclusions drawn from the trial. Additionally, it discusses the importance of patient-reported outcomes (PROs) in capturing patients' perspectives on treatment effects and quality of life while

X. Yang (✉)
Statistics and Decision Sciences, Johnson & Johnson Innovative Medicine, R&D, Shanghai, China
e-mail: xyang36@its.jnj.com

S. Sun
Statistics and Decision Sciences, Johnson & Johnson Innovative Medicine, R&D, Raritan, NJ, USA
e-mail: ssun@its.jnj.com

J. Wei
Advanced Methodology and Data Sciences, Novartis Institutes for Biomedical Research Co., Shanghai, China
e-mail: jiawei.wei@novartis.com

E. Degtyarev
Advanced Quantitative Sciences, Novartis Pharma AG, Basel, Switzerland
e-mail: evgeny.degtyarev@novartis.com

Z. Huang
Quantitative Science and Evidence Generation, Astellas Pharma Inc., Shanghai, China
e-mail: zhiyue.huang@astellas.com

D. Lu
Data Sciences, Akeso Biopharma Co., Ltd, Beijing, China
e-mail: dongmei.lu@akesobio.com

J. Wei et al. (eds.), *Estimands in Clinical Trials*, Springer Series in Pharmaceutical Statistics, https://doi.org/10.1007/978-3-032-02192-2_7

addressing issues related to missing data. The need for alignment between clinical questions and statistical analyses, as outlined in the ICH E9(R1) guideline, is also emphasized. In conclusion, this chapter underscores the vital role of the estimand framework in enhancing the understanding of treatment effects in oncology and hematology, offering insights for researchers and clinicians to navigate the complexities of cancer treatment and improve patient outcomes.

7.1 Introduction

The application of the estimand framework in oncology and hematology presents unique challenges due to the complex nature of diseases in these fields. This complexity arises from various factors, such as the intricate biology of cancer and blood disorders, the presence of multiple comorbidities in patients, and the difficulty or even impossibility of achieving a cure in many cases. These factors make it challenging to define clear trial objectives and establish reliable estimands, as the treatment outcomes can be influenced by a multitude of variables. Furthermore, the wide range of available treatments in oncology and hematology, including numerous drugs, treatment modalities, and treatment regimens, adds another layer of complexity. This diversity of treatment options can lead to heterogeneity in the patient population, making it challenging to estimate treatment effects and draw meaningful conclusions from clinical studies. Therefore, it is imperative to design trials with clear estimands and conduct appropriate statistical analyses to ensure that the results are reliable, interpretable, and applicable to the diverse patient population in oncology and hematology fields.

The cross-industry Oncology Estimand Working Group was established to promote a shared understanding and consistent implementation of the estimand framework in oncology clinical trials, see Sect. 6.4 in Chap. 6 of this book for details. In this chapter, we review carefully selected case studies to illustrate a diverse range of challenges, encompassing renal cell carcinoma (RCC), patient-reported outcomes (PROs) in oncology trials, chimeric antigen receptor T-cell (CAR-T) therapy, and non-Hodgkin lymphoma (NHL). Additionally, Sect. 18.6 in Chap. 18 discusses a case study on acute lymphoblastic leukemia patients. These examples, each representing different disease types, treatment modalities, and endpoints, serve to elucidate specific complexities inherent to oncology and hematology research. It is essential to note that this chapter's key messages revolve around these examples, illustrating how the practical application of estimands addresses well-identified questions within these complex contexts.

Moreover, the definitions of estimands in each case study will be clearly outlined, including the choice of specific intercurrent event strategies for each estimand, accompanied by their clinical rationales, as well as a detailed explanation of the statistical analysis methods employed to address these estimands. Finally, a comprehensive summary and discussion of the results will be presented, facilitating a deeper understanding of the implications and limitations of the findings. These case studies adhere to the principles and thought processes outlined in Chaps. 1, 2, and 3. It is important to note that the case studies in Sects. 7.2, 7.3, and 7.5 were conducted before the release of the ICH E9(R1) guideline. As such, the retrospective exercise of implementing the framework of estimands is intended solely for illustrative purposes.

By delving into these case studies, we aim to contribute to the expanding knowledge base on the practical application of estimands in the fields of oncology and hematology. The insights derived from these studies will not only enhance our understanding of the diseases and treatment modalities but also serve as valuable references for future research endeavors and clinical practices in these domains. These case studies will particularly highlight the unique challenges and thought processes involved in implementing the estimands framework in oncology and hematology. We hope that future studies can benefit from these insights and better understand how to apply estimands in these fields.

7.2 Renal Cell Carcinoma

7.2.1 Background

Renal cell carcinoma (RCC) is the most common type of kidney cancer in adults, with nearly 300,000 new cases diagnosed globally each year (Ravaud et al., 2016). About 16% of RCC patients have localized disease, and the standard treatment is nephrectomy, followed by surveillance (Ravaud et al., 2016). RCC is a malignant tumor that originates from the renal tubular epithelium and is the second most common malignancy in the urological system, accounting for over 90% of all kidney tumors (Siegel et al., 2020). The etiology of renal cancer is still unknown, but its occurrence may be related to smoking, obesity, occupational exposure (such as asbestos and leather), genetic factors (such as loss of tumor suppressor genes), etc. The incidence of renal cancer is highest between the ages of 50 and 70, and the male-to-female ratio is 2:1 (Siegel et al., 2020). Clear cell carcinoma accounts for 85% of all renal cancers (Padala & Kallam, 2023). Overall, locoregional disease is diagnosed in 16% of patients with renal cell carcinoma, and up to 40% of these patients have a relapse with metastasis after nephrectomy. The five-year survival rate is 53% for locoregional (stage III) disease and 8% for metastatic disease (Ravaud et al., 2016). Therefore, adjuvant therapy after surgery plays an important role in preventing recurrence and improving survival in patients with renal cell carcinoma (Ravaud et al., 2016).

7.2.2 Trial Objective and Design

S-TRAC (ClinicalTrials.gov identifier: NCT00375674) is a randomized, double-blind, phase III trial designed to compare the adjuvant effect of sunitinib with that of placebo in localized, high-risk, clear cell RCC patients (Ravaud et al., 2016). The

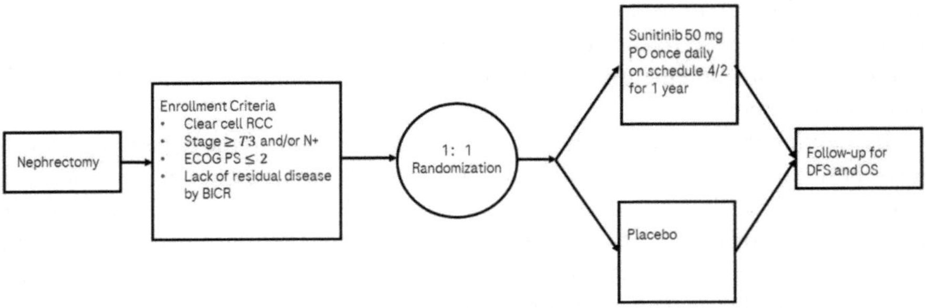

Fig. 7.1 S-TRAC trial design
Note: *RCC*: renal cell carcinoma, *ECOG*: Eastern Cooperative Oncology Group, *PS*: performance status, *BICR*: blinded independent central review, *PO*: per oral, *DFS*: disease-free survival, and *OS*: overall survival

purpose of the trial is to answer this question of clinical interest: Compared to placebo, will the use of sunitinib after surgery prolong disease-free survival (DFS) of the RCC patients if further anticancer therapy is not available to patients and regardless of dose adjustment due to intolerance and discontinuation of study treatment?

The trial design is shown in Fig. 7.1. Patients who meet the eligibility criteria are stratified and randomized equally to placebo and sunitinib. The stratification factors include the high-risk group defined by the University of California Los Angeles Integrated Staging System (UISS), the Eastern Cooperative Oncology Group (ECOG) score (<2 versus 2), and country of residence. They receive either oral sunitinib (50 mg daily) or placebo for a continuous period of one year on a four-week on, two-week off schedule. Dose adjustments (treatment interruption or dose reduction to 37.5 mg daily) due to intolerance are allowed. Study treatment is discontinued in case of relapse, death, diagnosis of second primary cancer, unacceptable toxicity, or withdrawal of consent.

During the treatment period, the tumor is assessed by computed tomography (CT) (≤5 mm slice thickness) or magnetic resonance imaging of the chest, abdomen, pelvis, and other applicable sites, conducted at screening, every 12 weeks during the first three years, and every six months thereafter, until disease recurrence or occurrence of metastasis, whichever is determined first until the time of final analysis.

7.2.3 *Estimand Considerations*

The primary objective of this trial is to demonstrate the superiority of oral sunitinib over placebo in patients with localized renal cell carcinoma in terms of the hazard ratio for DFS. The treatment effect of primary interest is regardless of dose adjustments due to intolerance or discontinuation of treatment and had further anticancer therapy not been available to patients. In the following part, we define the estimand, with a detailed description of its five attributes.

(a) Population
Patients diagnosed with localized renal cell carcinoma (stage III or higher tumor, regional lymph node metastasis, or both) and diagnosed based on a modified UISS criteria.

(b) Variable
DFS, defined as the time from randomization to the occurrence of relapse, death, or diagnosis of second primary cancer, whichever comes first. The exact definition of DFS varies among different studies due to the clinical trial objectives. This reflects the different strategies (implicitly) adopted by different studies for addressing intercurrent events. For example, in S-TRAC, due to the adoption of a composite strategy for diagnosis of second primary cancer, DFS is defined as the time from randomization to the earliest occurrence of progression, death, or diagnosis of a second primary cancer based on the blinded independent central review (BICR). The consideration could be that the onset of a second primary cancer reflects the failure of treatment. However, in another RCC trial, PROTECT (ClinicalTrials.gov identifier: NCT01235962), the diagnosis of a second primary cancer is addressed by treatment policy strategy, so it is not composited in the definition of DFS (Motzer et al., 2017). It implies that the onset of a second primary cancer does not directly reflect the failure of treatment, although the second primary cancer may impact the onset time of the occurrence of progression or death.

(c) Treatment
Oral sunitinib (50 mg daily) or placebo for a continuous period of one year on a four-week on, two-week off schedule, regardless of dose adjustments due to intolerance or discontinuation of study treatment and had further anticancer therapy not been available to patients. Dose interruptions or dose reductions to 37.5 mg per day are allowed, depending on the type and severity of toxicity. Treatment continues until disease recurrence, diagnosis of a second primary cancer, unacceptable toxic effects, or consent withdrawal.

(d) Intercurrent Events
Dose adjustments due to intolerance and study treatment discontinuation are common in oncology trials. The treatment policy strategy is adopted to reflect this medical practice in the clinical question of interest, see the treatment attribute above. Meanwhile, diagnosis of a second primary cancer is also identified as an intercurrent event, and a composite strategy is adopted, being defined as a DFS event in the variable. Another identified intercurrent event is the initiation of a new antineoplastic therapy prior to the confirmation of relapse adjudicated by blinded independent central review. It is addressed by a hypothetical strategy to reflect the clinical question of interest, see the treatment attribute above.

In S-TRAC, a patient may experience a series of intercurrent events from the start of treatment to the endpoint events. First, the patient may undergo a dose adjustment due to drug intolerance. Such intercurrent events reflect clinical practice and are, therefore, addressed using a treatment policy strategy. The efficacy at the population level includes the impact of dose adjustment due to drug intolerance. Second, the patient may discontinue study treatment early for any reason, but according to the protocol, the patient would continue to be followed up until an endpoint event occurred or the trial ended. Since there were no other options for adjuvant treatment at that time, the untreated outcome after study treatment discontinuation reflects clinical reality and is consistent with the trial objectives, so it is addressed using a treatment policy strategy. Therefore, the efficacy at the population level also includes the impact of early treatment discontinuation. Third, before the BICR, the investigator may diagnose a patient with progression and initiate a new antineoplastic treatment for the patient. Since the new antineoplastic treatment is not included in the trial objectives, a hypothetical strategy is adopted.

(e) Population-Level Summary
The summary measure used to quantify the treatment effect on disease-free survival is the conditional hazard ratio, adjusting for all stratification factors.

7.2.4 *Statistical Analysis*

7.2.4.1 Analysis Set and Data Collection

The analysis set is defined as including all randomized patients. In order to estimate the primary estimand, the data of a patient should be collected from the randomization date until the occurrence of relapse, death, diagnosis of second primary cancer, initiation of a new antineoplastic therapy prior to the confirmation of relapse adjudicated by BICR or the data cutoff date, whichever is earlier.

7.2.4.2 Statistical Model, Hypothesis, and Method of Analysis

A Cox proportional hazard regression model stratified by the UISS high-risk group is used to estimate the hazard ratio between sunitinib and placebo. A log-rank test stratified by the UISS high-risk group (significance level 0.05) is used to test the difference in efficacy between sunitinib and placebo. The Kaplan–Meier method is used to estimate survival functions, the median DFS derived from them, and its Brookmeyer–Crowley 95% confidence interval.

7.2.4.3 Handling of Missing Data

With consideration of the intercurrent event strategy, DFS is defined as the time from randomization to the earliest occurrence of a BICR-evaluated recurrence, death, or second primary cancer diagnosis. Because the start of a subsequent antineoplastic treatment before the BICR evaluation will be addressed by the hypothetical strategy, if a patient starts subsequent antineoplastic treatment before the centrally reviewed blind independent evaluation, the DFS will be censored at the start of the subsequent treatment under the assumption that this patient is similar to those who do not start a subsequent treatment.

In addition, if a patient's DFS event occurs after at least two missing tumor assessments, the DFS will be censored at the last non-missing tumor evaluation before the DFS event occurred. This censoring rule is not related to the intercurrent event strategy because missing tumor evaluation is not an intercurrent event; it reflects the consideration that a DFS event might happen during the period of missing tumor assessments and the assumption that the missing tumor assessments are not related to the hazard of the occurrence of DFS events, i.e., censoring at the last non-missing tumor evaluation before the DFS event occurs is independent.

7.2.4.4 Sensitivity Analysis

Three sensitivity analyses are considered. First, the investigator-assessed data is used to evaluate the robustness of the central review method for evaluating disease recurrence. For example, the benefit of sunitinib on investigator-assessed DFS is studied. Investigator-assessed DFS is defined as the time from randomization to the earliest occurrence of investigator-assessed recurrence, death, or second primary cancer diagnosis; therefore, the measurement approach of the variable attribute of the estimand is changed.

Second, due to the treatment policy strategy, any events occurring after study treatment discontinuation are used in the time-to-event analysis. However, there exists a tendency that patients are more likely to withdraw from the trial or miss tumor assessment due to noncompliance once they discontinue study treatment. Therefore, the independent censoring assumption used in the primary analysis may not be realistic. To evaluate the impact of informative missing data on the efficacy evaluation, S-TRAC uses a reference-based imputation method as sensitivity analysis, which specifies that the hazard for experimental patients who discontinued lies between the hazard for experimental patients who continued and the hazard for the reference control patients (Lu et al., 2015).

Third, when in the primary analysis, the DFS is censored at the last non-missing tumor assessment if there are two or more consecutive missing tumor assessments before a DFS event, it assumes that the missing tumor assessments are independent of the DFS. That is, the censoring rule for the two or more consecutive missing tumor assessments is independent. To assess the robustness of the analysis results of such an independent censoring assumption, in the sensitivity analysis, the DFS event after two missing tumor assessments is used (i.e., no censoring).

7.2.4.5 Supplementary Analysis

Other clinical questions are of interest, such as "Compared to placebo, will the use of sunitinib after surgery prolong DFS of the RCC patients, regardless of further use of anticancer therapy, dose adjustment due to intolerance, and study treatment discontinuation?" In this supplementary analysis, all other attributes remain unchanged except for the intercurrent event strategy for the start of subsequent anticancer treatment, which is changed to the treatment policy strategy.

7.2.5 *Summary and Discussion*

This case study involves some unique considerations under the estimand framework in the field of oncology. Based on different clinical questions of interest, different intercurrent event strategies are used, such as the composite variable strategy in S-TRAC and the treatment policy strategy in PROTECT for the diagnosis of the second primary cancer and the treatment policy strategy in the primary estimand and the hypothetical strategy in the supplementary estimand in S-TRAC.

We also describe sensitivity analyses based on different clinical assumptions, for example, the use of investigator-assessed DFS as a sensitivity analysis to the DFS used by the BICR. We also discuss sensitivity analyses to assess the robustness of the primary analysis in terms of its censoring rule for study withdrawal or multiple missing tumor assessments after an intercurrent event (study treatment discontinuation) and any multiple missing tumor assessments. Casey et al. (2021) provided a detailed comparison of the estimand used in S-TRAC compared to other studies in RCC patients.

7.3 Patient-Reported Outcomes in Oncology Trials

7.3.1 *Background*

Patient-reported outcomes (PROs) play an important role in oncology clinical trials. PRO results can reflect patients' perceptions, functional status of body parts, improvement in disease-related symptoms, and quality of life. In the process of developing cancer drugs, PROs can be used to support the overall evaluation of the benefit–risk ratio for patients. Regulatory agencies also consider PRO results when approving cancer drugs. PRO data could be summarized in the label of oncology drugs to substantiate the evidence if the data is well-collected in the trial. In addition, PRO measures attract the attention of various stakeholders (such as health insurance agencies) and provide data on patients' quality of life to support their decisions.

The thinking of the estimand framework (ICH, 2019) can also help describe estimands for PROs. The US Food and Drug Administration (FDA) drafted a guideline on incorporating clinical outcome assessments into the endpoints for regulatory decision-making; one of the difficulties of PRO data is the missing data handling, which should align with the estimand of interest (FDA, 2023a). The Chinese National Medical Product Agency (NMPA) drafted a guideline on the application of

PRO in drug clinical trials (NMPA, 2022), indicating that the PRO estimand should be clearly defined when a PRO is used as a primary or key secondary endpoint.

According to the 2020 global cancer statistics (Sung et al., 2021), breast cancer is the most common cancer in women and has the highest mortality rate among female cancers. Therefore, there have been many studies on the quality of life and symptom burden of breast cancer patients. A trial of 1513 patients showed that patients with metastatic breast cancer had lower quality of life and the greatest symptom burden compared to all other groups of patients with breast cancer. Patients under the age of 50 and with early or locally advanced breast cancer also have lower quality of life and higher symptom burden, including fatigue, depression, and irritability, compared with all other age groups. Patients treated with chemotherapy or selective estrogen receptor modulators also had a higher symptom burden compared to those not on the treatment, and the quality of life of patients treated for 2–10 years after treatment is lower than that of patients treated for over 10 years (Hamer et al., 2017). PRO measures can, therefore, be quite meaningful for evaluating a breast cancer patient's quality of life.

7.3.2 *Trial Objective and Design*

This hypothetical trial is a double-blind, randomized, placebo-controlled trial conducted in patients with hormone receptor-positive or progesterone receptor-positive, human epidermal growth factor receptor 2 (HER2)-negative metastatic breast cancer who progressed on first-line treatment. The patients are recruited with a high functional status, with an ECOG score of 0 or 1. Patients are randomized equally across the two arms and according to the following stratification factors: geographic region (America versus Europe versus others), the number of previous lines of chemotherapy (one versus two), and the ECOG score (0 versus 1). The experimental arm, in which patients receive an experimental drug orally plus standard hormone therapy, is compared against the control arm, in which patients receive placebo plus standard hormone therapy (Fiero et al., 2020).

In this section, we focus on PROs, although the primary efficacy endpoint in oncology trials is often progression-free survival (PFS) or overall survival. PRO measures are a standard tool for measuring physical and emotional functioning and will be collected at each treatment visit until death or the end of the trial. In clinical trials, three analysis approaches are typically examined: as a continuous variable, to compare whether there is a difference in the mean change from baseline between treatment arms at a certain time point; as a categorical variable, to compare the proportion of treatment arms that achieve the clinical improvement; as a time-to-achieving clinical improvement variable, whether hazard ratio could be used to examine the difference between treatment arms.

7.3.3 Estimand Considerations

The primary objective of this trial is to demonstrate the superiority of the experimental arm over the control arm in patients with hormone receptor-positive or progesterone receptor-positive, HER2-negative metastatic breast cancer who progressed on first-line treatment. The treatment effect of primary interest is assessed in terms of the mean change in physical function score from baseline at week 28 after randomization or at the last assessment prior to death (whichever occurs first), regardless of disease progression, discontinuation of study treatment, and initiation of subsequent anticancer therapy. Next, we define the estimand, with a detailed description of its five attributes.

(a) Population: Patients with hormone receptor-positive or progesterone receptor-positive, HER2-negative metastatic breast cancer who progressed on first-line treatment.
(b) Variable: Mean change in physical function score from baseline to week 28 after randomization or at the last assessment prior to death (whichever occurs first).
(c) Treatments: Experimental drug, orally daily, or placebo on top of standard hormonal therapy, regardless of disease progression, study treatment discontinuation, or initiation of subsequent anticancer therapy.
(d) Intercurrent events are displayed in Table 7.1. Few death events are expected to occur as patients are expected to have long survival times in this specific cancer setting. Some authors argue that in these settings, different strategies can be used, such as using a while alive strategy or a hypothetical strategy for the intercurrent event of death (Lawrance et al., 2020). Using a while alive strategy to address death as an intercurrent event implies that we are interested in the effect on PROs until death and that the last observation prior to death data may be used to analyze if patients die prior to the time of interest (i.e., week 28 in our case).
(e) Population-level summary: Difference in mean change from baseline in physical function scores between the experimental arm and control arm at week 28.

Table 7.1 Proposed estimand strategies

Intercurrent events	Strategies	Comments
Study treatment discontinuation, subsequent anticancer therapy, and disease progression	Treatment policy strategy	Reflects the clinical question of interest that the effect of study treatment discontinuation, subsequent anticancer therapy, or disease progression is considered as part of the overall treatment strategy; see the treatment attribute
Death	While alive	The strategy focuses on the treatment difference while alive; see the population attribute. Few death events are expected to occur as patients are expected to have long survival times in this specific cancer setting

7.3.4 Statistical Analysis

7.3.4.1 Analysis Set and Data Collection

The analysis set is defined as all patients who meet the eligibility criteria and are randomized. For patients who discontinued study treatment or started subsequent anticancer therapy after disease progression or for whom the disease progressed before week 28, we continue to collect the data after these intercurrent events occurred. The available data at week 28 are used based on the treatment policy strategy. For patients who die before week 28, the last valid physical function score before death is used for the primary analysis.

7.3.4.2 Statistical Model, Hypothesis, and Method of Analysis

An analysis of covariance (ANCOVA) model is used to compare the differences between the experimental arm and the control arm and to estimate the mean of the difference in change in physical function scores from baseline at week 28 and the corresponding 95% confidence interval. The covariates include the geographic region, the number of previous lines of chemotherapy, and the ECOG score. The assumptions of the ANCOVA model include variance homogeneity and that the observations are independent and follow a normal distribution.

7.3.4.3 Handling of Missing Data

Missing data at week 28 due to reasons other than death are imputed by the multiple imputation method (Rubin, 1987). The model includes the following covariates: age, physical function score at baseline, geographic region, the number of previous lines of chemotherapy, and the ECOG score. We assume that the mechanism of missing data is missing at random.

7.3.4.4 Sensitivity Analysis

Two sensitivity analyses are considered. First, for the primary analysis, the physical function score data at week 28 is missing due to reasons other than death, and we assume that the data is missing at random. To evaluate the robustness of the primary analysis and the assumptions of missing data mechanism, a mixed-effect models for repeated measures model is used to compare the mean of the difference in change in physical function scores from baseline between the treatment arm and control arm as sensitivity analysis. The missing data does not need to be preprocessed using this method. The dependent variable is the change from baseline in physical score, and the independent variables in the model are the baseline values of physical function score, time (planned visit time point), the treatment arm, and the interaction of time with the treatment arm. The assumptions of the model are that the repeated measurements of a patient follow a multinormal distribution and that the variance structure of the multinormal distribution reflects the correlation of physical function scores among patients. The unstructured variance is chosen for this sensitivity analysis. The least square mean of change from baseline in physical score at week 28 and standard deviation are provided for each arm, and the difference of least square mean between the treatment arm and the control arm and the corresponding 95% confidence interval are estimated.

Second, for the primary analysis under a missing-at-random assumption, a reference-based multiple imputation under a missing-not-at-random assumption could be provided as a sensitivity analysis. Several reference-based imputation methods can be considered, including jump to reference, copy reference, copy increments in reference, and last mean carried forward; see, for example, Carpenter et al. (2013) for details. We only specify the jump to reference method here, where patients with missing data after study treatment discontinuation behave similarly to those in the control arm. In the imputation model, we include the geographic region, the number of previous lines of chemotherapy, the ECOG score, the baseline value of the physical function score, and time (planned visit time point) as covariates, and the analysis model is the same as the primary analysis. We perform 100 imputations and then combine the imputed results using Rubin's rule (Rubin, 1987).

7.3.4.5 Supplementary Analysis

If a relatively large percentage (greater than 30%) of physical score data at week 28 cannot be collected due to poor quality of data collection, the analysis set could be changed and defined as the patients randomized with evaluable physical score data at week 28. The analysis method is the same as the primary analysis.

7.3.5 Summary and Discussion

In conclusion, the application of the estimand framework provides a clear and structured approach to defining and handling PROs in clinical trials. The guidelines from the FDA (2023a) and the NMPA (2022) underscore the importance of clearly defining PRO estimands, aligning missing data handling with the estimand of interest, and properly incorporating clinical outcome assessments into regulatory decision-making. This hypothetical case provides a preliminary idea on how to apply the estimand framework for PROs in oncology trials.

One challenge of using PROs in clinical trials is the high proportion of missing data. The use of electronic devices can improve the efficiency and convenience of data collection as well as patients' compliance, in addition to the missing data handling under the estimand framework, leading to a more robust treatment effects estimate. The integration of PRO measures within clinical trial designs, alongside a clear consideration of the estimand framework, ensures that the patient's voice is effectively captured and evaluated. This holistic approach not only enriches our understanding of treatment impacts on patients' quality of life but also advances the overall credibility and applicability of clinical research in oncology and beyond.

7.4 Non-Hodgkin Lymphoma with CAR-T Therapy

7.4.1 Background

Non-Hodgkin lymphoma (NHL) is a heterogeneous malignant tumor. NHL is classified into various subtypes based on the cell lineage and derivation of precursor or mature lymphocytes, among which diffuse large B-cell lymphoma (DLBCL) is the most common type in NHL and is a highly heterogeneous and invasive malignant tumor in terms of clinical presentation and prognosis. DLBCL accounts for 30–40% of adult NHL in Europe and the United States and approximately 35–50% in China. The clinical course presents as a rapidly growing mass. About one-third of the patients have B symptoms (e.g., fever, drenching night sweats, and unexpected weight loss), and more than half of the patients have elevated lactate dehydrogenase (LDH) levels. Approximately 50% of the patients are diagnosed at stage III or IV. At the time of the trial design of this case study (Degtyarev et al., 2019), the most commonly used first-line treatment for newly diagnosed DLBCL and other B-cell invasive NHL in Europe and the United States is the R-CHOP regimen (rituximab combined with cyclophosphamide, doxorubicin, vincristine, and prednisone). However, due to the heterogeneity of DLBCL, approximately 35–50% of the patients still experience disease recurrence or refractory disease. How to prolong the survival of patients with refractory DLBCL and improve their prognosis has become a research hotspot. For salvage treatment after first-line treatment failure, generally, non-cross-resistant chemotherapy or personalized regimens are selected, such as hematopoietic stem cell transplantation after chemotherapy if the patient meets the transplantation criteria and reaches remission. If the patient does not meet the transplantation criteria or does not achieve remission after treatment, a clinical trial or the best supportive care is recommended. However, the prognosis of patients with refractory DLBCL is poor, with less than 50% of the patients responding to second-line treatment, a three-year overall survival rate of only about 30%, and a high mortality rate. Lenalidomide, combined with rituximab, ibrutinib, and other drugs, are the commonly used choices in clinical practice, but these regimens have low response rates and limited duration of response. Therefore, there is still a lack of effective and safe treatment options for these patients, and most guidelines recommend participation in clinical research.

7.4.2 Trial Objective and Design

This case study is a global phase III, multicenter, randomized, open-label trial that aims to compare chimeric antigen receptor T-cell (CAR-T) therapy with standard therapy (autologous stem cell transplantation (ASCT)) in the second-line treatment of relapsed or refractory invasive B-cell NHL. Due to the complexity of the two treatment options, the oncologist expects that the patient may encounter a complex journey in each treatment option, as shown in Fig. 7.2.

As shown in Fig. 7.2, patients in the standard treatment arm initially receive salvage chemotherapy. The best standard of care after the first-line therapy with R-CHOP at the time of the trial design is high-dose salvage chemotherapy, followed by autologous stem cell transplantation for those who achieve deep remission after salvage chemotherapy. If deep remission is not achieved after the first salvage chemotherapy (approximately 6 weeks after two to three cycles), a new salvage therapy (second salvage) will be offered, with the goal of achieving deep remission,

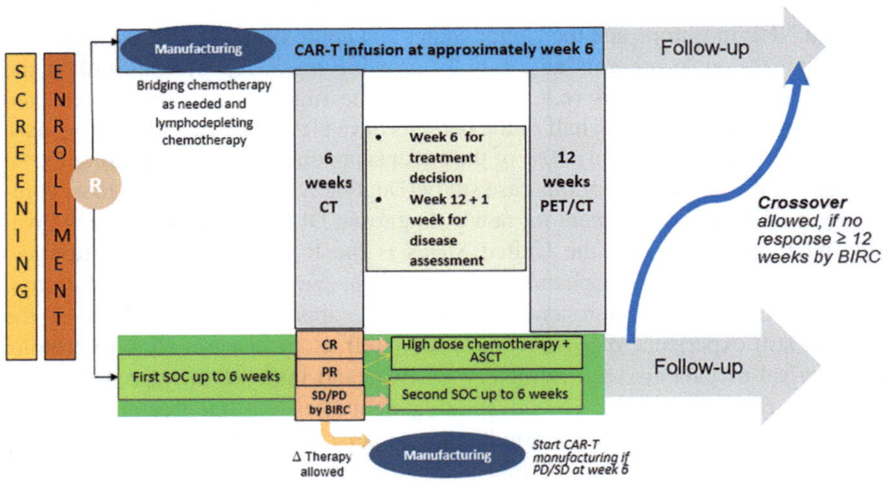

Fig. 7.2 The CAR-T therapy phase III trial designAfter screening and leukapheresis, patients are randomly assigned to one of the two treatment strategies: CAR-T or standard of care (SOC). In the CAR-T arm, patients may receive bridging chemotherapy during the manufacturing period, before a single CAR-T infusion. Patients are then observed for tumor progression from week 12 onward. In the SOC arm, patients receive up to two salvage chemotherapies, with the aim of receiving autologous stem cell transplantation (ASCT) when the disease responds to chemotherapy. If no sufficient response to the first round of chemotherapy is achieved in SOC patients, CAR-T is manufactured in parallel to the patient receiving a new round of chemotherapy. This enables investigators to offer a crossover to CAR-T should a lack of response be confirmed at week 12, after the second round of chemotherapy

Note: *BIRC*: blinded independent review committee, *CR*: complete response, *CT*: computed tomography, *DLBCL*: diffuse large B-cell lymphoma, *PD*: progressive disease, *PET*: positron emission tomography, *PR*: partial response, *R*: random assignment, *SD*: stable disease, and *SOC*: standard of care

followed by transplantation. Hence, tumor assessment after the first salvage is necessary to guide future treatment. If the disease has not improved after two salvage therapies (approximately 12 weeks later), standard treatment will be considered a failure. In this case, CAR-T therapy can be offered as a crossover, as it was approved as a third-line-and-above treatment at the time of trial conduct.

Patients in the CAR-T arm receive treatment through a single infusion. However, first, T-cells are collected from the patient's peripheral blood to manufacture CAR-T. Then, the patient may need bridging chemotherapy to control the disease and prevent rapid tumor progression during the approximately 4–6-week period required for CAR-T manufacture and delivery. In the week before the infusion of CAR-T, the patient receives lymphodepletion chemotherapy. Although a response is possible after bridging chemotherapy and before lymphodepletion chemotherapy, there is also a low probability of rapid deterioration of the patient's health or failure of CAR-T manufacture, which may delay or prevent the use of CAR-T.

From the perspective of the researchers, comparing the two treatment regimens in a randomized clinical trial presents a significant challenge due to the different courses that patients experience in each treatment regimen, which makes it challenging to determine the research questions of interest and the treatment that we want to estimate the efficacy of. To design a scientifically sound and interpretable trial, several challenges need to be addressed.

- First, the comparison is between two treatment regimens, not simply two different treatments. Both regimens are complex, involving multiple interventions and decision points, and patients may not receive all components of each regimen. The standard treatment regimen includes the first or second course of salvage therapy, depending on the tumor response to first-line therapy; after this, patients may or may not receive ASCT, depending on the tumor response to each salvage therapy. CAR-T therapy also has its complexity, as not all patients randomized to the CAR-T arm will receive CAR-T therapy. Some patients may die, or their status may significantly deteriorate, preventing the CAR-T infusion. Additionally, CAR-T manufacturing may fail, resulting in patients not receiving treatment.
- Second, during CAR-T manufacturing, patients may receive bridging therapy, and their tumors may progress or respond to bridging therapy, but the tumor response status before CAR-T infusion is irrelevant to the decision of whether or not to infuse CAR-T. This is different from the autologous stem cell transplantation that requires a response to chemotherapy as a prerequisite. Therefore, the disease assessment after bridging therapy does not reflect the outcome of CAR-T treatment strategy, as the patient can subsequently benefit from treatment if CAR-T is infused, even if disease progression is observed after bridging therapy. In the standard treatment regimen, an absence of response after the first course of salvage therapy does not constitute the final negative outcome of standard treatment but determines the next step in the process.
- Third, at the start of the individual patient journey, the two treatment arms are expected to have similar outcomes. This is because the bridging therapy given before CAR-T infusion is similar to the salvage therapy in the standard treatment

regimen. Therefore, the treatment effect of CAR-T therapy is not expected to be fully realized during the waiting period compared to the standard treatment regimen.
- Finally, CAR-T can be administered after standard treatment regimen failure. For patients receiving standard treatment, once second-line salvage therapy is ineffective, they become eligible for CAR-T therapy. This means that patient outcomes observed later in the standard treatment arm may reflect not only the effect of the standard regimen but also the effect of this crossover therapy.

7.4.3 Estimand Considerations

The estimand framework helps address the challenges posed by the complexity of patient journeys in different treatment regimens. Based on the estimand framework, researchers are able to provide a more precise definition of the treatment effect of interest. The trial is to compare CAR-T therapy with the ASCT arm in patients with relapsed or refractory invasive B-cell NHL. The primary objective is to demonstrate superiority between the two arms in hazard ratio of the event-free survival (EFS). The treatment effect of primary interest is regardless of manufacturing failure in the CAR-T arm or failing to receive ASCT in the standard-of-care (SOC) arm or stable/progressive disease at week 6, had a new cancer therapy before observing EFS event not been available. The following is a definition of the estimand, with a detailed description of the five attributes.

(a) Population
The population of interest includes all patients who are eligible to receive CAR-T or standard treatment regimens, with further clarification of appropriate inclusion and exclusion criteria. Eligible patients should be 18 years of age or older with histologically confirmed aggressive B-cell lymphoma that is refractory (lack of complete response) or relapsed after the receipt of a first-line anti-CD20 antibody and anthracycline-containing regimen within 12 months after the last dose. Patients have to be eligible for autologous hematopoietic stem cell transplantation (HSCT) according to the investigator's assessment and have an Eastern Cooperative Oncology Group (ECOG) performance-status score of 0 or 1 (on a five-point scale, with higher numbers indicating greater disability) and adequate organ function.

(b) Variable
In this disease environment, the primary variable or endpoint is EFS, which represents the time from randomization to treatment failure. Failure is defined as the first recorded disease progression, disease stabilization, or death for any reason at any time. However, the description of patient journeys indicates that the assessment of the tumor is premature after the first cycle of bridge or salvage therapy, making it impossible at this early stage to determine the outcome of the treatment regimen. Disease progression or stabilization is relevantly

assessed as a treatment failure if observed at or after the 12-week evaluation, which is the time frame used to consider disease progression or stabilization as an endpoint for EFS. The 6-week evaluation is only used for treatment decisions, so it is not included in the EFS calculation. However, death represents the most informative and decisive outcome in both treatment regimens; it represents an event as part of the composite EFS endpoint, regardless of when it occurs.

(c) Treatment
The intent of the trial is to evaluate the efficacy of the CAR-T and ASCT regimens, including all possible interventions in each treatment regimen, had a new cancer therapy not been available before observing an EFS event. Patients randomized undergo several steps over different time periods once they decide to receive CAR-T or standard treatment regimens. Patients who are excluded due to insufficient response may still benefit from CAR-T treatment, which cannot be reflected in the estimand. Therefore, it seems more meaningful to compare the full content of the two treatment regimens, including all possible paths in patient journeys, had a new cancer therapy before observing an EFS event not been available (as these are not part of the treatment strategy). This is consistent with clinical practice, where not all patients receive all parts of a treatment regimen.

(d) Intercurrent Events
Intercurrent events are displayed in Table 7.2.

(e) Population-Level Summary
In trials comparing two treatments, the hazard ratio is commonly used to quantify the relative treatment effect on EFS, assuming that the treatment effect does not vary over time (proportional hazards assumption). However, in this trial, it can be anticipated that the difference in treatment effect during the stage of similar bridging or salvage therapy may be limited or even nonexistent. Additionally, both CAR-T and ASCT regimens are potentially curative therapies, and therefore, some patients may have similar outcomes after being cured. These situations violate the proportional hazards assumption, and the hazard ratio may not be an appropriate population-level summary. Other summaries for quantifying treatment effects in the presence of nonproportional hazards are being investigated.

Table 7.2 Proposed estimand strategies

Intercurrent events	Strategies	Comments
Manufacturing failure in the CAR-T arm or failing to receive ASCT in the SOC arm	Treatment policy strategy	Intrinsic to the treatment strategy; these events reflect the clinical reality of the treatment strategy
New cancer therapy before observing the EFS event	Hypothetical strategy	Not part of the treatment strategy and affecting the observation and interpretation of further assessments
Stable or progressive disease at week 6	Treatment policy strategy	Does not reflect an outcome of the treatment strategy; only used for treatment decision in the SOC arm; not used for the CAR-T arm

7.4.4 *Statistical Analysis*

7.4.4.1 Analysis Set and Data Collection

The analysis set is defined as including all randomized patients, regardless of whether they received all or part of the randomized treatment and the dose received. All data after the manufacturing failure in the CAR-T arm or after failing to receive ASCT in the SOC arm and stable or progressive disease at week 6 are collected and used for analysis.

7.4.4.2 Statistical Model, Hypothesis, and Method of Analysis

The final analysis of EFS is based on the observed data in the analysis set, until the data cutoff date, based on the required number of EFS events. If the one-sided p-value from the stratified log-rank test performed in the final analysis of EFS (stratified by the randomization stratification factors) is less than or equal to 0.025, the trial will be considered positive.

The survival distribution of EFS is estimated using the Kaplan–Meier method and plotted by the treatment arm. The median EFS and its 95% confidence interval are reported by the treatment arm. A stratified Cox regression model is used to estimate the hazard ratio of EFS and its 95% confidence interval, stratified by the randomization stratification factors.

The intercurrent event of a new anticancer therapy is addressed using a hypothetical strategy, and consequently, EFS will be censored at the last disease assessment prior to the start of a new therapy in the analysis.

7.4.4.3 Handling of Missing Data

If no EFS event is observed before the earliest censoring event, EFS will be censored at the latest available disease assessment. Censoring events include a loss to follow-up, withdrawal of consent, and data cutoff date.

7.4.4.4 Sensitivity Analysis

Further sensitivity analyses can be performed based on the handling of missing data. For example, the extended time without assessment just prior to observing an event could introduce some bias. For example, what if a patient dies 2 years after the last available disease assessment? Assigning the date of the event on the day of death could overestimate the true EFS in such a case, as the patient possibly progressed during the two-year period with missing data. Therefore, predefined sensitivity analyses can help understand the robustness of the primary analysis with regard to missing data. One typically used approach is to censor events occurring after two or more missing assessments.

7.4.4.5 Supplementary Analysis

Two possible supplementary analyses could be performed, considering different strategies for the intercurrent event of a new anticancer therapy. First, it is of interest to compare two treatment regimens, including possible subsequent treatments (i.e., treatment policy strategy). In this analysis, EFS events are counted, even if they occur after the start of a new anticancer therapy, and it implicitly considers the effect of randomized treatment regimen on the choice and efficacy of subsequent therapy. Second, the new anticancer therapy itself, even in the absence of documented disease progression, can be viewed as a bad outcome and considered an EFS event. This would correspond to the composite strategy and compare two treatment strategies with regard to the delay of progression, death, and start of a new anticancer therapy.

7.4.5 Summary and Discussion

Cancer patients typically go through different trajectories in clinical trials, and researchers need to consider this diversity when determining the treatment effect of interest in clinical trials. Various accompanying events that occur after randomization may affect the assessment and interpretation of the related treatment effect. The estimand framework provides a structured approach to transparently discuss and explain different patient trajectories. The estimand can help us define the scientific question of interest more precisely and make the trial design and data analysis more targeted. Especially when comparing complex treatment regimens involving multiple interventions and decision points, the use of the treatment attribute is particularly important.

7.5 Non-Hodgkin Lymphoma

7.5.1 Background

As introduced in Sect. 7.4, NHL encompasses a diverse group of diseases, with over 60 subtypes identified. Among them, follicular lymphoma (FL) is the second most common subtype of NHL worldwide, accounting for 20–33% of all NHL cases. The incidence rate is similar in males and females. FL shows an indolent course characterized by relapses and remissions, with 16–60% of cases transforming to aggressive lymphoma, most commonly DLBCL. Treatment options for NHL depend on disease progression rate and location, including chemotherapy, radiation therapy, immunotherapy, targeted therapy, bone marrow transplant, surgery, and watchful waiting. FL, originating from B-cells in the follicles, is diagnosed through histopathology and immunohistochemical analysis.

Sun et al. (2021) discuss the application of the estimand framework in hematologic oncology trials. Their work provides practical recommendations and strategies to incorporate the estimand framework into hematologic oncology clinical trials, especially in addressing common intercurrent events when designing a clinical trial for hematology malignancies. The article emphasizes the importance of ensuring alignment between the key questions of interest, analysis, and interpretation in clinical trials. It includes real examples, such as a clinical trial in FL patients, to illustrate the application of different estimand strategies. The authors also suggest template language for describing estimands in trial protocols and statistical analysis plans as a reference for statisticians.

In March 2023, the FDA conducted an Oncologic Drugs Advisory Committee (ODAC) meeting to address concerns regarding the POLARIX trial and the use of polatuzumab plus R-CHP for previously untreated large B-cell lymphoma (LBCL) patients (FDA, 2023b). The primary topics discussed by the FDA include the modest benefit in progression-free survival (PFS) observed with this combination, as well as overall survival results, other efficacy endpoints, and the heterogeneity of the trial population. Throughout this meeting, the FDA demonstrated the implementation of the estimand framework in their discussions.

This section primarily focuses on the case study of GALLIUM in FL patients discussed by Sun et al. (2021). Additionally, we will discuss the estimand framework used during the FDA's ODAC meeting regarding the POLARIX trial.

7.5.2 Trial Objective and Design

This is an open-label, international, multicenter, randomized, phase III trial of patients with previously untreated, advanced, indolent NHL to investigate the efficacy and safety of obinutuzumab (G) plus chemotherapy (G-chemo), followed by obinutuzumab maintenance therapy for responders (patients who demonstrate a complete or partial response), compared with rituximab (R) plus chemotherapy (R-chemo), followed by rituximab maintenance therapy for up to 2 years for responders (Marcus et al., 2016). The trial is referred to as GALLIUM and has been registered with the ClinicalTrials.gov identifier NCT01332968.

Approximately 1200 patients with follicular lymphoma and 200 patients with marginal zone lymphoma are planned to be recruited and randomly assigned either to the arm receiving G-chemo followed by G maintenance in responders or to the arm receiving R-chemo followed by R maintenance in responders in a 1:1 ratio. The trial is powered to detect statistically significant differences in PFS among patients with follicular lymphoma only. As a result, the presentation of the estimand

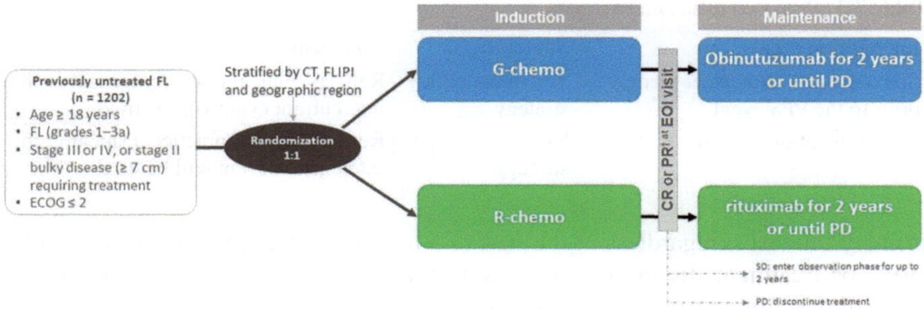

Fig. 7.3 GALLIUM trial design
Note: *FLIPI:* follicular lymphoma international prognostic index, *EOI:* end of induction, *PD:* disease progression, *PR:* partial response, *CR:* complete response, and *SD:* stable disease

framework used in this case study focuses solely on the primary target patients with follicular lymphoma (Fig. 7.3).

The schedule for administration of R or G is dependent upon the accompanying chemotherapy regimen. In the control arm, six to eight doses of R at 375 mg/m^2 are administered by intravenous (IV) infusion with the accompanying chemotherapy regimen. In the experimental arm, eight to ten doses of G (including two additional doses of G on days 8 and 15 of cycle 1) at an absolute (flat) dose of 1000 mg are administered by IV infusion with the accompanying chemotherapy regimen. For patients who achieve a complete or partial response at the end of induction therapy, the treatment continues with R at 375 mg/m^2 or G at a flat dose of 1000 mg every two months until disease progression, with a maximum duration of two years. Patients who have stable disease (SD) at the end of induction therapy are monitored for progression for up to two years, following the same schedule of follow-up as patients who are responding (complete or partial response) and receiving maintenance (observation). If induction therapy is discontinued due to toxicity or any reason other than toxicity, patients are taken off the study treatment and enter the follow-up phase.

The primary trial objective is to evaluate the efficacy of G-chemo, followed by G maintenance therapy, compared with R-chemo, followed by R maintenance therapy, in patients with previously untreated advanced follicular lymphoma, as measured by investigator-assessed PFS, regardless of new anti-lymphoma treatments prior to experiencing a PFS event.

7.5.3 *Estimand Considerations (Primary)*

The primary objective of this trial is to demonstrate the superiority of G plus chemotherapy, followed by G maintenance therapy, over R plus chemotherapy, followed by R maintenance therapy, in patients with previously untreated advanced FL in terms of the hazard ratio of investigator-assessed PFS. The treatment effect of

Table 7.3 Proposed estimand strategies

Intercurrent events	Strategies	Comments
Start of a new anticancer therapy prior to the PFS event	Treatment policy strategy	Reflects clinical practice. Data after the intercurrent event will be used
Discontinuation of study treatment	Treatment policy strategy	Reflects clinical practice. Data after the intercurrent event will be used

primary interest is regardless of the start of a new anticancer therapy prior to a PFS event or treatment discontinuation. As follows, we define the estimand, with a detailed description of its five attributes.

(a) Population: Previously untreated late-stage FL patients.
(b) Variable: PFS, defined as the time from randomization to progression or death, whichever occurs first.
(c) Treatment: Patients receive six or eight cycles of induction chemoimmunotherapy (G or R plus chemotherapy), with the possibility of discontinuing study treatment or starting a new anticancer therapy, as needed, prior to a PFS event. Responding patients receive up to two years of monotherapy maintenance treatment (G or R).
(d) Intercurrent events are displayed in Table 7.3. Both types of intercurrent events are addressed using a treatment policy strategy, see the treatment attribute above. The reason for this approach is that in clinical practice, it is common to initiate a new anticancer treatment or discontinue study treatment before a PFS event takes place.
(e) Population-level summary: The conditional hazard ratio between the treatment arm and the control arm, adjusting for all stratification factors.

7.5.4 *Statistical Analysis (Primary)*

7.5.4.1 Analysis Set and Data Collection

The analysis set is defined as all randomized previously untreated patients. For the primary estimand, all data should be collected and used for analysis from the randomization date until the first occurrence of progression, relapse, or death from any cause; initiation of a new anticancer therapy prior to disease progression; or the data cutoff date, whichever is earlier.

7.5.4.2 Statistical Model, Hypothesis, and Method of Analysis

The primary analysis is to analyze the efficacy data, as assessed by the investigators. This analysis utilizes a stratified Cox proportional regression model stratified by the factors used in the randomization, with treatment as a sole explanatory variable. The stratification factors are the chemotherapy regimen (cyclophosphamide, doxorubicin, vincristine, and prednisone (CHOP); cyclophosphamide, vincristine, and prednisone (CVP); or bendamustine) and the Follicular Lymphoma International Prognostic Index (FLIPI) risk group (low, intermediate, or high). This approach assumes that all types of censoring are independent and that baseline risks differ across strata. Furthermore, it assumes that hazard functions within each stratum remain proportional over time.

7.5.4.3 Handling of Missing Data

PFS for patients without disease progression, relapse, or death is censored at the time of the last tumor assessment or, if no tumor assessments are performed after the baseline visit, on the date of randomization.

7.5.4.4 Sensitivity Analysis

The corresponding primary statistical analysis involves several assumptions and data limitations, the impact of which can be explored and evaluated via sensitivity analyses. The first sensitivity analysis uses PFS based on the independent review committee (IRC), which is considered less biased than the PFS based on the investigator's assessment in open-label studies, as the IRC reviewers typically performing their assessments in a blinded fashion. On the other hand, the IRC review may be subject to potential bias compared to the investigator's assessment, particularly when the investigator calls for disease progression before the IRC review, leading to nonrandom censoring. This sensitivity analysis corresponds to the same estimation objective as the primary analysis and is considered a sensitivity analysis that addresses the limitations of the disease assessment data.

Second, the assumption in the main statistical analysis that baseline risks differ across strata but hazard functions within each stratum are proportional over time may not hold, as it implies the same baseline risks across strata and that hazard functions within each stratum are proportional over time. The unstratified Cox regression analysis can be used under this assumption as a sensitivity analysis. This analysis corresponds to the same objective as the primary analysis and is designed to check the heterogeneity assumptions in the primary analysis and explore the robustness of the results. Note that this may be controversial because the estimate of treatment effect size based on unstratified analysis can be viewed as a marginal effect size, while the estimate based on stratified analysis can be viewed as a conditional effect size. In this sense, the analysis can be viewed as a supplementary analysis.

Third, when the assumption of independent censoring in the primary statistical analysis may not be valid, imputing the PFS for patients with nonindependent censoring can be performed to assess the impact on treatment effect. This includes imputation of nonrandom dropouts (e.g., dropouts due to adverse events) based on a plausible missing mechanism (e.g., reference-based imputation). This is to check the impact of violations of independent censoring assumptions and assess the robustness of the main estimator.

Fourth, in cases where two or more consecutive disease assessments are missing before the occurrence of the PFS event, one may question whether the true disease progression occurred in the missing disease assessment interval. This situation is not specifically addressed by the primary analysis method, which simply assumes that no disease progression occurred during the missing disease assessment interval. If it is considered that disease progression may have occurred in patients during consecutive missing assessment intervals, the timing of disease assessment indicating the event of interest may not reflect the truth; therefore, censoring PFS at the last disease assessment prior to the missing assessment could be a reasonable approach. This sensitivity analysis considers the two or more consecutive missing assessments as if there is an administrative termination and examines the robustness of the overall results under the assumption of no disease progression during the missing disease assessment interval.

7.5.4.5 Supplementary Analysis

Three supplementary analyses are considered. First, the per-protocol set (PPS) analysis method is aimed at a different estimand as the population attribute is changed; more specifically, it aims to estimate the treatment effect in the ideal world in which patients can follow the protocol perfectly. The definition of the PPS population usually depends on the treatment outcome, such as completion of at least six cycles of treatment. This analysis was traditionally performed in the past as a supplementary/sensitivity analysis. However, the ICH E9(R1) guideline discourages such analyses due to the questionable interpretability of PPS analysis.

Second, if it is believed that the subsequent therapy may impact the interpretation of the treatment effect, a hypothetical strategy can be adopted for the intercurrent event of the start of a new anticancer therapy prior to the PFS event. Since this method corresponds to a different estimand, which aims to estimate the treatment effect as if a new anticancer therapy is not available, we consider it a supplementary analysis. This estimand can be estimated by censoring the PFS at the last evaluation before the start of subsequent anticancer therapy, which gives an unbiased estimate only if we assume that the time to subsequent therapy and progression are independent of each other.

Third, the primary estimand typically addresses a scientific question related to the marginal treatment effect, which can be answered using a Cox regression model, with the treatment as the only covariate. However, if the scientific question of interest pertains to estimating the conditional treatment effect where patients' covariates are at their mean value, a Cox regression model with prognostic baseline covariates can be employed (Hougaard, 2012).

Table 7.4 Proposed estimand strategies

Intercurrent events	Strategies	Comments
Start of a new anticancer therapy before death	Treatment policy strategy	Reflects clinical practice. Uses the overall survival time regardless of the occurrence of the intercurrent event
Discontinuation of study treatment	Treatment policy strategy	Reflects clinical practice. Data after the intercurrent event is used

7.5.5 *Estimand Considerations (Secondary)*

In most oncology clinical trials, overall survival is defined as the time from randomization until death from any cause and is the key efficacy endpoint. Overall survival is considered the gold standard cancer endpoint and is typically analyzed based on survival data collected for all patients in the trial. The overall survival analysis is presented here as an example to demonstrate how it can be analyzed within the framework of estimands. The following is a definition of the estimand, with a detailed description of the five attributes.

(a) Population: Previously untreated late-stage FL patients.
(b) Variable: Overall survival, defined as the time from randomization till death from any cause.
(c) Treatment: Patients receive six or eight cycles of induction chemoimmunotherapy (G or R plus chemotherapy), with the possibility of discontinuing study treatment or starting a new anticancer therapy before death. Responding patients receive up to two years of monotherapy maintenance treatment (G or R).
(d) Intercurrent events are displayed in Table 7.4.
(e) Population-level summary: The conditional hazard ratio between the treatment arm and the control arm, adjusting for all stratification factors.

7.5.6 *Statistical Analysis (Secondary)*

7.5.6.1 Analysis Set and Data Collection

The analysis set is defined as all randomized previously untreated patients. All data from randomization till death from any cause are collected and used for analysis.

7.5.6.2 Statistical Model, Hypothesis, and Method of Analysis

The primary analysis is to analyze the overall survival data using a stratified Cox proportional regression model, with treatment as a sole explanatory variable, with the implicit assumptions that all types of censoring are independent and that baseline risks differ across strata but that hazard functions within each stratum are proportional over time.

7.5.6.3 Handling of Missing Data

For overall survival, patients for whom death has not been documented have their observations censored on the last date on which they were known to be alive.

7.5.6.4 Sensitivity Analysis

The statistical analysis corresponding to the estimand and its assumptions and limitations can be explored and evaluated via the following sensitivity analysis. A loss to follow-up leads to missing data, which may affect the evaluation of treatment effect if the reason for the loss to follow-up is not independent of the treatment arm. Before analyzing the survival data, the missing data can be imputed (Zhao et al., 2014), for example, by resampling patients with follow-up data in each arm. Tipping point analysis can be used to evaluate the impact of missing data.

7.5.6.5 Supplementary Analysis

Two supplementary analyses are considered. First, if in analogy to the second supplementary analysis, in PFS, it is believed that a new anticancer therapy will affect the interpretation of overall survival, then a clinical interest is the treatment effect if there is no new anticancer therapy. Therefore, a hypothetical strategy can be adopted for the intercurrent event of starting a new anticancer therapy before death. This strategy can be estimated by censoring the overall survival at the start of subsequent treatments anticancer. It aimed at a different clinical question with a different estimand, which used a different strategy for the intercurrent event.

Second, if there is sufficient evidence to demonstrate the significant efficacy of the experimental arm compared to the control arm (such as the favorable result of PFS), ethical considerations often allow for the choice of switching to the experimental arm treatment for patients in the control arm who experience disease progression. A different scientific question may be of interest, such as the treatment effect if patients in the control arm are not allowed to receive the experimental treatment regimen after disease progression. Accordingly, this corresponds to a different estimand, which adopts a hypothetical strategy to deal with the intercurrent event of treatment switching. The Rank Preserving Structural Failure Time (RPSFT) method (Robins & Tsiatis, 1991; Branson & Whitehead, 2002), the Inverse Probability of Censoring Weighting (IPCW) method (Robins & Finkelstein, 2000), and the two-stage method (Latimer et al., 2017) are the commonly used statistical approaches to address treatment switching in clinical trials. However, as they differ in their underlying assumptions and methodologies, we further introduce these methods hereafter.

We also refer to Sect. 22.5 in Chap. 22 of this book for more discussions on applying the estimand framework in settings with treatment switching.

7.5.6.5.1 RPSFT Method

This method assumes a common treatment effect, regardless of when the treatment is administered. In other words, this method assumes that the observed and counterfactual failure times are comparable, i.e., the treatment effect would have been the same for a patient, regardless of the treatment they actually received. The model also assumes that the treatment effect is constant over time and does not interact with the time-dependent status of a patient (e.g., whether they have experienced an event or are still at risk).

The RPSFT method provides an estimate of the treatment effect by relating a patient's observed event time to their counterfactual event time. The counterfactual event time is that which would have occurred if treatment switching had not occurred. The model treats the potential counterfactual outcome as a baseline characteristic, which is balanced between the randomized arms, and thus, the treatment effect estimation is based on finding a treatment effect that achieves a balance in the potential counterfactual outcome.

7.5.6.5.2 IPCW Method

The key assumption is that there are no unmeasured confounders. More specifically, the method assumes that all relevant variables influencing both treatment assignment and the switching decision are adequately measured and included in the analysis. Unmeasured confounding could bias the estimated treatment effects. There are other assumptions, such as the exchangeability assumption, which assumes that the distribution of potential outcomes for patients who switch treatments is similar to the distribution for those who do not switch, given their observed covariates.

The IPCW method involves artificially regarding patients as dependently censored at the time of treatment switching. By assigning weights that represent the inverse probabilities of not switching treatments, a pseudo-population is constructed, which is a hypothetical population that would have been observed if treatment switching had not occurred.

7.5.6.5.3 Two-Stage Method

This method assumes no unmeasured confounders at the secondary baseline, defined as a time point where patients are at a similar stage of disease and prior to which switching cannot occur. Other assumptions include the no carryover effect, which implies that the efficacy or impact of the first treatment does not persist in the period when patients switch to the second treatment, and the homogeneity of treatment effects, which means that treatment effects are homogeneous across patients, both before and after treatment switching.

The two-stage method is implemented as follows:

- Stage 1: An accelerated failure time model (such as a Weibull model) is fitted to the data of the control arm patients who switch to the experimental treatment after disease progression. This model includes covariates measured at the secondary baseline and a time-varying covariate indicating treatment switch.
- Stage 2: Counterfactual survival times are obtained using the estimated treatment effect from Stage 1. These counterfactual survival times allow for a comparison of the treatment options and are used to estimate the overall treatment effect.

The choice of method depends on the specific trial design, available data, and assumptions that are reasonable for the given context. Violations of these assumptions can affect the accuracy and reliability of the treatment effect estimates. Sensitivity analyses and robustness checks are often performed to evaluate the impact of potential violations on the results.

In general, regulatory agencies often favor a treatment policy strategy because it aligns with subsequent therapies that typically mirror clinical practice. However, a hypothetical strategy may be a viable option if the treatment switch or subsequent therapy is unique to the current trial and does not align with standard clinical practice. For a more comprehensive discussion on the appropriateness of each strategy in various scenarios, please refer to the paper authored by Manitz et al. (2022). Additionally, it is worth noting that the secondary estimand implicitly involves treatment policy strategy for the intercurrent event of treatment switching. If it is expected that such intercurrent events may occur, it is recommended to reflect them using the estimand framework.

7.5.7 Summary and Discussion

We utilize the GALLIUM trial in this section to explore the application of commonly used efficacy endpoints, PFS and overall survival, within the estimand framework in hematologic oncology trials. In the context of hematologic oncology trials, the framework has proven to be particularly valuable in addressing the unique challenges associated with treatment complexity, intercurrent events, and diverse patient populations.

One of the key takeaways from this trial is the importance of therapeutic knowledge and drug mechanisms in determining the estimand of interest and trial design. The framework has provided a transparent way to specify each objective of a trial, ensuring alignment with the selected estimator/analysis method. By doing so, it has facilitated the identification and application of the most appropriate methods for primary and sensitivity analyses.

This case study illustrates the utility of the estimand framework in addressing common challenges, including intercurrent events, in hematologic oncology trials, highlighting how different strategies for addressing intercurrent events can lead to distinct scientific questions, emphasizing the need for mutual agreement on estimand descriptions between trial sponsors and regulatory agencies.

Furthermore, the discussion has shed light on the significance of sensitivity and supplementary analyses in understanding the impact of treatment interventions. These analyses, targeting the same estimand, have proven instrumental in assessing the robustness of statistical inferences and exploring different assumptions of the statistical methods.

It is evident that the estimand framework has the potential to minimize ambiguity in the interpretation of trial results. By ensuring consistency between the scientific question and the definition of trial objectives, the framework promotes transparency, even in unfavorable yet unavoidable situations in clinical trials.

In March 2023, the FDA hosted an ODAC meeting to discuss a supplemental biologics license application for polatuzumab vedotin-piiq (POLIVY) for injection. The purpose of this meeting was to evaluate the benefit–risk profile of POLIVY in combination with R-CHOP for a specific patient population with LBCL, including patients with DLBCL, not otherwise specified, based on the findings of the POLARIX trial.

According to the applicant, POLARIX demonstrated that patients receiving treatment with POLIVY in combination with R-CHOP experienced a 27% reduction in risk of disease progression, disease relapse, or death compared to patients treated with R-CHOP (hazard ratio of 0.73 with a 95% confidence interval of [0.57,0.95] and a p-value of $p = 0.0177$). However, the FDA has expressed concerns regarding the magnitude of this benefit and the heterogeneity observed in the treatment effect. To assess the robustness of the PFS results within the framework of estimands, the FDA conducted various sensitivity and supplementary analyses. The details can be found in the ODAC briefing documents (FDA, 2023b).

The FDA provided a demonstration on how to align clinical questions with analysis approaches for clinical trials. It emphasizes the importance of clear alignment between a clinical question and the analysis approach, as outlined in the ICH E9(R1) guideline. The clinical question of interest should guide the selection of the estimand strategy. In the briefing document, two estimands with different strategies are proposed for the intercurrent event of start of a new anti-lymphoma treatment (NALT). One estimand applies the treatment policy strategy, which ignores whether or not NALT was given to patients. This estimand is estimated by not censoring for NALT or more than two consecutive missed disease assessments and focuses solely on evaluating the effect of experimental treatment, regardless of subsequent therapy. The other estimand applies the hypothetical strategy, which addresses the clinical question of a treatment effect if NALT had not been administered, estimated by censoring NALT. This case study also highlights the importance of considering both estimands, as they answer different clinical questions and lead to different assumptions in the analysis, and both are important to consider when analyzing clinical trial data. Overall, this case study serves as an informative resource for researchers and clinicians seeking a better understanding of how to estimate treatment effect in clinical trials in a manner that aligns with the clinical question of interest for NHL.

7.6 Concluding Remarks

In conclusion, this chapter has shed light on the complexities and challenges inherent in the practical application of estimands in oncology and hematology. The diverse case studies presented have illustrated the critical importance of defining clear trial objectives and establishing reliable estimands to ensure that treatment outcomes are accurately assessed and interpreted.

The examples discussed have highlighted the unique considerations and thought processes involved in implementing the framework of estimands in oncology and hematology research. The comprehensive summary and discussion of the results have provided valuable insights into the implications and limitations of the findings, emphasizing the need for robust statistical analyses and sensitivity analyses to ensure the reliability and applicability of the results.

Furthermore, this chapter has underscored the significance of therapeutic knowledge, drug mechanisms, and patient trajectories in determining the estimand of interest and trial design. It has also emphasized the importance of aligning clinical questions with analysis approaches, as outlined in the ICH E9(R1) guideline, and the need for mutual agreement on estimand descriptions between trial sponsors and regulatory agencies.

The practical application of estimands in oncology and hematology plays a significant role in advancing our understanding of diseases and treatment approaches. It provides a foundation for future research and clinical practices and may ultimately benefit the diverse patient populations within these fields. The discussions in this chapter aim to contribute to the growing body of knowledge and serve as a resource for researchers and clinicians seeking to apply estimands in these complex areas. Additionally, readers are encouraged to explore Part IV of this book, which describes statistical analyses under the estimand framework for various endpoints, including continuous endpoints (Chap. 15), binary endpoints (Chap. 16), recurrent event endpoints (Chap. 17), and time-to-event endpoints (Chap. 18), offering more details on methodologies and considerations for analyzing these endpoints.

References

Branson, M., & Whitehead, J. (2002). Estimating a treatment effect in survival studies in which patients switch treatment. *Statistics in Medicine, 21*(17), 2449–2463.

Carpenter, J. R., Roger, J. H., & Kenward, M. G. (2013). Analysis of longitudinal trials with protocol deviation: A framework for relevant, accessible assumptions, and inference via multiple imputation. *Journal of Biopharmaceutical Statistics, 23*(6), 1352–1371.

Casey, M., Degtyarev, E., Lechuga, M. J., Aimone, P., Ravaud, A., Motzer, R. J., et al. (2021). Estimand framework: Are we asking the right questions? A case study in the solid tumor setting. *Pharmaceutical Statistics, 20*(2), 324–334.

Degtyarev, E., Zhang, Y., Sen, K., Lebwohl, D., Akacha, M., Hampson, L. V., et al. (2019). Estimands and the patient journey: Addressing the right question in oncology clinical trials. *JCO Precision Oncology, 3*, 1–10.

FDA. (2023a). Patient-focused drug development: Incorporating clinical outcome assessments into endpoints for regulatory decision-making. Guidance for Industry [draft].

FDA. (2023b). Oncologic Drugs Advisory Committee (ODAC) Meeting. Accessed March 9, 2023. https://www.fda.gov/advisory-committees/advisory-committee-calendar/march-9-2023-meeting-oncologic-drugs-advisory-committee-meeting-announcement-03092023

Fiero, M. H., Pe, M., Weinstock, C., King-Kallimanis, B. L., Komo, S., Klepin, H. D., et al. (2020). Demystifying the estimand framework: A case study using patient-reported outcomes in oncology. *The Lancet Oncology, 21*(10), e488–e494.

Hamer, J., McDonald, R., Zhang, L., Verma, S., Leahey, A., Ecclestone, C., et al. (2017). Quality of life (QOL) and symptom burden (SB) in patients with breast cancer. *Supportive Care in Cancer, 25*, 409–419.

Hougaard, P. (2012). *Analysis of multivariate survival data*. Springer.

ICH. (2019). *ICH E9(R1) addendum on estimands and sensitivity analysis in clinical trials to the guideline on statistical principles for clinical trials*.

Latimer, N. R., Abrams, K. R., Lambert, P. C., Crowther, M. J., Wailoo, A. J., Morden, J. P., et al. (2017). Adjusting for treatment switching in randomised controlled trials–A simulation study and a simplified two-stage method. *Statistical Methods in Medical Research, 26*(2), 724–751.

Lawrance, R., Degtyarev, E., Griffiths, P., Trask, P., Lau, H., D'Alessio, D., et al. (2020). What is an estimand & how does it relate to quantifying the effect of treatment on patient-reported quality of life outcomes in clinical trials? *Journal of Patient-Reported Outcomes, 4*(1), 1–8.

Lu, K., Li, D., & Koch, G. G. (2015). Comparison between two controlled multiple imputation methods for sensitivity analyses of time-to-event data with possibly informative censoring. *Statistics in Biopharmaceutical Research, 7*(3), 199–213.

Manitz, J., Kan-Dobrosky, N., Buchner, H., Casadebaig, M. L., Degtyarev, E., Dey, J., et al. (2022). Estimands for overall survival in clinical trials with treatment switching in oncology. *Pharmaceutical Statistics, 21*(1), 150–162.

Marcus, R. E., Davies, A. J., Ando, K., Klapper, W., Opat, S., Owen, C. J., et al. (2016). Obinutuzumab-based induction and maintenance prolongs progression-free survival (PFS) in patients with previously untreated follicular lymphoma: Primary results of the randomized phase 3 GALLIUM study. *Blood, 128*(22), 6.

Motzer, R. J., Haas, N. B., Donskov, F., Gross-Goupil, M., Varlamov, S., Kopyltsov, E., et al. (2017). Randomized phase III trial of adjuvant pazopanib versus placebo after nephrectomy in patients with localized or locally advanced renal cell carcinoma. *Journal of Clinical Oncology, 35*(35), 3916.

NMPA. (2022). *Guidance of Patient reported outcome application in drug development*. https://www.cde.org.cn/zdyz/listpage/9cd8db3b7530c6fa0c86485e563f93c7

Padala, S. A., & Kallam, A. (2023). *Clear cell renal carcinoma*. StatPearls [Internet].

Ravaud, A., Motzer, R. J., Pandha, H. S., George, D. J., Pantuck, A. J., Patel, A., et al. (2016). Adjuvant sunitinib in high-risk renal-cell carcinoma after nephrectomy. *New England Journal of Medicine, 375*(23), 2246–2254.

Robins, J. M., & Finkelstein, D. M. (2000). Correcting for noncompliance and dependent censoring in an AIDS clinical trial with inverse probability of censoring weighted (IPCW) log-rank tests. *Biometrics, 56*(3), 779–788.

Robins, J. M., & Tsiatis, A. A. (1991). Correcting for non-compliance in randomized trials using rank preserving structural failure time models. *Communications in statistics-Theory and Methods, 20*(8), 2609–2631.

Rubin, D. B. (1987). *Multiple imputation for nonresponse in surveys*. Wiley.

Siegel, R. L., Miller, K. D., & Jemal, A. (2020). R cancer statistics. *CA: a Cancer Journal for Clinicians, 70*(1), 7–30.

Sun, S., Weber, H. J., Butler, E., Rufibach, K., & Roychoudhury, S. (2021). Estimands in hematologic oncology trials. *Pharmaceutical Statistics, 20*(4), 793–805.

Sung, H., Ferlay, J., Siegel, R. L., Laversanne, M., Soerjomataram, I., Jemal, A., & Bray, F. (2021). Global cancer statistics 2020: GLOBOCAN estimates of incidence and mortality worldwide for 36 cancers in 185 countries. *CA: a Cancer Journal for Clinicians, 71*(3), 209–249.

Zhao, Y., Herring, A. H., Zhou, H., Ali, M. W., & Koch, G. G. (2014). A multiple imputation method for sensitivity analyses of time-to-event data with possibly informative censoring. *Journal of Biopharmaceutical Statistics, 24*(2), 229–253.

Chapter 8
Applying the Estimand Framework: Case Studies in Immunology and Inflammation

Leslie Meng, Peter Mesenbrink, Fan Wang, Chang Chen, and Hongjie Deng

Abstract This chapter illustrates the use of the estimand framework in clinical trials for four diseases in immunology and inflammation: generalized pustular psoriasis (GPP), rheumatoid arthritis (RA), atopic dermatitis (AD), and non-radiographic axial spondylarthritis (nraSpA). These diverse diseases necessitate varied trial designs to achieve specific treatment objectives. The estimand framework is crucial for trial design, addressing confounding factors, and examining key questions like symptom reduction, disease remission rates, maintenance, and flare control. Each case study includes a detailed trial design with clear objectives, well-defined estimands, and strategies for addressing intercurrent events. The description of the analysis approaches includes the statistical models and methods being used, often completed by sensitivity and supplementary analyses. These case studies highlight the complexities of applying the estimand framework in immunology and inflammation, emphasizing the importance of articulating clear trial objectives and estimands for interpretable treatment effects.

L. Meng (✉)
Boehringer Ingelheim Pharma GmbH & CO.KG, Biberach an der Riß, Germany
e-mail: leslie.meng@boehringer-ingelheim.com

P. Mesenbrink
Advanced Quantitative Sciences, Novartis Pharmaceuticals Corporation, East Hanover, USA
e-mail: peter_g.mesenbrink@novartis.com

F. Wang · C. Chen
Biostatistics and Research Decision Sciences, MSD R&D (China) Co., Ltd., Beijing, China
e-mail: fan.wang1@merck.com; chang.chen1@merck.com

H. Deng
Biostatistics and Data Sciences, Boehringer Ingelheim (China) Investment Co., Ltd., Shanghai, China
e-mail: hongjie.deng@boehringer-ingelheim.com

J. Wei et al. (eds.), *Estimands in Clinical Trials*, Springer Series in Pharmaceutical Statistics, https://doi.org/10.1007/978-3-032-02192-2_8

8.1 Introduction

Immunology encompasses a wide range of diseases, classified based on severity, prevalence, disease progression, and symptom chronicity. Some diseases involve chronic symptoms that worsen over time if untreated, leading to mortality or morbidity, while others are driven by flares, with the goal of treating active flares and preventing future ones. Autoimmune diseases occur when the immune system mistakenly attacks healthy cells, causing symptoms like fatigue, joint pain, inflammation, skin issues, digestive problems, recurring fever, swollen glands, and nausea. Each autoimmune disease is unique, and patients may present differently or even have multiple autoimmune diseases simultaneously.

There are at least 100 identified autoimmune diseases, and new ones are being identified every day. The most common autoimmune diseases can be grouped into the categories listed in Table 8.1. The most challenging feature of these diseases is that there is often not much that can be done to prevent the onset of many of these conditions unless there is an identified genetic marker which is known to increase the individual's risk.

Such a diverse set of diseases implies that a wide range of potential trial designs exist that can be tailored to the objectives of treating the underlying condition. Several key questions impact the type of clinical trial that will be designed and the potential confounding factors (i.e., intercurrent events) that could play a role in determining whether a specific investigational treatment could answer the key

Table 8.1 List of common autoimmune diseases

Disease category	Examples of common autoimmune diseases
Diseases of the joints, muscles, and bones	• Psoriatic arthritis • Ankylosing spondylitis • Rheumatoid arthritis • Polymyalgia rheumatica • Sjogren's syndrome • Systemic lupus erythematosus • Gout
Diseases of the digestive system	• Crohn's disease • Celiac disease • Ulcerative colitis
Diseases of the endocrine system	• Graves' disease • Hashimoto's thyroiditis • Addison's disease
Diseases of the skin	• Psoriasis • Atopic dermatitis • Vitiligo
Diseases of the nervous system	• Multiple sclerosis • Guillain-Barre syndrome
Other diseases	• Myasthenia gravis • Type 1 diabetes • Vasculitis

scientific question that is being asked as part of the estimand framework for the clinical trial. Clinical questions that are often asked in the design of such clinical trials include the following:

- Can patients with a specific disease who receive investigational treatment experience a reduction in the magnitude of severity of the signs and symptoms relative to patients with the disease who receive standard of care?
- Can patients with a specific disease who receive investigational treatment reduce the severity of signs and symptoms of the disease by xx% relative to patients with the disease who receive standard of care?
- Can patients with a specific disease who receive induction therapy with investigational treatment achieve disease remission over xx weeks at a rate higher than patients with the disease who receive standard of care?
- Can patients with a specific disease maintain disease remission at a higher rate over xx weeks with investigational treatment, when background therapy is withdrawn, than patients who receive standard-of-care treatment, who also have their background treatments for the disease withdrawn?
- Can patients who experience a disease flare be controlled and prevented from having a subsequent disease flare at a lower rate than patients receiving treatment with standard of care?

This chapter illustrates the estimand framework for four immunology clinical trials, each focusing on a different disease: generalized pustular psoriasis (GPP) (Sect. 8.2), rheumatoid arthritis (RA) (Sect. 8.3), atopic dermatitis (AD) (Sect. 8.4), and non-radiographic axial spondylarthritis (nraSpA) (Sect. 8.5).

8.2 Generalized Pustular Psoriasis

8.2.1 Background

Generalized pustular psoriasis (GPP) is a rare, potentially life-threatening autoimmune inflammatory neutrophilic skin disease characterized by widespread sterile visible pustules, with or without plaque psoriasis, and systemic inflammation. GPP is highly heterogeneous, with some patients experiencing frequent relapses, several times per year, while for others, flares may occur less frequently, potentially years apart. Acute GPP flares are associated with substantial morbidity and mortality if left untreated. Developing effective therapeutic interventions for GPP presents major challenges. First, GPP is a rare disease, which results in the challenge of conducting a large phase III trial to effectively answer the clinical question of interest. Second, the efficacy of interventions on GPP is difficult to evaluate due to the intermittent remission periods of the disease and the occurrence of spontaneously self-limiting episodic pustular flares. Third, there is no globally approved treatment for the prevention of acute GPP flares. Effective treatments with a rapid onset of action for acute GPP flares that can allow early control of skin inflammation and the prevention of complications are needed.

8.2.2 Trial Objective and Design

This trial is designed as a global, phase II, multicenter, randomized, double-blind, placebo-controlled trial with the use of spesolimab in patients with GPP presenting with an acute flare of moderate-to-severe intensity (Choon et al., 2021). The primary objective of this trial is to evaluate the efficacy, safety, and tolerability of a single dose of spesolimab in comparison to placebo at week 1/day 8.

Patients are randomized at a ratio of 2:1 to spesolimab and placebo, respectively, and evaluated daily until day 3. Clinical visits on days 4–7 are optional and not required if the patient has already achieved complete pustular clearance at the previous visit. At the week 1/day 8 visit, the primary endpoint and key secondary endpoints are assessed. At week 4, secondary endpoints are assessed. All randomized patients continue with the subsequent visits up to week 28 until the end of the trial.

In the trial, patients receive a single dose of spesolimab or placebo on day 1. If the severity and progression of the disease worsens within the first week, the investigator can treat the patient with a standard-of-care treatment of his/her choice as escape medication. If the disease condition remains stable, it is recommended to wait until the primary endpoint visit (week 1/ day 8) before prescribing an escape medication since there will be an option to administer open-label spesolimab at this time. If escape medication is administered within the first week, the patient is not eligible to receive treatment with open-label spesolimab on day 8. Restricted medications are prespecified in the protocol, and the use of restricted medication for purposes other than treating worsening of GPP is permitted and is not considered a treatment failure.

The primary endpoint is the achievement of the generalized pustular psoriasis physician global assessment (GPPGA) pustulation sub-score of 0 at week 1/day 8, where a sub-score of 0 indicates complete pustular clearance. An early efficacy endpoint is chosen, considering the unmet medical need of early skin flare control and the successful early performance of the GPPGA in a phase I trial. The primary endpoint of a GPPGA pustulation sub-score of 0 (clearance) at week 1 is considered clinically meaningful, as it represents disease remission/complete pustular clearance (Fig. 8.1).

8.2.3 Estimand Considerations

The trial compares spesolimab with placebo in patients with moderate-to-severe acute GPP flares. The primary objective is to demonstrate the superiority of spesolimab relative to placebo with respect to achieving complete pustular clearance at week 1, regardless of using restricted medication (not intended for GPP disease worsening) prior to week 1. Any use of escape medication or death prior to week 1 is considered a treatment failure at week 1. We define the estimand, with a detailed description of its five attributes as follows.

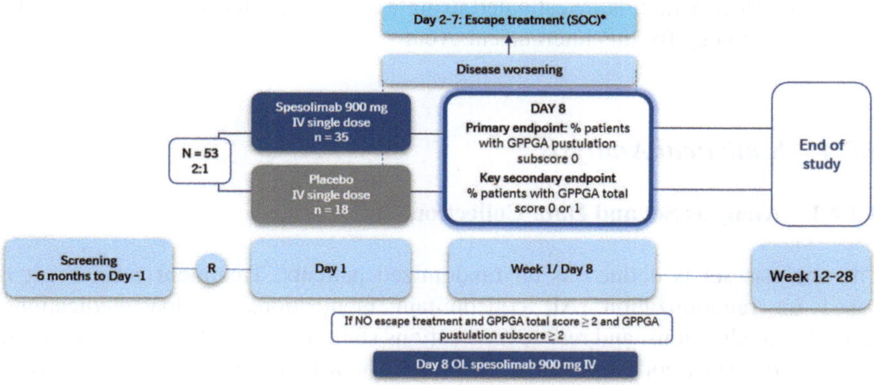

Fig. 8.1 GPP trial designNote: Days 2–7: Escape medication may be offered in case of disease worsening, defined as worsening of clinical status or GPP skin and/or systemic symptoms

(a) Population: Patients with moderate-to-severe acute GPP flare who meet the inclusion/exclusion criteria for the trial.
(b) Variable: GPPGA, where a pustulation sub-score of 0 at week 1 is defined as a response; if a patient dies or uses escape medication within the first week, the variable will be set to nonresponse.
(c) Treatment: Single intravenous injection of spesolimab or placebo, plus restricted medication (not intended for GPP disease worsening), as needed, prior to week 1.
(d) Intercurrent events: Death and intake of escape medication within the first week are addressed using a composite strategy (see the variable attribute above), while intake of restricted medication (not intended for GPP disease worsening) is addressed using the treatment policy strategy (see the treatment attribute above).
(e) Population-level summary: Absolute difference in response rate between spesolimab and placebo at week 1.

The intercurrent events in this trial include any use of escape medication within the first week, the open-label use of spesolimab at week 1/day 8, rescue medication with spesolimab after week 1, any use of restricted medication, and death. Since the interest is in the treatment effect at week 1 for the primary estimand, only intercurrent events within the first week are relevant. Intercurrent events that occur after week 1 are relevant to other secondary estimands, which are not discussed here.

Escape medication is taken for treating the underlying disease GPP, when the severity and progression of GPP worsen. Intake of escape medication and death indicate a treatment failure of the study treatment; therefore, a composite strategy is applied for these intercurrent events. Restricted medication taken for purposes other than treating the worsening of GPP is not considered to be treatment failure. Therefore, the treatment policy is applied for this intercurrent event. However, there is a suspicion that the use of restricted medication may have an impact on the treatment effect, which is investigated using a supplementary analysis, based on a composite strategy for this intercurrent event.

8.2.4 *Statistical Analysis*

8.2.4.1 Analysis Set and Data Collection

The analysis set is defined as all randomized patients. Treatment assignment is based on randomization. All concomitant medications, escape medications, restricted medications, and rescue medications should be recorded in the electronic case report forms. For all patients, the reason for withdrawal from the study treatment (such as adverse events or other diseases) or withdrawal from the whole trial must be documented. Patients who terminate the study drug early should be encouraged to follow all trial procedures and continue to complete all trial visits.

8.2.4.2 Statistical Model, Hypothesis, and Method of Analysis

This trial is designed to demonstrate the superiority of spesolimab over placebo for the primary endpoint (i.e., the achievement of the GPPGA pustulation sub-score at week 1). The null hypothesis being tested for the primary endpoint is that the effect of spesolimab on the proportion of patients achieving a GPPGA pustulation sub-score of 0 at week 1 is less than or equal to the effect in placebo, regardless of any use of restricted medication and considering death and intake of escape medication as treatment failure.

Given the small sample size, the Suissa–Shuster test (Suissa & Shuster, 1985) is used to assess the statistical significance of the treatment effect at an overall one-sided significance level of 0.025 since Fisher's exact test may be unnecessarily conservative. In the primary analysis, if there is any use of escape medication or death occurring prior to week 1, a composite strategy is applied, and be the primary endpoint/variable is considered as nonresponse. If there is any use of restricted medication for treating diseases other than GPP prior to week 1, the treatment policy strategy is applied, and the primary endpoint as observed at the week 1 time point is used.

8.2.4.3 Handling of Missing Data

Since restricted medication is addressed by the treatment policy strategy, data will be collected and used after that; however, missing data can also occur due to patients' early withdrawal from the trial or other reasons. Nonresponse imputation is performed to handle missing data for binary endpoints under a missing-at-random assumption. The nonresponse imputation is conducted in the following way: Since the GPPGA sub-score is measured at multiple visits, if there are observed data in the visits before and after the visit with the missing outcome, the missing outcome is imputed as a response only if the outcomes in both neighboring visits represent a response because there is sufficient confidence and information to assume that efficacy is sustained in the visit with the missing outcome. Otherwise, the missing outcome will be imputed as a nonresponse.

8.2.4.4 Sensitivity Analysis

Two sensitivity analyses are used to assess the impact of missing data on the primary estimator: the best response imputation and the exhaustive method (enumeration method). For the best response imputation under a missing-at-random assumption, the missing data is imputed based on the best response observed in the visits prior to the occurrence of the missing data. If no data is observed at all for the patient, the primary endpoint/variable is imputed as a nonresponse. The exhaustive method assumes data to be missing completely at random. If fewer than three patients have missing data on the primary endpoint, then all possible treatment differences will be generated, whereby each of the potential responses (response and nonresponse) will be imputed for each patient in an exhaustive manner.

8.2.4.5 Supplementary Analysis

The use of restricted medication for treating diseases other than GPP may potentially impact the treatment effect. A supplementary estimand is defined to consider the impact of restricted medication by applying a composite strategy for the intercurrent event of restricted medication. This means that the primary endpoint/variable is considered a nonresponse if this intercurrent event occurs. Other intercurrent events, including the intake of escape medication and death, are addressed in the same way as part of the primary estimand.

8.2.5 Summary and Discussion

In this case, the estimand is defined based on the trial objective with five attributes. Since the primary endpoint is at week 1/day 8, only the intercurrent events occurring before week 1 are considered in the primary estimand. To evaluate the robustness of the primary analysis, an exhaustive method is performed as a sensitivity analysis. Multiple imputation is not performed, considering the small sample size of the trial and potentially limited number of intercurrent events. When handling missing data, imputation is conducted only at the binary level (e.g., endpoint level). The GPPGA total score itself is not imputed, although the binary endpoint is derived based on this score.

8.3 Rheumatoid Arthritis

8.3.1 Background

Rheumatoid arthritis (RA) is an autoimmune ailment that primarily manifests as erosive arthritis (Aletaha, 2018). The main symptoms include morning joint stiffness, swelling, and pain during the early stages. In severe cases, it leads to joint deformity, affecting close to 24.5 million people as of 2015, with a prevalence rate of about 0.5–1% in the developed world. Genetics play a significant role, with females accounting for about 80% of the patients (Smolen, 2016). Currently, RA is incurable, and the disease-modifying treatments aim to achieve disease remission, reduce disability rates, and improve patients' quality of life (Saag et al., 2008). Besides laboratory and imaging diagnoses, common diagnostic criteria include the disease activity score in 28 joints (DAS28) and the American College of Rheumatology 20% response criteria (ACR20) (Pincus et al., 2004). The DAS28 combines the number of swollen joints (28-joint count), the number of tender joints (28-joint count), the patient's global assessment of disease activity (using a visual analog scale), and the measurement of erythrocyte sedimentation rate (ESR) or C-reactive protein (CRP) levels, which are markers of inflammation. Both DAS28-ESR and DAS28-CRP are continuous variables. ACR20 evaluates whether there is an improvement of more than 20% in ACR joint pain and joint swelling score and whether at least three indicators in the remaining five indicators of ACR have an improvement of more than 20%.

Current treatment for RA includes drug therapy and surgery. The first-line treatment approved by regulatory agencies is the use of disease-modifying antirheumatic drugs (DMARDs). The most common conventional synthetic DMARD is methotrexate (MTX) (Donahue et al., 2019). Currently, clinical development focuses on patients who have an inadequate response to DMARDs and other biological therapies. If a patient's symptoms do not improve significantly with a single DMARD, combination therapy with biologic DMARDs or targeted synthetic DMARDs, such as tocilizumab and baricitinib, may be considered (add-on trials). Surgical treatment is typically considered after the unsuccessful use of DMARDs.

Several authors have discussed the estimand framework and provided relevant case studies (Ratitch et al., 2020; Casey et al., 2021; Lipkovich et al., 2020); see also Part I of this book. Ratitch et al. (2020) introduced a hypothetical confirmatory trial of a biological agent for MTX-inadequate-responder patients, illustrating the intercurrent events expected during the trial and how they can be addressed so as to be consistent with the study objectives. To avoid similarity with existing articles, this section introduced a phase III therapeutic equivalence clinical trial of a biosimilar in RA as an example to illustrate the estimand framework and related statistical considerations.

8.3.2 Trial Objective and Design

Tocilizumab is a monoclonal immunoglobulin antibody, which has been approved by the European Medicines Agency (EMA) as an add-on treatment to MTX for adult patients with moderate-to-severe active RA. MSB11456 is a biosimilar candidate to tocilizumab, which needs a therapeutic equivalence trial to show the similarity of efficacy and safety relative to the branded drug.

A multicenter, randomized, active-controlled, double-blind, multiple fixed-dose, multinational, two-arm clinical trial compares the efficacy, safety, and immunogenicity of the proposed biosimilar MSB11456 versus tocilizumab in patients with moderate-to-severe active RA (ClinicalTrials.gov identifier: NCT04512001). This case study is inspired by the estimand section of the trial protocol, with some adaptations where appropriate.

Patients are randomized at the beginning of the trial to receive either MSB11456 or tocilizumab once a week (QW). After 24 weeks, patients who have received tocilizumab are re-randomized to either continue receiving tocilizumab QW or switch to receive MSB11456 QW. Investigators may use protocol-defined prohibited therapy according to the patient's status. Patients who discontinue treatment before week 24 are asked to return for all planned assessment visits before and at week 24. The trial schema is displayed in Fig. 8.2.

8.3.3 Estimand Considerations

This trial compares biosimilar MSB11456 and tocilizumab in patients with moderate-to-severe active RA. The primary objective is to demonstrate therapeutic equivalence between the two arms as measured by the difference in mean change from baseline of DAS28-ESR (see Sect. 8.3.1 for its definition) at week 24. The treatment effect is of interest regardless of treatment discontinuation due to any reason, use of prohibited medications as defined in the protocol, dosage modification of MTX after the first dose, and coronavirus disease (COVID-19) vaccination during or after the first dose prior to week 24. In the following, we define the estimand, with a detailed description of its five attributes.

(a) Population: Patients with moderate-to-severe active RA as defined by the inclusion/exclusion criteria.
(b) Variable: Absolute change of DAS28-ESR from baseline at week 24.
(c) Treatment: Subcutaneous injection of MSB11456 versus tocilizumab, regardless of treatment discontinuation due to any reason, use of prohibited medications as defined in the protocol, dosage modification of MTX after the first dose, and COVID-19 vaccination during or after the first dose prior to week 24. Note that prohibited medications, as defined in this protocol, may be referred to as rescue medication in other protocols.
(d) Intercurrent events are displayed in Table 8.2.

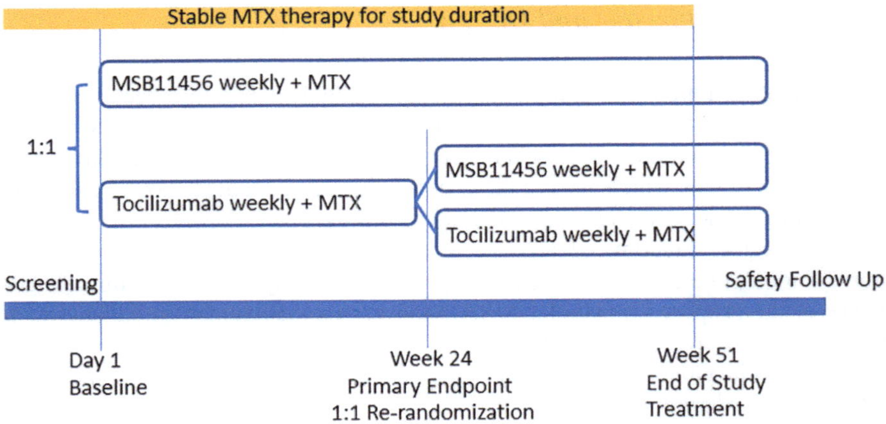

Fig. 8.2 Trial schema. (Adapted from the original protocol)

Table 8.2 Proposed estimand strategies

Intercurrent event	Strategies	Comment
Treatment discontinuation due to any reason, including adverse events and lack of efficacy	Treatment policy strategy	The strategies reflect clinical practice All available information at week 24 is included in the analysis. The intercurrent events are considered a part of the treatment regimen of interest
Use of prohibited medications, as defined in the protocol, prior to week 24	Treatment policy strategy	
Dosage modification of MTX after the first dose and prior to week 24	Treatment policy strategy	
COVID-19 vaccination during or after the first dose	Treatment policy strategy	

(e) Population-level summary: The mean difference between MSB11456 and tocilizumab at week 24.

8.3.4 *Statistical Analysis*

8.3.4.1 Analysis Set and Data Collection

The analysis set includes all randomized patients with moderate-to-severe active RA who have an inadequate response to at least one disease-modifying antirheumatic drug and who are currently receiving a stable dose of MTX. According to the protocol and the treatment policy strategy, patients who discontinue the study treatment before week 24 are requested to return for the week-24 visit to ensure data collection after the intercurrent event occurrences.

8.3.4.2 Statistical Model, Hypothesis, and Method of Analysis

The objective of this trial is to demonstrate therapeutic equivalence of MSB11456 and tocilizumab at DAS28-ESR at week 24. Change from baseline at week 24 of DAS28-ESR is analyzed using an analysis of covariance model, with treatment and prior medication of RA as fixed effects and baseline DAS28-ESR as a covariate. The method of difference between treatments uses the least squares mean difference between MSB11456 and tocilizumab, along with a two-sided 90% confidence interval. As a therapeutic equivalence trial, the timing of the primary efficacy analysis at week 24 is consistent with the primary endpoint of tocilizumab phase III clinical trials, on which the assumptions for the equivalence margin and sample size are based.

8.3.4.3 Handling of Missing Data

Missing values for the DAS28-ESR score are imputed by a multiple imputation procedure at each post-baseline visit when using the treatment policy strategy. For non-monotone missing data, intermittent missing DAS28-ESR scores are imputed under a missing-at-random assumption. Under this assumption, the missing outcomes would be similar to those of patients with similar baseline and previous post-baseline values in their treatment arm. For monotone missing data (i.e., missing DAS28-ESR scores due to patient lost-to-follow-up), the multiple imputation is based on the observations from those patients in the same treatment arm who continue in follow-up after the intercurrent events.

8.3.4.4 Sensitivity Analysis

To evaluate the robustness of the missing-at-random assumption for the primary analysis, a tipping point analysis is performed as a sensitivity analysis for the primary endpoint. Missing values of changes from baseline for DAS28-ESR at week 24 are imputed by considering the treatment arm, randomization stratum, and the baseline DAS28-ESR as a continuous covariate. Patients with missing baseline values are excluded from the analysis.

8.3.4.5 Supplementary Analysis

In the primary estimand, for imperfect compliance due to various reasons (such as discontinuation of treatment, use of prohibited drugs predefined by the protocol, change to other drug or dosage of antirheumatic drugs, and COVID-19 vaccination), the sponsor regards them as a part of the assessed treatment regimen and broadens the treatment regimens under evaluation. The combined treatment effect is available in the primary estimand. These intercurrent events are also in line with general clinical practice, so the efficacy data observed after the intercurrent events is still used. In addition, as a therapeutic equivalence trial, the estimand framework of the primary endpoint needs to refer to the objective of the brand drug to maintain the similarity of treatment effect, which is a combined effect of the initial randomized treatment and the modified treatment because of intercurrent event(s).

However, the ICH E9 guideline (ICH, 1998) also states that equivalence trials are not conservative in nature. Due to small differences in the treatment effect of treatment arms, the treatment policy strategy may bias the results toward equivalence conclusions. It is difficult to demonstrate the treatment effect of the experimental arm without any confounding factors in the trial, thus reducing the reliability of the trial. Therefore, for equivalence trials, ICH (1998) mentions the importance of the minimization of protocol violations and noncompliance. Further estimand considerations for non-inferiority and equivalence trials can be found in Chap. 22.

In this trial, besides the primary objective, both the regulatory agency and the sponsor focus on the scientific question of the worst treatment effect of MSB11456 and tocilizumab; i.e., any rescue therapies during or after treatment are regarded as treatment failure. Composite strategies can be used for this scientific question. For intercurrent events like treatment discontinuation due to a lack of efficacy or adverse events, as well as after the use of a prohibited medication or a dosage modification of MTX, they can use a composite strategy to validate the robustness of the result for the primary endpoint. In this strategy, these intercurrent events are classified as failures for the target treatment regimen, which no longer benefit from treatment. Measurement of DAS28-ESR is assigned as a worst-case scenario, i.e., the value of the composite endpoint for the patient returns to baseline measurements after the intercurrent event. The objective is changed to estimate the therapeutic equivalence of treatment effect under a composite strategy where the discontinuation of treatment due to lack of efficacy or adverse event as well as use of prohibited medication or dosage modification of MTX defined as non-response and no change from baseline at week 24. For the composite strategy, the week-24 data after intercurrent events is set to be the baseline value, whether missing data exists or not.

8.3.5 Summary and Discussion

This section provides the estimand consideration for a therapeutic equivalence trial of a biosimilar in RA. The estimand framework for the primary trial objective is used such that it aligns with what was previously used with the branded drug. It should be noted that due to small differences in the treatment effects between treatment arms, the treatment policy strategy may bias the results toward equivalence conclusions. Demonstrating the treatment effect of the experimental arm without accounting for the confounding factors within the trial is challenging, thereby reducing the trial's reliability. Consequently, for equivalence trials, ICH (1998) emphasizes the importance of minimizing protocol violations and noncompliance. Further considerations regarding estimands for non-inferiority and equivalence trials are discussed in Chap. 22.

8.4 Atopic Dermatitis

8.4.1 Background

Atopic dermatitis (AD), also known as atopic eczema, is the most common, highly prevalent, chronic, life-long inflammatory skin condition (Weidinger et al., 2018). As stated in the Global Report on Atopic Dermatitis from 2022, AD affects up to 20% of children and up to 10% of adults, and its disease burden ranks number one for skin conditions (GADA, 2022). The disease etiology of AD is still under investigation to be fully elucidated (Sideris et al., 2022; GADA, 2022). Factors associated with AD include immune system dysfunction, skin barrier disruption, and genetic (e.g., family history) and environmental (e.g., living in regions with low ultraviolet light exposure or dry climatic conditions) factors (Sideris et al., 2022; GADA, 2022).

AD flare substantially impacts patients' or even caregivers' physical (e.g., sleep disruption, work, and school performance) and emotional (e.g., embarrassment and self-confidence) well-being and quality of life (Zuberbier et al., 2006). The most common symptom of AD is itching, and the skin damage gets worse over time due to the itch–scratch–itch cycle (i.e., the intensity of itch leads to repeated scratching to relieve the itch, and it causes more itch). There are many patient-reported outcomes (PROs) developed to assess different AD-associated symptoms and/or quality of life, such as the numerical rating scale (NRS), pruritus; verbal rating scale (VRS), pruritus; night time itch scale (NTIS); patient-oriented eczema measure (POEM); patient global assessment (PGA); dermatological quality of life index (DLQI), or children's DLQI; pruritus and symptoms assessment for atopic dermatitis (PSAAD), hospital anxiety and depression scale (HADS); and many others (Vakharia et al., 2018; Thyssen et al., 2022; Reich et al., 2022).

In the following, we use peak pruritus NRS (PP-NRS) as a valid and reliable PRO that is commonly used in AD (Thyssen et al., 2022; Reich et al., 2022). PP-NRS assesses the AD-associated severity of itch. It is a univariate instrument recorded on a daily basis by asking about the worst itching over the past 24 hours with a score range of 0–10 (0 means no itch, and 10 means the worst itch imaginable) (Yosipovitch et al., 2017). As suggested by its user manual, the weekly summary score is computed as the average of observed daily measurements within a week (i.e., on a seven-day duration basis) and is used to derive different types of endpoints. A weekly average score of PP-NRS can be computed if there are at least four days of observed measurements within a prespecified week; otherwise, the corresponding week will be imputed as missing. The weekly average of PP-NRS is a continuous score, and it can be dichotomized (e.g., response to a four-point improvement) and evaluated as a time-to-event endpoint (e.g., time to four-point improvement), depending on the trial objectives. In this case, we focus on the binary endpoint of PP-NRS.

8.4.2 Trial Objective and Design

We consider a phase III, randomized, double-blind, double-dummy, head-to-head clinical trial (ClinicalTrials.gov identifier: NCT04345367) to compare the efficacy and safety of abrocitinib versus dupilumab in adult patients on background topical therapy with moderate-to-severe AD (Reich et al., 2022). The trial consists of a four-week screening period, a 26-week double-blind treatment period, and a four-week off-treatment follow-up period (see Fig. 8.3). Seven hundred and twenty-seven patients are randomized. During the 26-week double-blind treatment period, patients receive abrocitinib 200 mg orally once every day with dupilumab-matching placebo through subcutaneous injection every two weeks (per label guidelines) or 300 mg dupilumab through subcutaneous injection every two weeks with abrocitinib-matching placebo orally once daily.

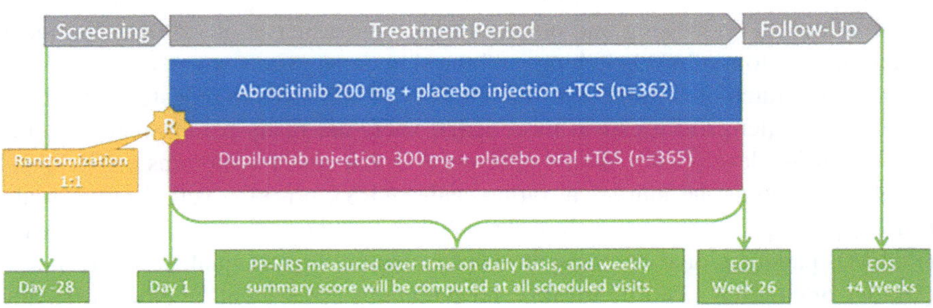

Fig. 8.3 Adapted trial schema from Reich et al. (2022), with special focus on PP-NRSNote: *TCS*: topical corticosteroids, as stated in the trial protocol; *EOT*: end of trial; *EOS*: end of study; *R*: randomization; *mg*: milligram; and *n*: number of randomized patients

The trial has two co-primary objectives: early itch reductions (as measured by achieving at least a four-point improvement from baseline in the severity of PP-NRS response at week 2) and disease signs (as measured by achieving at least 90% improvement in the eczema area and severity index (EASI-90) response at week 4). These two co-primary objectives assess the efficacy of abrocitinib versus dupilumab in adults with moderate-to-severe AD (Reich et al., 2022). This case study focuses on the estimand considerations of PP-NRS. Note that the estimand considerations discussed in the following section also apply to the co-primary endpoint, EASI-90. Since the scope of this case study focuses on the PRO, EASI-90 will not be discussed.

8.4.3 Estimand Considerations

The primary objective of this trial is to demonstrate the superiority of abrocitinib plus topical corticosteroids (TCS) over dupilumab plus TCS in patients with moderate-to-severe AD. The treatment effect of primary interest is assessed in terms of the response rate difference, where clinical response is defined as a composite of achieving at least a four-point improvement from baseline in the severity of PP-NRS at week 2, with treatment discontinuation due to any reason or the use of rescue therapies considered to be a nonresponse. In the following, we define the estimand, with a detailed description of its five attributes.

(a) Population: Patients with moderate-to-severe AD as defined by the inclusion criteria to reflect the targeted population.
(b) Variable: Response defined as achieving at least a four-point improvement from baseline in the severity of PP-NRS at week 2, with the discontinuation of treatment for any reason and the use of rescue therapies defined as nonresponse.
(c) Treatment: Abrocitinib 200 mg once daily plus TCS or dupilumab 300 mg every two weeks (per label dosing guidelines) plus TCS.
(d) Intercurrent events: Treatment discontinuation for any reason and use of rescue therapy are captured through the variable definition.
(e) Population-level summary: Difference in response rate between abrocitinib and dupilumab.

The above-defined estimand is the primary estimand stated in the trial. The two intercurrent events, treatment discontinuation for any reason and the use of rescue therapies, are addressed by the composite strategy, which is reflected through a variable definition. That is, the response is then defined as nonresponse after the occurrence of the event. By applying the composite strategy, the variable of interest becomes the composite of the use of rescue therapies (nonresponse), the discontinuation of treatment due to any reason (nonresponse), and the measures of the clinical outcome of interest (PP-NRS response at week 2).

8.4.4 Statistical Analysis

8.4.4.1 Analysis Set and Data Collection

The analysis set is defined as all randomized patients receiving at least one dose of trial intervention, with a baseline PP-NRS score of at least 4. Patients are analyzed based on their randomized treatments, not the actual received treatments, and the actual stratum, i.e., baseline disease severity and moderate or severe investigator global assessment (IGA). Patients are required to have non-missing baseline PP-NRS scores of at least 4.

8.4.4.2 Statistical Model, Hypothesis, and Method of Analysis

The proportion of responders by treatment arm and differences are presented between the two arms with 95% confidence intervals. The superiority test is conducted for the four-point improvement of PP-NRS response at week 2. The Cochran–Mantel–Haenszel test, adjusting for baseline disease severity (moderate or severe IGA), is employed to test the hypothesis of no or negative difference in binary responses. The difference in proportions is summarized based on a weighted average of stratum estimates (moderate or severe IGA), obtained from the Cochran–Mantel–Haenszel test.

8.4.4.3 Handling of Missing Data

The scoring algorithm stated in the trial statistical analysis plan suggests that PP-NRS (weekly summary score) can be calculated if there are at least four days of observed scores within a seven-day duration; otherwise, the PP-NRS and its corresponding binary outcome are considered missing and can be imputed by statistical methods. Based on the primary estimand, patients who discontinue the trial treatment for any reason or initiate rescue therapies are defined as nonresponders after that point and, thus, should have the non-missing response value.

8.4.4.4 Supplementary Analysis

A supplementary estimand is also considered. The supplementary objective is to demonstrate the superiority between two arms in response rate difference, where clinical response is defined as a composite of achieving at least a four-point improvement from baseline in the severity of PP-NRS at week 2, with treatment discontinuation due to any reason defined as nonresponse.

This supplementary estimand adopts the treatment policy strategy to address the use of rescue therapies rather than the composite strategy; thus, related information is captured in the treatment definition. In other words, the treatment attribute of the estimand is defined as abrocitinib plus TCS plus rescue therapies as compared with dupilumab plus TCS plus rescue therapies. By applying the treatment policy strategy on the use of rescue therapies, it is believed that the intercurrent event is included in the treatment regimen of interest.

The supplementary analysis is performed based on the supplementary estimand. By applying the treatment policy strategy, data is assessed regardless of the intercurrent event, and missing values are addressed by multiple imputation. For monotone missing data, multiple imputation under the missing-at-random assumption and multiple imputation based on retrieved dropout data (Wang & Hu, 2022) are both considered.

PRO instruments can result in various endpoints in a single trial, revealing the fact of having multiple PRO-related clinical questions. In this trial, another supplementary clinical question based on PP-NRS is about the difference in time course of the severity of itch score improvement (as measured by the time from baseline to achieve at least a four-point improvement in the severity of PP-NRS scale) between the two arms in patients with moderate-to-severe AD if all patients maintain the same treatment. A hypothetical strategy is applied to address the intercurrent events by assuming that they have not occurred and are censored at the occurrence of the intercurrent event. It is assumed that future hazards for patients with intercurrent events are the same as for patients without them. The underlying assumption is reasonable, as the potential improvements of rescue therapies are ignored or removed, and it is unlikely to approach a four-point improvement after treatment discontinuation. Therefore, intercurrent events are captured in the treatment effect of abrocitinib as compared to dupilumab if all patients maintain the same treatment.

8.4.5 Summary and Discussion

This section provides the estimand considerations of binary PROs based on a clinical trial of assessing the safety and efficacy of abrocitinib versus dupilumab in adults with AD. Two intercurrent events (discontinuation of treatment for any reason and the use of rescue therapies) are addressed, with different strategies applied for the binary PP-NRS endpoint using composite and treatment policy strategies.

PRO derivations could consist of a two-step computation: First, calculate the PRO average score using the instrument's scoring algorithm, and second, derive the binary endpoint based on the calculated continuous score. The scoring algorithm is clearly defined in its user manual but still results in missing data and, thus, advanced statistical techniques (e.g., multiple imputation and others) are needed to further address. In this case, a binary endpoint of four-point improvement at a specific visit is then derived based on the computed PP-NRS weekly average score to comprehensively understand the improvement of patients' experience of the peak pruritus.

8.5 Non-radiographic Axial Spondyloarthritis

8.5.1 Background

Axial spondyloarthritis (SpA) is a chronic inflammatory disease of the spine, which includes non-radiographic axial SpA (nraSpA) and ankylosing spondylitis (AS). Differences in the disease subtypes of SpA are determined based on whether there exists X-ray evidence of structural damage in the sacroiliac joints and/or the spine. Patients with nraSpA differ from AS patients relative to their lack of radiographic evidence of sacroiliitis. The two subpopulations are similar with respect to their symptoms of disease burden, which include inflammatory back pain in the pelvis and lower back, morning stiffness, nocturnal awakening, fatigue, and reduced spinal mobility (Deodhar et al., 2021).

The prevalence of nraSpA is reported to be ~0.1–0.4% in the general population, more prevalent in women, and ~ 16–37% in patients with inflammatory back pain. The epidemiology of nraSpA continues to evolve due to the heterogeneity in definition, slow progression, and diagnostic delays.

The reported rate of progression from nraSpA to AS varies from ~10% to 40% of patients over 2–10 years, with a lifetime risk of progression of ~50%. Early diagnosis of nraSpA is important for the management of disease symptoms and to potentially limit the amount of damage that is done to the spine. The Assessment of SpondyloArthritis international Society (ASAS) criteria have been developed for the classification of axial SpA and include patients with early disease, with or without radiographic evidence of sacroiliitis.

Nonsteroidal anti-inflammatory drugs (NSAIDs) are recommended as first-line therapy in patients with nraSpA by all of the rheumatology professional societies (Reich et al., 2022; Saag et al., 2008). Biological disease-modifying drugs are recommended in patients with active disease and clear signs of inflammation (e.g., elevated CRP level and/or evidence of sacroiliitis on magnetic resonance imaging (MRI)) while being treated with NSAIDs. Interleukin-17 (IL-17) has an important role in the progression of axial SpA, contributing to inflammation, enthesitis, and structural damage. According to the 2019 update of the ACR/SAA/SPARTAN treatment guidelines (Ward et al., 2019), IL-17 inhibitors are the preferred therapy compared to using a second tumor necrosis factor inhibitor (TNFi) agent in patients with AS with an initial inadequate response to the first TNFi treatment.

Secukinumab, a human monoclonal antibody that directly works to block IL-17A, has provided significant and sustained improvement in the signs and symptoms of AS, as evidenced in the phase III MEASURE trials.

PREVENT is a unique phase III trial that is designed to evaluate the efficacy, safety, and tolerability of secukinumab 150 mg, with or without loading doses, in patients with active nraSpA. It is unique in that the design is flexible enough to have two different sets of estimands to meet the regulatory requirements for the United States (US) and European Union (EU). Details of these special features are described further in the subsequent subsections.

8.5.2 Trial Objective and Design

PREVENT (ClinicalTrials.gov identifier: NCT02696031) is a phase III, placebo-controlled, multicenter trial evaluating the efficacy and safety for up to two years with secukinumab 150 mg (with and without loading) in patients with nraSpA. This trial serves as an exemplary case. It is required to have different analysis strategies for the EMA and the US Food and Drug Administration (FDA), given that the primary efficacy analysis time point is at week 16 for the EMA and at week 52 for the FDA. These differences are necessary because, in consultation with the FDA on the trial design, it is suggested that in the population that is being studied, it is possible for patients not receiving investigational treatment to have a spontaneous resolution of symptoms and then flare up again. Therefore, a week-52 endpoint would be more reflective of the true treatment effect of secukinumab. Following these primary efficacy analyses, patients are allowed to be considered for an optional dose escalation to 150 mg or 300 mg of secukinumab for up to another two years, which will be outside the scope of this example. Figure 8.4 shows the trial design for the first 52 weeks, as it is presented in the trial protocol available on ClinicalTrials.gov.

For the EU analysis plan (referred to going forward as Analysis Plan A, as opposed to Analysis Plan B for the US), the primary objective is to demonstrate that patients treated with secukinumab 150 mg (with loading regimen) have a superior response rate in the ASAS relative to placebo in tumor-necrosis-factor-naïve patients at week 16. ASAS40 is defined as an improvement of at least 40% and at least two units on a scale of 10 in at least three of the four main domains and no worsening in the remaining domain. The ASAS response measures consist of the following assessment domains (Sieper et al., 2009):

- Patient global assessment of disease activity measured on a visual analog scale.
- Patient assessment of back pain, represented by either total or nocturnal pain scores, both measured on a visual analog scale.
- Function, as measured by the Bath ankylosing spondylitis functional index (BASFI) average of ten questions related to performing specific tasks and reported on visual analog scales.
- Inflammation reported as the mean duration and severity of morning stiffness by averaging the last two questions of the Bath ankylosing spondylitis disease activity index (BASDAI), as measured by visual analog scales.

8.5.3 Estimand Considerations

This section focuses on the definition of the estimand for the primary endpoint for Analysis Plan A and Analysis Plan B. Two different estimand strategies are necessary for the primary efficacy endpoint in the EU and US regulatory approvals because of the following:

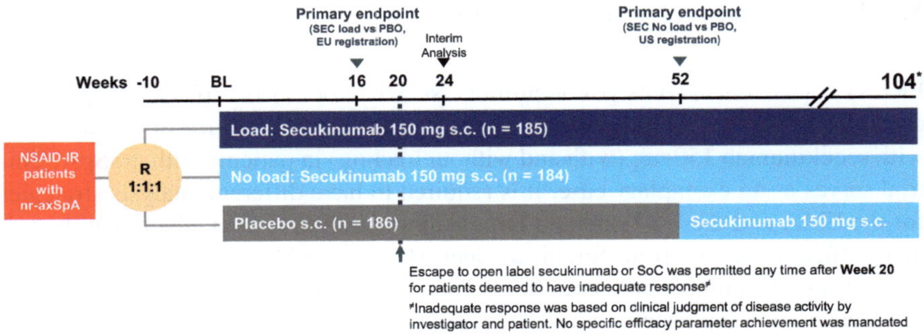

Fig. 8.4 PREVENT trial design for the first 104 weeks. (Adapted from the clinical trial protocol. (ClinicalTrials.gov identifier: NCT02696031))

1. The different time points at which the primary efficacy endpoint is evaluated (week 16 versus week 52).
2. Patients are not allowed to be rescued prior to the primary efficacy endpoint in the EU, whereas patients are allowed to be rescued with open-label secukinumab from week 20 onward, which could potentially confound the interpretation of the primary endpoint at week 52. In addition, changes or new NSAIDs and/or disease-modifying antirheumatic drugs could be initiated from week 16. It is also possible for someone to start a new biological treatment other than secukinumab after a 12-week washout.
3. Two separate teams exist for the conduct of these statistical analyses to maintain the integrity of Analysis Plan B, which has both week-16 and week-52 endpoints in the testing hierarchy

8.5.3.1 Primary Estimand for the EU Regulatory Approval (Analysis Plan a)

The following is a definition of the estimand for the EU regulatory approval, with a detailed description of the five attributes.

(a) Population: Patients with nraSpA, as defined by the inclusion/exclusion criteria.
(b) Variable: Patients remaining in the trial and on randomized treatment through week 16 and achieving ASAS40 response at week 16 are defined as responders. Discontinuing from the trial or the study treatment resulted in a patient being classified as a nonresponder. Note that a rescue treatment with open-label secukinumab was not permitted prior to the evaluation of the primary efficacy endpoint at week 16.

(c) Treatment: Secukinumab 150 mg subcutaneous injection administered every 4 weeks (without loading) or secukinumab 150 mg subcutaneous injection administered weekly for the first 4 weeks and every 4 weeks thereafter (with loading) versus placebo subcutaneous injection administered weekly for the first 4 weeks and every 4 weeks thereafter.
(d) Intercurrent events: Discontinuation of study treatment is addressed by a composite strategy, as captured in the variable definition above. Discontinuations of study treatment usually coincide with receiving escape/rescue treatment, but per protocol, this is not allowed to occur until week 16.
(e) Population-level summary: Odds ratio of ASAS40 response proportions between the secukinumab treatment regimens and the placebo.

8.5.3.2 Primary Estimand for the US Regulatory Approval (Analysis Plan B)

The following is a definition of the estimand for the US regulatory approval, with a detailed description of the five attributes.

(a) Population: Patients with non-radiographic axial spondylarthritis, as defined by the inclusion/exclusion criteria.
(b) Variable: Patients remaining in the trial and on randomized treatment through 52 weeks and achieving ASAS40 response at week 52 are defined as responders. Discontinuing from the trial or the study treatment resulted in a patient being classified as a nonresponder.
(c) Treatment of interest: Secukinumab 150 mg subcutaneous injection administered every 4 weeks (without loading) or secukinumab 150 mg subcutaneous injection administered weekly for the first 4 weeks and every 4 weeks thereafter (with loading) versus placebo subcutaneous injection administered weekly for the first 4 weeks and every 4 weeks thereafter (to maintain the blind to the two secukinumab regimens).
(d) Intercurrent events: Discontinuation of study treatment is addressed by a composite strategy, as captured in the variable definition above. Discontinuations of study treatment usually coincide with receiving escape/rescue treatment, but per protocol, this is not allowed to occur until week 20. This results in a large percentage of placebo-arm patients switching to active treatment at week 20. NSAIDs and DMARDs could be modified or added at week 16 to treat signs and symptoms. Patients could also switch to biological treatments other than secukinumab from week 20 after a 12-week washout.
(e) Population-level summary: Odds ratio of ASAS40 response proportions between the secukinumab treatment regimens and the placebo.

8.5.4 Statistical Analysis

8.5.4.1 Primary Analysis Plan for the EU Regulatory Approval

8.5.4.1.1 Analysis Set and Data Collection

The full analysis set comprises all patients with non-radiographic axial spondylarthritis, as defined by the inclusion/exclusion criteria, and the analyzable patients from the randomized set to whom study treatment has been assigned. Following the intent-to-treat principle, patients are evaluated according to the treatment assigned at randomization, but the actual stratum (CRP+/MRI+, CRP+/MRI-, or CRP-/MRI+) is used in analysis in the event that, at the time of randomization, a patient is randomized to the incorrect subgroup within the stratification factors.

8.5.4.1.2 Statistical Model, Hypothesis, and Method of Analysis

The primary analysis for ASAS40 response at week 16 is conducted via logistic regression, with the treatment arm and stratification factor (CRP+/MRI+, CRP+/MRI-, or CRP-/MRI+) as factors and weight as a covariate. Odds ratios and 95% confidence intervals are presented comparing each secukinumab regimen to placebo.

8.5.4.1.3 Handling of Missing Data

Missing data for the ASAS40 response at week 16 and other binary secondary endpoints at week 16 are handled as follows:

- Patients who prematurely discontinue from the trial for any reason are considered nonresponders from the time that they prematurely discontinue from the trial through week 16 (composite strategy).
- Patients who do not have the required data to compute responses (e.g., ASAS components) are classified as nonresponders at week 16.

8.5.4.2 Primary Analysis Plan for the US Regulatory Approval

8.5.4.2.1 Analysis Set and Data Collection

The full analysis set comprises all patients with nraSpA, as defined by the inclusion/exclusion criteria, and the analyzable patients from the randomized set to whom study treatment has been assigned. Following the intent-to-treat principle, patients are evaluated according to the treatment assigned at randomization but actual stratum (CRP+/MRI+, CRP+/MRI-, or CRP-/MRI+) is used in analysis.

8.5.4.2.2 Statistical Model, Hypothesis, and Method of Analysis

The primary analysis for ASAS40 response at week 52 is conducted via logistic regression, with the treatment arm and stratification factor (CRP+/MRI+, CRP+/MRI-, or CRP-/MRI+) as factors and weight as a covariate. Odds ratios and 95% confidence intervals are presented comparing each secukinumab regimen to placebo.

8.5.4.2.3 Handling of Missing Data

Missing data for the ASAS40 response at week 52 and other binary secondary variables at week 16/52 are handled as follows:

- Patients who prematurely discontinue from the trial for any reason are considered nonresponders from the time that they prematurely discontinue from the trial through week 16/52 (composite strategy).
- Patients who do not have the required data to compute responses (e.g., ASAS components) are classified as nonresponders at week 16/52.

8.5.4.2.4 Handling of Data Post-Treatment Switch

Within Analysis Plan B, the statistical testing hierarchy has endpoints at week 16 and week 52, which is different from Analysis Plan A (all testing hierarchy endpoints are at week 16), and it is permitted for all patients to escape to open-label biological treatment starting at week 20.

- For binary endpoints, a composite strategy is applied (this is covered by the discontinuation of the study treatment for any reason), and this includes even those patients who escape from secukinumab-randomized treatment regimens. All such patients would be considered nonresponders for the week-52 primary and secondary endpoints if this occurs.
- For continuous endpoints in the testing hierarchy at week 52 in Analysis Plan B, a composite strategy is applied after switching to open-label treatment, and the data after the switch is set to the most unfavorable value.

8.5.5 Summary and Discussion

This section describes the estimands for a very special example from a phase III trial in nraSpA, where there are two different analysis plans, one for the EU registration and one for the US registration. It also shows the evolution of the estimand framework since it first began appearing in the statistical analysis plan in 2015/2016. Since these estimands are defined and implemented, we have increased our knowledge with respect to endpoint definition and distinguishing between what should be considered an intercurrent event and what is part of the endpoint definition and how should missing data not due to intercurrent events be addressed. In addition, the summary measure based on odds ratios that is used as the summary measure for both analysis plans would likely not be used if this analysis is going to be executed today; instead, a summary measure that incorporates some form of risk differences would likely be used as the summary measure. The influence of intercurrent events related to changes in the study treatment after week 16 in Analysis Plan B (for the US registration) adds to the complexities in constructing the estimand because it is allowed from week 20 to escape to open-label secukinumab treatment for all patients, requiring a composite endpoint strategy to be applied for all endpoints evaluated after week 16 as well as changes to the background therapy, which begins at week 16. This is a problem for which awareness is needed in the future in the design of immunology clinical trials, where the regulatory requirements may be different in certain parts of the world, especially if it is not believed that the patients who are randomized to the control arm can remain on this treatment for the full duration of the double-blind period.

8.6 Concluding Remarks

In conclusion, this chapter has highlighted the complexities and challenges involved in applying estimands in immunology. The diverse case studies presented underscore the essential role of defining clear trial objectives and establishing reliable estimands to accurately assess and interpret treatment outcomes. We discuss and summarize specific features of immunology trials in this section.

In immunology trials, true placebo arms are rare, as background treatments like NSAIDs, oral steroids, or other immunosuppressants are common. Patients are stabilized on these drugs before the trial to set a baseline. Maintaining stable background medication is crucial for valid comparisons. Changes in background medication are considered intercurrent events unless they are part of the endpoint. Management of these changes depends on the availability of approved therapies. In the absence of approved treatments, adding a new one may require a treatment policy strategy despite the potential for confounding. For diseases typically treated with steroids, tapering schedules test whether the investigational treatment works without them. If relapse occurs, the control arm generally shows a higher relapse rate than the investigational arm.

Composite endpoints are usually considered primary endpoints in immunology clinical trials, where they capture various dimensions of the disease, recognizing that patients may improve differently in each area. These endpoints, used in diseases like rheumatoid arthritis and psoriatic arthritis, often allow for some worsening in one component if overall improvements are significant. This complexity necessitates addressing intercurrent events both at the component and the composite level to maintain the integrity of efficacy assessments. Robust considerations of supplementary estimands are essential to ensure the robustness of the primary analysis.

Patients with chronic immunological diseases may require both short-term and long-term management to maintain treatment response and prevent future flares. During trials, numerous intercurrent events—such as the need for rescue medication, the use of prohibited drugs, adverse events, or patient noncompliance—can confound the treatment effect interpretation. When long-term efficacy is the key, it may be necessary to simulate scenarios involving intercurrent events before unblinding to understand their impact and plan additional trial design features or statistical analyses, such as incorporating external controls.

Given the myriad potential sources of complications in immunology trials, a collaborative approach is crucial. Teams must work together to define estimands that best address the scientific questions and trial objectives.

References

Aletaha, D. (2018). Diagnosis and management of rheumatoid arthritis: A review. *Journal of the American Medical Association, 320*(13), 1360–1372.

Casey, M., Degtyarev, E., Lechuga, M. J., et al. (2021). Estimand framework: Are we asking the right questions? A case study in the solid tumor setting. *Pharmaceutical Statistics, 20*(2), 324–334.

Choon, S. E., Lebwohl, M. G., Marrakchi, S., et al. (2021). Study protocol of the global Effisayil 1 Phase II, multicentre, randomised, double-blind, placebo-controlled trial of spesolimab in ss with generalized pustular psoriasis presenting with an acute flare. *BMJ*.

Deodhar, A., Blanco, R., Dokoupilová, E., Hall, S., Kameda, H., Kivitz, A. J., Poddubnyy, D., van de Sande, M., Wiksten, A. S., Porter, B. O., Richards, H. B., Haemmerle, S., & Braun, J. (2021). Improvement of signs and symptoms of nonradiographic axial Spondyloarthritis in patients treated with secukinumab: Primary results of a randomized, placebo-controlled phase III study. *Arthritis Rheumatology, 73*(1), 110–120.

Donahue, K. E., Schulman, E. R., Gartlehner, G., et al. (2019). Comparative effectiveness of combining MTX with biologic drug therapy versus either MTX or biologics alone for early rheumatoid arthritis in adults: A systematic review and network meta-analysis. *Journal of General Internal Medicine, 34*(10), 2232–2245.

GADA. (2022). *Global report on atopic dermatitis 2022*. global-report-on-atopic-dermatitis-2022.pdf (eczemacouncil.org).

Lipkovich, I., Ratitch, B., & Mallinckrodt, C. H. (2020). Causal inference and estimands in clinical trials. *Statistics in Biopharmaceutical Research, 12*(1), 54–67.

Pincus, T., Sokka, T., & Kavanaugh, A. (2004). Relative versus absolute goals of therapies for RA: ACR 20 or ACR 50 responses versus target values for "near remission" of DAS or single measures. *Clinical and Experimental Rheumatology, 22*(5 Suppl 35), S50–S56.

Ratitch, B., Goel, N., Mallinckrodt, C., et al. (2020). Defining efficacy estimands in clinical trials: Examples illustrating ICH E9(R1) guidelines. *Therapeutic Innovation & Regulatory Science, 54*(2), 370–384.

Reich, K., Thyssen, J. P., Blauvelt, A., Eyerich, K., Soong, W., Rice, Z. P., et al. (2022). Efficacy and safety of abrocitinib versus dupilumab in adults with moderate-to-severe atopic dermatitis: A randomised, double-blind, multicentre phase 3 trial. *The Lancet, 400*(10348), 273–282.

Saag, G., Teng, G., Patkar, M., et al. (2008). American College of Rheumatology 2008 recommendations for the use of nonbiologic and biologic disease-modifying antirheumatic drugs in rheumatoid arthritis. *Arthritis and Rheumatism, 59*(6), 762–784.

Sieper, J., Rudwaleit, M., & Baraliakos, X. (2009). The Assessment of Spondylarthritis International Society (ASAS) handbook: A guide to assess spondylarthritis. *Annals of the Rheumatic Diseases, 68 Suppl 2*, ii1–i44.

Sideris, N., Paschou, E., Bakirtzi, K., Kiritsi, D., Papadimitriou, I., Tsentemeidou, A., et al. (2022). New and upcoming topical treatments for atopic dermatitis: A review of the literature. *Journal of Clinical Medicine, 11*(17), 4974.

Smolen, J. S. (2016). Rheumatoid. *Lancet, 388*(10055), 2023–2038.

Suissa, S., & Shuster, J. J. (1985). Exact unconditional sample size for the 2 X 2 binomial trial. *Journal of the Royal Statistical Society Series A (General), 148*(4), 317–327.

Thyssen, J. P., Yosipovitch, G., Paul, C., Kwatra, S. G., Chu, C. Y., DiBonaventura, M., et al. (2022). Patient-reported outcomes from the JADE COMPARE randomized phase 3 study of abrocitinib in adults with moderate-to-severe atopic dermatitis. *Journal of the European Academy of Dermatology and Venereology, 36*(3), 434–443.

Vakharia, P. P., Cella, D., & Silverberg, J. I. (2018). Patient-reported outcomes and quality of life measures in atopic dermatitis. *Clinics in Dermatology, 36*(5), 616–630.

Wang, S., & Hu, H. (2022). Impute the missing data using retrieved dropouts. *BMC Medical Research Methodology, 22*(1), 82.

Ward, M. M., Deodhar, A., Gensler, L. S., Dubreuil, M., Yu, D., Khan, M. A., Haroon, N., Borenstein, D., Wang, R., Biehl, A., Fang, M. A., Louie, G., Majithia, V., Ng, B., Bigham, R., Pianin, M., Shah, A. A., Sullivan, N., Turgunbaev, M., & Oristaglio, J. (2019). 2019 update of the American College of Rheumatology/Spondylitis Association of America/Spondyloarthritis Research and Treatment Network Recommendations for the Treatment of Ankylosing Spondylitis and Nonradiographic Axial Spondyloarthritis. *Arthritis Care & Research, 71*(10), 1285–1299. https://doi.org/10.1002/acr.24025

Weidinger, S., Beck, L. A., Bieber, T., Kabashima, K., & Irvine, A. D. (2018). Atopic dermatitis. *Nature Reviews Disease Primers, 4*(1), 1. https://doi.org/10.1038/s41572-018-0001-z. PMID: 29930242.

Yosipovitch, G., Reaney, M., Mastey, V., et al. (2017). Validation of the peak pruritus numerical rating scale: Results from clinical studies of dupilumab in adult patients with moderate to severe atopic dermatitis: 5063. *Journal of the American Academy of Dermatology, 76*, AB278.

Zuberbier, T., Orlow, S. J., Paller, A. S., Taïeb, A., Allen, R., Hernanz-Hermosa, J. M., et al. (2006). Patient perspectives on the management of atopic dermatitis. *Journal of Allergy and Clinical Immunology, 118*(1), 226–232.

Chapter 9
Applying the Estimand Framework: Case Studies in Neuroscience

Hans Ulrich Burger, Nikolaos Sfikas, Baldur Magnusson, Mette Krog Josiassen, Peter Quarg, Annabelle Monnet, Judith Anzures-Cabrera, Nima Shariati, and Paul Delmar

Abstract Neuroscience is a heterogeneous therapeutic area with many different facets and challenges. Different types of endpoints are utilized in neuroscience, and many different problems arise, especially with intercurrent events and missing data. The estimand framework is, therefore, helpful in many neuroscience indications, as it allows a structured approach to address such challenges. This chapter focuses on several typical neuroscience indications, including multiple sclerosis (MS), pain and migraine, Parkinson's disease (PD), and Alzheimer's disease (AD). It discusses and explains typical challenges arising in these heterogeneous diseases and, for each one, lays out a path forward based on the estimand framework. As expected, the strategies for addressing intercurrent events are the central focus and will be specifically discussed. A treatment policy strategy is frequently proposed and justifiable but not always. There are also examples where a composite variable strategy, a hypothetical strategy, or even a principal stratum strategy seems reasonable.

H. U. Burger (✉)
Medical University Graz, Basel, Switzerland
e-mail: hans_ulrich.burger@roche.com

N. Sfikas · P. Quarg
Advanced Quantitative Sciences, Novartis Pharma AG, Basel, Switzerland
e-mail: nikolaos.sfikas@novartis.com; peter.quarg@novartis.com

B. Magnusson
Biometrics & Quantitative Sciences, UCB, Basel, Switzerland
e-mail: baldur.magnusson@ucb.com

M. K. Josiassen
Biostatistics & Data Science, Lundbeck, Copenhagen, Denmark
e-mail: MKJO@lundbeck.com

A. Monnet · N. Shariati · P. Delmar
Data & Statistical Sciences, F. Hoffmann-La Roche AG, Basel, Switzerland
e-mail: annabelle.monnet@roche.com; nima.shariati@roche.com; paul.delmar@roche.com

J. Anzures-Cabrera
Data & Statistical Sciences, Roche Products, Welwyn, UK
e-mail: judith.anzures-cabrera@roche.com

J. Wei et al. (eds.), *Estimands in Clinical Trials*, Springer Series in Pharmaceutical Statistics, https://doi.org/10.1007/978-3-032-02192-2_9

9.1 Introduction

Neuroscience is one of the major therapeutic areas with a high unmet medical need. For many of its indications, it is characterized by two major challenges: a limited biological understanding of the underlying root causes of a disease and a lack of robust, objective endpoints. The biological level of understanding varies by disease. Some indications are well-understood, while others lack insights into the pathophysiology of the disease. Sometimes, the diagnosis of a disease is only possible based on an assessment of symptoms. Many endpoints in neuroscience are based on clinician- or patient-rated questionnaires with a high subjective component and a substantial lack of sensitivity to measure relevant treatment effects. In addition, clinical outcome data collection is often challenging in neuroscience clinical trials, especially after study treatment discontinuation. This can lead to a substantial amount of missing data in many studies. All this makes the development of new therapies challenging in neuroscience. At the same time, there remains a high unmet medical need in many neuroscience diseases, such as in neurodevelopmental and psychiatric disorders (e.g., depression or schizophrenia), neurodegenerative disorders (e.g., Parkinson's disease (PD) or Alzheimer's disease (AD)), pain and migraine, and neuroimmunological disorders (e.g., multiple sclerosis (MS)). In addition, many rare diseases are of neurological origin and are increasingly becoming a research focus.

All these challenges in the development of new therapies in neurological disorders make the use of the estimand framework particularly fruitful, although its implementation still poses some challenges and requires careful consideration. In addition, trials require long follow-up, which increases the risk of observing intercurrent events, study withdrawal, and subsequent missing data problems. The estimand framework facilitates the discussion around endpoints, which, as noted, tend to be subjective with high variability between patients. The estimand framework also provides guidance on how to handle uncertainty in the characterization of the underlying trial population and how to address intercurrent events and missing data. An introduction to the estimand framework is given in Part 1 of this book, see also Mészáros et al. (2023) and Polverejan et al. (2023).

In many neurological diseases, the main analyses are based on longitudinal continuous outcomes. For more than a decade, a mixed model for repeated measures (MMRM) approach was the de facto standard for the primary efficacy analysis for such outcomes (Mallinckrodt et al., 2008). The MMRM approach implicitly handles missing data under a missing-at-random (MAR) assumption. However, MAR assumptions do not distinguish whether (missing) data is collected before or after study withdrawal. Also, no distinction is made between intermittent or monotone missing data. To ensure better alignment between the targeted estimand and the missing data assumptions, statistical approaches such as multiple imputation are increasingly used. These approaches can accommodate more flexible missing data assumptions, including retrieved dropout models and other models based not only on the MAR assumption but also on reference-based missing data assumptions. We refer to Chap. 15 on continuous endpoints for a more in-depth discussion of these methods.

This chapter illustrates the application of the estimand framework in various typical neuroscience indications. There are different considerations for each of the four examples presented, such as the types of endpoints, longitudinal data with short-term follow-up, longitudinal endpoints with long-term follow-up, or time-to-event endpoints. Taken together, all four examples should provide an overview of the implementation of the estimand framework in many indications of neuroscience.

We start with a discussion of multiple sclerosis in Sect. 9.2, where a time-to-event endpoint is used to measure disease progression. This section also includes an in-depth example in secondary progressive multiple sclerosis (SPMS). In Sect. 9.3, we continue with migraine as another set of neurological disorders, which has a longitudinal endpoint of rather short-term duration. The discussion on estimands in indications with longitudinal endpoints requiring long-term follow-up focuses on Parkinson's disease in Sect. 9.4 and Alzheimer's disease in Sect. 9.5.

9.2 Multiple Sclerosis

9.2.1 Background

Multiple sclerosis (MS) is a chronic, immune-mediated, demyelinating, and degenerative disease of the central nervous system, ultimately leading to severe disability. It affects nearly one million people in the United States and more than 2.8 million people worldwide (Walton et al., 2020).

At the time of diagnosis, approximately 85% of adult MS patients present with relapsing-remitting MS (RRMS). RRMS is characterized by MS relapses, such as by recurrent episodes of acute neurological dysfunction, severely affecting the quality of life of patients. Relapses are caused by acute inflammation of the central nervous system, with resulting edema, conduction blocks, and demyelination. Each relapse is followed by a period of complete or partial clinical recovery from symptoms and is associated with the risk of accumulation of residual deficits and permanent worsening of disability (Lublin et al., 2022; Chitnis et al., 2020). Historically, the primary treatment goal in RRMS patients was the prevention of relapses. Additional treatment goals are the suppression of subclinical disease activity (e.g., MS white matter lesion formation as visible on magnetic resonance imaging) and the slowing of the accumulation of disability, called confirmed disability progression (CDP).

Most RRMS patients eventually transition to secondary progressive MS (SPMS), which is characterized by the gradual worsening between or in the absence of clinical relapses. Primary progressive MS (PPMS) is characterized by disability progression with a low rate of relapses. Today, the primary treatment goal in patients with progressing MS (PPMS or SPMS) is the slowing of confirmed disability progression.

The definition of confirmed disability progression is based on the Expanded Disability Status Scale (EDSS). EDSS is an ordinal scale used for assessing neurological impairment in MS based on a standardized clinician-administered neurological examination (Kurtzke, 1983). The EDSS assessment is rather complex and can be time-consuming and is, therefore, more commonly used in clinical trials than in clinical practice. It consists of examination scores in each of the seven functional scores and one ambulation score that are then combined to determine the EDSS total score, ranging from 0 (neurologically normal) to 10 (death due to MS) in 0.5-step increments between 1 and 10 (a score of 0.5 does not exist). Disability progression is defined by a clinically meaningful change in EDSS and needs to be confirmed by a subsequent assessment to form an event of confirmed disability progression (CDP).

9.2.2 Trial Objective and Design

The primary clinical endpoint in RRMS phase III trials is often the annualized relapse rate (EMA, 2011), such as the mean number of relapses experienced by a cohort of patients, standardized to one year. In clinical trials, relapses typically require confirmation, where, for example, the patients' reported symptoms are objectified based on neurological examination using EDSS.

The key objective in MS is, however, to slow down or halt the disease progression and preserve function. Therefore, as noted across the spectrum of MS, the key clinical endpoint is the accumulation of disability. In RRMS trials, disability is typically a secondary endpoint (with relapse prevention being the primary), while in trials in progressive MS, disability progression is the primary endpoint. Two mechanisms of disability have been described in literature: a stepwise accrual of disability either through incomplete recovery from relapse and the accumulation of residual neurological deficits (i.e., relapse-associated worsening) or through gradual disability progression independent of relapse activity. For this overview, we will not go into further details here but concentrate on the objective of a trial to slow down or halt all-cause CDP.

Trials in progressive MS are generally randomized and double-blind, comparing a new therapy to a standard therapy or placebo, with the time to CDP as the primary endpoint. Since MS is a chronic disease, patients typically have to be followed up for a minimum of 2 years due to slow changes in the disease over time. Specific for MS is the confirmation assessment in order to document a progression event, usually done either 3 or 6 months after the initial observation of an event. This confirmation assessment is needed to exclude variability in the underlying EDSS assessment and exclude the possibility of transient worsening from the definition of progression.

In the following sections, we will focus on trials in patients with progressive MS and CDP as the primary endpoint. We first provide recommendations for estimands in PPMS trials and present a case study in the last section that focuses on SPMS.

9.2.3 Estimand Considerations

In a trial, it is important first to describe the estimand, or the target of estimation. This includes the population included in the trial, the variable used to capture the treatment effect, the treatment conditions of interest, any intercurrent events not captured by these three attributes, and a population summary, see Chap. 2 in this book. In the following, we propose an estimand for confirmed disability progression for a typical phase III trial in patients with progressive MS and provide a detailed description of the five attributes.

(a) Population
In general, the target population in a clinical trial comprises patients who satisfy the inclusion and exclusion criteria in the clinical trial protocol. The eligibility criteria for a confirmatory trial should mirror the targeted population in clinical practice and be broad enough to assess the impact of potentially influential factors on the effect of treatment (e.g., the treatment effect in progressive MS patients with or without prior relapses).

(b) Variable
The variable or endpoint measures aspects of an individual patient's outcome with the aim of addressing the primary research question. The time to the first CDP endpoint is intended to address the scientific question of interest, such as whether a new therapy delays the time to the first disability progression after randomization, as compared to the control treatment. For the time-to-CDP endpoint, the date of randomization should be identified as the reference point, and the event date should be defined as the date of the initial disability progression (i.e., the first time the disability progression was observed and not the time of the confirmation assessment). For patients without a CDP, the censoring time is defined as the date of the latest follow-up, depending on the chosen estimand strategy for intercurrent events. If a composite variable strategy is used to accommodate study treatment withdrawal due to a lack of efficacy or death, then the variable attribute should reflect this.

(c) Treatment
The treatment is the investigational drug or the control treatment. The investigational drug may be given as monotherapy or as a combination therapy. If given as a combination therapy, this would need to be defined as part of the treatment attribute of the estimand. Importantly, predefined dose modifications or rescue therapy schemes could be part of the treatment attribute. This also includes the possibility of study treatment withdrawal and the start of another therapy if a treatment policy strategy is used.

(d) Intercurrent Events
Table 9.1 summarizes the intercurrent events that may occur in MS clinical studies with all-cause CDP as the primary variable, including the proposed estimand strategies. Generally, these proposed estimand strategies should be

Table 9.1 Proposed estimand strategies

Intercurrent events	Strategies	Comments
Study treatment withdrawal due to a lack of efficacy	Composite variable strategy (recommended) or treatment policy strategy (alternative)	The composite endpoint may accurately reflect clinical practice when patients have alternative treatment options
Study treatment withdrawal for reasons other than a lack of efficacy	Treatment policy strategy	The probability of CDP is considered unrelated to the intercurrent event
Start of other therapy due to a lack of efficacy	Treatment policy strategy (recommended) or Composite variable strategy (alternative)	The treatment policy approach would be appropriate if no therapy with proven efficacy exists in the target population. The intercurrent event of study treatment withdrawal due to a lack of efficacy would precede this intercurrent event and could be regarded as the lead intercurrent event, such that the strategy there should be followed
Start of other therapy due to reasons other than a lack of efficacy	Treatment policy strategy (recommended) or Hypothetical strategy (alternative)	The intercurrent event of study treatment withdrawal due to other reasons than a lack of efficacy would likely precede this intercurrent event, and the corresponding strategy could be followed. The assumption for using the treatment policy strategy is that the other therapy would not have a strong impact on the endpoint of interest. Alternatively, the hypothetical estimand would aim to exclude the influence of the newly started treatment in case the other therapy may have a strong impact on the variable of interest
Death	Composite variable strategy	Death can be expected to be rare in MS clinical trials. As a rare intercurrent event, it could also be ignored, as it would anyhow have only a minimal impact on the interpretation of the trial results

discussed at the trial planning stage with health agencies to confirm their regulatory acceptance.

Study treatment withdrawal and the start of another therapy are common intercurrent events not specific to MS. For both types of intercurrent events, differentiation by the reason of the event (due to a lack of efficacy or for reasons other than a lack of efficacy) is justified, as the implications of the intercurrent event for the disability outcome of interest (time to first CDP) are likely to differ. Patients who discontinue from the study treatment based on a perceived lack of efficacy might be at a higher risk of progression than either patients who do not discontinue from treatment or patients who discontinue for other reasons (e.g., liver enzyme elevations).

For each type of intercurrent event, an appropriate intercurrent event strategy needs to be defined such that the statistical population summary measure allows a meaningful interpretation and addresses the clinical research question. Sometimes, there is more than one possible strategy for a particular intercurrent event, and this needs to be discussed. Importantly, different strategies change the clinical interpretation of the treatment effect. The choice of strategy may also depend on the frequency of the occurrence of the different intercurrent events. In some cases, it is useful to apply one intercurrent event strategy in the primary analysis but another one in supplementary analyses to provide additional insights into the treatment effect.

(e) Population-Level Summary

A population-level summary of the variable should be used to quantify the effect of the experimental versus the control treatment in the recruited population. The overall treatment effect of a time-to-event analysis is usually captured by the hazard ratio between the new therapy and the control treatment. The hazard ratio quantifies the treatment effect of the test treatment relative to the control as a single number under the proportional hazard assumption. Proportional hazard means that the test treatment reduces the risk of a disability progression by a constant factor (or percentage) relative to the control treatment at all time points.

9.2.4 Statistical Analysis

The statistical analysis is usually based on Kaplan–Meier estimates and Cox regression for estimation and log-rank test and Cox regression for testing. As long as patients stay in the trial, even after study treatment withdrawal or the start of rescue therapy, thereby providing full data, these standard analyses are sufficient for estimating a treatment policy estimand. However, patients may also decide to leave the trial, in which case further follow-up information is not available. Often, such missing data is preceded by intercurrent events like study treatment withdrawal or start of rescue therapy. Handling such missing data should, therefore, follow the intercurrent event strategies laid out in the estimand definition. Ultimately, the estimation of different estimands has to take the missing data into account, and the specific strategy will drive the implementation of the analysis, including the handling of missing data.

For different intercurrent event strategies, different statistical methods should be used. Importantly, for a time-to-event endpoint, censoring missing information is only appropriate if censoring is independent of the outcome, i.e., if loss to follow-up is independent of the patient's disease status, which is often not the case. When deciding on a composite variable strategy to address the intercurrent event, we basically take the time of the intercurrent event as an event time. When deciding on a hypothetical strategy, we would need to estimate future EDSS assessments, although this is rarely done in practice. Multiple imputation methods of events as an alternative to censoring and event imputation could serve as meaningful sensitivity analyses.

On occasion, different types of intercurrent events may occur in the same patient. Depending on how this is addressed, the analysis may become quite complex. One simplifying option is to specify a leading intercurrent event (e.g., typically, the one that occurs first within a patient), which would then define the handling of all subsequent data.

There is one more aspect when estimating the estimand in an MS trial, which is important to discuss. As already mentioned, an initial disability progression event needs to be confirmed either 12 or 24 weeks later by a second assessment indicating progression in order to constitute a CDP. Sometimes, patients drop out of the trial after an initial event, and the status of the CDP remains unknown. This is a special case of treatment withdrawal due to a lack of efficacy, as the lack of efficacy is very much documented by the initial progression event, and a missing confirmation event is usually driven by previous treatment and trial withdrawal. In this case, censoring may be an inappropriate strategy, as it essentially replaces the missing information with the totality of patients who have not yet progressed or experienced an initial disability progression. However, the presence of an initial disability progression itself clearly indicates an increased likelihood that the event would have been subsequently confirmed had the patient remained in the trial. Imputing an event may also not be straightforward, as there is a risk of imputing a CDP as confirmed, which would not have been confirmed had the data been available. The appropriate strategy should be carefully discussed, weighing the likelihood of a confirmation on the basis of patients who stayed in the trial after the initial assessment. One can anticipate that the likelihood of a confirmation of the event is higher in patients who withdraw than in patients who remain in the trial, but such evaluations should always be addressed with caution. Generally, in PPMS or SPMS, there is an agreement that the imputation of an event makes sense, whereas in RRMS populations, the confirmation rate is much lower, and censoring is preferred. In any case, both analyses should be presented, accompanied by supplementary multiple imputation analyses or a tipping point analysis.

9.2.5 Case Study: A Principal Stratum Estimand in Secondary Progressive Multiple Sclerosis

The following is an example of a trial in SPMS and is different from what we have discussed so far, as it is an application of a principal stratum estimand.

9.2.5.1 Trial Objective and Design

The EXPAND trial (Kappos et al., 2018) was a multicenter, randomized, double-blind, parallel-group, placebo-controlled trial with variable treatment duration (expected range of 23–42 months). The main purpose of the trial was to confirm the efficacy of siponimod relative to placebo in delaying the time to three-month confirmed disability progression as measured by the EDSS. A total of 1651 SPMS patients aged 18–60 years (EDSS score of 3–6.5) were randomized to siponimod or placebo in a 2:1 ratio. The trial achieved its goal, with an estimated hazard ratio of the main estimand of 0.79 (95% confidence interval: 0.65–0.95).

The primary endpoint in the trial was all-cause disability progression of SPMS, which is a combination of progressive disability independent of relapses and accumulated disability due to incomplete recovery after relapses. Although relapses are relatively rare in SPMS, approximately 13% of patients did experience relapses during the trial, and the EDSS score would increase during relapses without confirmation of CDP. Therefore, from a scientific perspective (understanding the overall treatment effect) and a regulatory perspective (supporting label discussions), the question of whether the occurrence of relapses (intercurrent events) affects the treatment effect of the study drug is of interest. To answer this scientific question, a supplementary estimand was defined.

9.2.5.2 Estimand Considerations

A supplementary estimand was defined in the trial with the attempt to quantify the effect of siponimod on disability progression, independent of its effect on relapses. The preferred approach was to focus on patients who would be considered highly unlikely to experience a relapse in a given time frame. More precisely, this estimand would quantify the treatment effect in patients who would not relapse in a given period of time, regardless of their treatment assignment. This corresponds to the principal stratum estimand in ICH (2019). The application of other estimands is discussed by Magnusson et al. (2019).

The following is a definition of the principal stratum estimand, with a detailed description of the five attributes.

(a) Population: Patients with SPMS who did not experience relapses during a specific time period in treatment (e.g., up to 12, 18, or 24 months post-randomization), regardless of which treatment arm they were assigned to (non-relapse principal stratum).
(b) Treatment: Once-daily oral siponimod or placebo.
(c) Variable: Occurrence of three-month confirmed disability progression within the specific time period.
(d) Intercurrent events and strategies: Relapses during a specific time period addressed by the principal stratum strategy, reflected in the population definition. Although there may be other intercurrent events in this trial, they are not discussed in this case.
(e) Population-level summary: Risk ratio of siponimod compared to the placebo arm.

This estimand is justified through the characteristics of the employed principal stratum strategy:

1. Patients in each stratum defined by the principal stratum strategy are not subject to treatment allocation confounding, so causal inference of drug efficacy can be made in the non-relapse stratum.
2. Since each patient can only observe their relapse status under one treatment assignment, patients in each stratum cannot be directly identified and require inference.

Note that the principal stratum strategy is fundamentally different from subgroup analyses, where subgroups are defined based on the occurrence of relapses after randomization, with patients divided into two groups: those who experienced relapses and those who did not. Subgroup analysis is often influenced by confounding factors, especially in this case, where intercurrent events (relapses) may be affected by the drug. Therefore, causal conclusions cannot be drawn in such subgroup analyses. Patients in each stratum defined by the principal stratum strategy cannot be directly identified and require inference.

9.2.5.3 Statistical Analysis

Given the complexity of statistical methods, only the main characteristics of the statistical analysis for the principal stratum estimand are listed here.

After applying the principal stratum strategy, patients are divided into four mutually exclusive strata:

1. Non-relapsing stratum: patients who would not experience relapses regardless of their treatment allocation.
2. Definite-relapsing stratum: patients who would experience relapses regardless of their treatment allocation.
3. Benefiting stratum: patients who would experience relapses if allocated to the placebo arm but not if allocated to the siponimod arm.
4. Harmed stratum: Patients who would not experience relapses if allocated to the placebo arm, but would if allocated to the siponimod arm.

Each patient has a pair of potential outcomes, but only one can be observed, i.e., the outcome corresponding to the actual treatment arm assignment; therefore, patients in each stratum cannot be directly identified and require inference. In a randomized trial, potential outcomes are independent of treatment arm assignment, so causal inference of drug efficacy can be made in the non-relapse stratum.

In order to obtain estimates of treatment effects in each principal stratum, some assumptions are needed, and different statistical methods may have different assumptions, which are often unverifiable. For example, a common assumption of the principal stratum analysis is the monotonicity assumption, which states that if a patient assigned to the placebo does not relapse, then that patient would also not relapse had they been assigned to the active treatment arm. Assuming monotonicity allows us to classify some patients to exactly one principal stratum (e.g., a patient assigned to placebo who does not experience a relapse must belong to the non-relapsing stratum).

Relying only on randomization and the monotonicity assumption, we are able to fully identify the denominator of our estimand (the placebo probability of CDP in the non-relapsing stratum). For patients assigned to the placebo arm, the probability of confirmed disability progression is estimated using data from patients who did not relapse but had confirmed disability progression. However, the estimand numerator (the siponimod probability of CDP in the non-relapsing stratum) is not identifiable without further assumptions. This is because patients who did not relapse may belong to either the non-relapsing principal stratum or the benefiting principal stratum, and the analysis of how to estimate the probability of confirmed disability progression is more complex.

An analysis using the Bayesian framework was, therefore, conducted to draw inference about the target estimand. The Bayesian model specified a likelihood factorized into a disability progression model, a relapse model, and a joint prior for all model parameters. The monotonicity assumption was built into the model using a strongly informative prior on the existence of the harmed principal stratum, and the sensitivity to this assumption was assessed by gradually relaxing the prior toward the common prior for all principal strata. Prior distributions for all model parameters were constructed based on clinical considerations in order to focus sampling on plausible regions of the parameter space. Key covariates were included in the context of handling missing data. Inference was drawn for time periods from randomization to 12, 18, and 24 months post-randomization. For more details on the analysis approach, we refer to Magnusson et al. (2019).

9.2.5.4 Summary and Discussion

The principal stratum strategy for addressing intercurrent events is discussed in ICH (2019) and is related to the population attribute. The experience of using the principal stratum strategy to estimate targets is limited, especially in statistical analysis methods. We refer to Chap. 19 in this book for more details.

For our case study, the principal stratum estimand approach was received positively by regulatory agencies, and comments and questions focused on medical rationale, assumptions, and modeling decisions. The work was helpful both to better understand the efficacy of siponimod in non-relapsing patients and to illustrate the potential utility of a principal stratum estimand in a randomized confirmatory trial setting.

9.2.6 Summary and Discussion

This section addresses estimand considerations and statistical analysis for phase III trials in progressive multiple sclerosis, focusing on CDP as the primary endpoint. It highlights the importance of defining clear estimands. Key intercurrent events, such as the start of other therapy due to a lack of efficacy, may be addressed by the treatment policy strategy if a therapy with proven efficacy exists in the target population; otherwise, a composite variable strategy might be considered. The SPMS example explores the application of a principal stratum strategy in the supplementary estimand to address questions regarding the origin of disability progression and the impact of relapse.

Statistical analysis methods employ Kaplan–Meier estimates and Cox regression models, with handling of missing data aligned to estimand strategies. Sensitivity analyses, including multiple imputation, are essential to address potential biases. The challenge of confirming disability progression, especially in patients withdrawing from the trial after an initial event, is underscored, requiring careful consideration to ensure valid and meaningful results.

9.3 Migraine Prevention

9.3.1 Background

Migraine is characterized by recurrent headaches lasting 4–72 h and is often accompanied by nausea, vomiting, and hypersensitivity to light (photophobia) and sound (phonophobia). Many such headaches are preceded by nonspecific prodromes, sensory warning symptoms immediately prior to the headache attack (aura), and a nonspecific postdrome phase that can last for a number of days. A headache day is classified as a migraine day if the symptoms captured with the headache fulfill a specific set of requirements according to the International Headache Society (IHS, see Tassorelli et al., 2018; Headache Classification Committee of the International Headache Society 2018 and Abu-Arafeh et al. 2019).

Migraine is typically categorized based on the frequency of migraine days per month. Episodic migraine is defined as fewer than 15 headache days per month (Katsarava et al., 2012); however, in clinical prevention trials, a threshold of at least four migraine days per month is often chosen to reflect patients in need of preventive treatment. Chronic migraine is defined as 15 or more headache days per month, at least eight of which are typical migraine days (Tassorelli et al., 2018).

In general, migraine is treated with an agent(s) for the acute headache attacks, typically with nonspecific (symptomatic) agents such as nonsteroidal anti-inflammatory drugs and/or migraine-specific abortive medications such as triptans (less frequently, ergotamine derivatives). Patients experiencing, on average, one or more migraines a week often require prevention (Silberstein et al., 2012; Evers et al., 2009) in addition to acute medications. Several therapeutic options are available for migraine prevention.

Migraine prevention is intended to reduce the frequency, suffering, and disability associated with migraine attacks.

9.3.2 Trial Objective and Design

The primary treatment goal in a migraine prevention trial is a reduction in the monthly migraine frequency over a three- or six-month period compared to baseline. A typical phase II or III trial in migraine prevention has a double-blind, placebo-controlled, parallel-group design, and the duration of treatment is three to six months, in line with the regulatory requirement of at least a three-month duration (EMA, 2007, FDA, 2018).

Generally, patients who are admitted to such trials are diagnosed with chronic migraine, as defined by Tassorelli et al. (2018). The data on headaches and whether the headaches qualify as migraines are captured daily in an electronic diary (eDiary). Measures are taken across the prospective baseline phase (at least 4 weeks) and the treatment phase. Patients must have had a frequency of at least 15 headache days per 4 weeks, of which at least eight must be classified as migraine headaches.

With migraine, an essential part of the trial is the eDiary, where we collect data on headaches daily. Monthly migraine days (MMDs) are calculated for a four-week interval (28 days) using the data captured in the eDiaries on headaches and symptoms across the 4 weeks. The primary endpoint most often used is a change from baseline in MMDs, comparing the MMDs from the 4 weeks prior to baseline with the MMDs from either weeks 1–12 or weeks 9–12 after baseline.

9.3.3 Estimand Considerations

In this section, we present a proposal for estimands in a phase III migraine prevention trial. The primary objective of such trials is to demonstrate the superiority of an investigational drug over placebo in patients with chronic migraine, with or without the use of other preventive medications. The treatment effect of primary interest is assessed in terms of the change from baseline in MMDs (weeks 1–12), regardless of study treatment discontinuation due to adverse events, a lack of efficacy, or other reasons. In the following, we define the estimand, with a detailed description of its five attributes.

(a) Population
    The population attribute comprises adult patients diagnosed with chronic migraine.

(b) Variable
The primary variable used to assess the clinical benefit is the change from baseline in MMDs (weeks 1–12 or the change from baseline in MMDs (weeks 9–12), where MMD is defined as the number of days during a 28-day interval where the participant records a migraine according to the IHS criteria, including days where acute migraine medication is used to treat a headache. The characteristics of a headache day should meet the definition from the IHS (Tassorelli et al., 2018; Diener et al., 2020) to be classified as a migraine. This guideline defines several combinations of symptoms that classify a headache as a migraine. Its definition of a migraine day also includes the use of acute migraine medication, specifying that a day with a headache that is successfully treated with a triptan, ergotamine, or other migraine-specific acute medication should be considered a migraine day (Tassorelli et al., 2018). Thus, the guideline's endpoint definition addresses the potential intercurrent event of acute migraine medication intake by including it in the definition of a migraine on the individual-day level.

(c) Treatment
Treatment includes the investigational drug or placebo, with or without the use of other preventive migraine medications and regardless of study treatment discontinuation due to adverse events, a lack of efficacy, or other reasons.

(d) Intercurrent Events
Table 9.2 summarizes intercurrent events that may occur in migraine prevention trials, including proposals of strategies to address these intercurrent events.

The event of using acute medication has already been addressed implicitly via the definition of a migraine day and is thus covered by the definition of the endpoint of interest, see the variable attribute above. The use of other preventive migraine medications is addressed using a treatment policy strategy, assessing the treatment effect with or without the use of other preventive migraine medications. Likewise, study treatment discontinuations addressed with the treatment policy strategy are captured by the treatment attribute, see the treatment attribute above.

Table 9.2 Proposed estimand strategies

Intercurrent events	Strategies	Comments
Use of acute medication	(implicit) hypothetical strategy	Definition of a migraine day by Tassorelli et al. (2018) includes how to interpret the use of acute medication for migraine and, thus, is built into the definition of MMDs (see variable attribute)
Use of other preventive migraine medications	Treatment policy strategy	Treatment effect is of interest with and without the use of other preventive migraine medication (see treatment attribute)
Study treatment discontinuation due to adverse events, a lack of efficacy, or other reasons	Treatment policy strategy	It is relevant to assess the effect on a population level, supporting the use of a treatment policy strategy (see treatment attribute)

Protocols of migraine prevention trials should encourage the continued collection of data into the eDiary, even after a patient discontinues the study treatment (unless a patient decides to withdraw consent). Data collected after study treatment discontinuation will support the estimation based on the treatment policy strategy.

(e) Population-Level Summary
The population-level summary is the difference between the treatment means in change from baseline in MMDs for weeks 1–12 or weeks 9–12.

9.3.4 *Statistical Analysis*

Driven by the use of a treatment policy strategy, the sponsors would need to commit to reducing the occurrence of missing data and to make the best efforts to collect all clinical outcome data despite any intercurrent event occurrence. Ideally, trial clinical outcome data would also have been collected after the withdrawal of treatment, and the data could then be used to estimate the treatment effect. For example, an MMRM approach is often used that includes baseline MMDs, month, treatment arm, and country as fixed effects, along with the month by baseline MMDs and month by treatment interactions. With no or very limited missing data, the MMRM approach should result in an unbiased estimate since the underlying assumption requiring the missing data to be MAR would be reasonable in this case.

In most trials, data will not have been collected for some patients after study treatment discontinuation. If data were collected for a large proportion of the patients, options could exist for using the non-missing data to impute the missing data across similar patients (Wang et al., 2023). Based on our experience, there may only be a small proportion of patients with data collected after their study treatment discontinuation; however, in combination with the fact that the proportion of patients that discontinue treatment may be limited in migraine prevention trials, it may not be possible to base imputations on the data observed after discontinuation. Thus, a method that does not rely on observing data from all patients may be the most realistic option for an estimator, but then, it will require more assumptions and should be accompanied by suitable sensitivity analyses.

One option for an estimator is to use reference-based multiple imputation. To be conservative, for instance, the assumption can be that patients who discontinue from the active treatment arm would follow a trajectory similar to patients who are on placebo (jump-to-reference assumption), while patients who discontinue from the placebo arm would continue with a trajectory similar to those who are still on placebo (MAR assumption). Any patients with missing data after treatment discontinuation would then be imputed using multiple imputation under these assumptions.

9.3.5 Summary and Discussion

This section discusses estimand considerations and statistical analysis in migraine prevention trials. The proposed estimands focus on assessing the change from baseline in MMDs over 12 weeks, considering the population of adults with chronic migraine. Intercurrent events, such as the use of acute and preventive medications and study treatment discontinuation, are managed using strategies like the treatment policy approach, which evaluates the treatment effect on a population level.

To handle missing data, we emphasize reducing its occurrence and propose using an MMRM approach, assuming the missing data are missing at random. However, since data collection may be incomplete post-treatment discontinuation, reference-based multiple imputation is suggested, assuming different trajectories for placebo and active treatment discontinuations. Sensitivity analyses should be considered to evaluate the robustness of statistical inference.

9.4 Early Parkinson's Disease

In this section, we propose two estimands for trials in early Parkinson's disease using two different types of endpoints. The first example is for an estimand based on a continuous endpoint, which is recommended for phase II trials only. The second example is for an estimand based on a time-to-event endpoint, which can be used in either phase II or III trials. The use of symptomatic treatment is an important difference between both estimands.

9.4.1 Background

Parkinson's disease (PD) is a chronic, slowly progressive, and currently incurable neurodegenerative disorder affecting more than ten million patients worldwide (Parkinson's Disease Foundation, 2019). Prevalence data compiled in 2016 estimates that, overall, 1.43 million individuals were living with the disease across Europe (GBD, 2016, Parkinson's Disease Collaborators, 2018). In the United States, nearly 90,000 new cases are reported every year (Parkinson's Disease Foundation, 2023). Worldwide, 4% of patients are diagnosed with PD before 50 years of age, and it is estimated that 1% and 4% of individuals aged at least 60 and 80, respectively, are affected (He et al., 2018; Parkinson's Disease Foundation, 2019). Mortality does not increase in the first decade after disease onset but increases thereafter, eventually doubling compared to the general population (Pinter et al., 2015). The cause of PD is unknown, and the incidence seems to vary within subgroups defined by race, ethnicity, genotype, or environment (Poewe et al., 2017).

PD is a disorder of the central and peripheral nervous systems with typical neuropathological features and clinically presenting with characteristic motor signs, such as bradykinesia, rigidity, resting tremors, postural instability, and a plethora of debilitating non-motor symptoms. Typically, the cardinal symptoms begin on one side of the body and affect the other side over time (Fahn 2008). Disease progression from early to advanced stage is marked by the appearance of motor complications and fluctuations (Luquin et al. 2017).

Clinical examination, along with rating scales administration by a neurologist, is the convention for the diagnosis of a patient and is based upon the identification of motor symptoms, which typically reflect the dopaminergic deficit in the area of the brain facilitating movement. Indeed, progressive loss of dopaminergic innervation of the striatum leads to reduced local dopamine release, which is associated with the onset and progression of motor signs.

Generally speaking, for a clinical trial targeting early PD, patients should have been diagnosed with idiopathic PD less than 36 months prior to inclusion in the trial. They should present with bradykinesia and at least one other cardinal sign of PD (resting tremor or rigidity), be at Hoehn and Yahr stage I or II, and be either treatment-naïve or on symptomatic monotherapy without motor complications.

As there is currently no objective clinical test to support a definitive diagnosis (Postuma et al. 2016), misdiagnosis is common in the early stages of the disease (Poewe and Wenning 2002, Atik et al. 2016).

9.4.2 *The Movement Disorder Society (MDS)-Sponsored Unified Parkinson's Disease Rating Scale (UPDRS)*

PD rating scales assess the symptoms of the condition and the quality of life of a patient and help evaluate treatment and management strategies (EPDA, 2017). Several rating scales are used in PD to assist clinical management and research.

The revision of the Unified Parkinson's Disease Rating Scale (UPDRS) published by the Movement Disorder Society (MDS), termed MDS-UPDRS, is the most widely used clinical rating scale for PD (Goetz et al. 2008). It is a comprehensive assessment tool designed to monitor the burden and extent of PD across the longitudinal disease course and provide endpoints in interventional trials. It is composed of four parts: Part I assesses non-motor experiences of daily living, Part II assesses motor experiences of daily living completed by the patient, Part III assesses motor signs of PD administered by the rater, and Part IV assesses motor complications only if the patient is on levodopa.

The scale is composed of 65 items (questions), with responses scored from 0 to 4 for each question. Each question is assigned a numeric score between 0 and 4, where 0 represents normal, 1 slight, 2 mild, 3 moderate, and 4 severe impairments. The total score is 260 points. Each of the four subscales is determined by summing the numerical values of each question. Part I contains two components of six questions focusing on complex behaviors and another seven questions on the non-motor experiences of daily living. The Part II total score is a subscale consisting of 13 items, ranging from 0 to 52. The Part III total score contains 33 scores on 18 items, ranging from 0 to 132. The Part IV total score ranges from 0 to 24 based on 6 items. Higher scores indicate greater impairment.

The MDS-UPDRS scale is currently used as the standard endpoint in PD clinical trials. In longitudinal trials, the MDS-UPDRS is used as an indicator of disease progression, i.e., worsening of the disease as measured by the scale. This definition of progression provides the alternative of using a time-to-event endpoint in clinical trials, where interest lies in understanding the time that it takes for a patient to reach a certain worsening in the MDS-UPDRS scale.

9.4.3 Symptomatic Treatment

Current treatments for PD primarily target motor symptoms of the disease to improve the quality of life, mainly through the use of dopamine replacement therapy (i.e., levodopa), dopamine receptor agonists (both ergot and non-ergot), catechol-O-methyl transferase (COMT) inhibitors (e.g., entacapone and tolcapone), or monoamine oxidase type B inhibitors. The available symptomatic treatments can improve the score of motor-related scales (such as MDS-UPDRS Part II and Part III) commonly used in PD (Holden et al., 2018).

The usage of symptomatic treatments could be particularly problematic in clinical trials evaluating the possible treatment effect of new drugs on slowing or halting disease progression, as it adds complexity, both in terms of the ability to detect an effect and its meaningfulness. Indeed, the development of new drugs in early-stage PD has been hampered by the difficulties in conducting trials in real-life populations, for example, patients on standard of care. Most trials are undertaken in treatment-naïve patients. Even in this early population, where patients often start treatment relatively soon after the diagnosis, strategies need to be developed to keep patients from initiating symptomatic treatment as well as analytical strategies to mitigate the impact of change in therapy on motor-related endpoints. It is, therefore, necessary to identify an outcome that accounts for the intercurrent event of starting or changing a symptomatic therapy.

Here, we propose two different scenarios for using the estimand framework in PD trials. The first scenario is used in a trial using a continuous endpoint, whereas the second one uses a time-to-event endpoint. Different strategies are used for different intercurrent events. We follow the process defined by Polverejan et al. (2023) to describe the estimand, see also Chap. 3 in this book.

9.4.4 Estimand Considerations (Continuous Endpoint)

The clinical context of the estimand proposed below assumes that the experimental treatment is disease-modifying. In this example, the sponsor is interested in assessing the effect of the new treatment in a world where symptomatic treatment does not exist and the experimental treatment has a similar effect, irrespective of the duration of administration. This is a treatment effect commonly estimated in phase II proof-of-concept trials.

In the following, we consider a parallel, double-blind, placebo-controlled, randomized trial. The clinical question of interest is what the expected effect of the experimental treatment on disease progression at week 52 would be, compared to placebo, for patients with PD who are naïve to any symptomatic treatment, assuming they take the assigned treatment as indicated and do not initiate symptomatic medication. In the following, we define the estimand, with a detailed description of its five attributes.

(a) Population
The target population is early PD as measured by the Hoehn and Yahr scale (stages I and II), who are untreated with symptomatic medication.

(b) Variable
The variable of interest is the change from baseline in MDS-UPDRS score at week 52.

(c) Treatment
Treatment includes experimental treatment or placebo, assuming that patients take the assigned treatment as indicated and do not initiate symptomatic medication. Note that placebo is selected as the comparator arm, as there are no approved disease-modifying treatments available in the market.

(d) Intercurrent Events
There are two main intercurrent events of interest: the start of symptomatic treatment and study treatment discontinuation for any reason. A hypothetical strategy is used for addressing both intercurrent events as it aligns the estimand with the clinical question of interest, see the treatment attribute above. For the hypothetical strategy, all the data generated after the start of the intercurrent event is ignored, assuming a scenario in which the intercurrent event does not exist.

The hypothetical strategy is selected for this phase II trial as it estimates a treatment effect in an ideal setting where patients take the drug as indicated and do not start symptomatic treatment. Other treatment effects can be estimated with supplementary estimands that assign a treatment policy strategy to treatment discontinuation and/or the start of symptomatic treatment. These treatment effects could be estimated using dropout models and reference-based imputation methods, as discussed by Noci et al. (2022) and Wolbers et al. (2022). In theory, different estimand strategies could be proposed for different reasons of treatment discontinuation. However, addressing this intercurrent event in such a way is not of interest to the clinical question. Nevertheless, such reasons should be collected and understood for the subsequent phase III trials.

(e) Population-Level Summary
The main summary to capture the treatment effect is the difference in means between the experimental treatment and the placebo, conditional on baseline attributes.

9.4.5 Statistical Analysis (Continuous Endpoint)

The implementation of the hypothetical estimand, ignoring the data after the initiation of symptomatic treatment, is not straightforward, and various points and assumptions should be considered during the implementation and analysis phases. Implementing this strategy requires the date of occurrence of each intercurrent event to be clearly documented in the electronic case report form. In addition, the MDS-UPDRS scores should be collected from baseline to the start of symptomatic treatment or treatment discontinuation. For the analysis, we use an MMRM approach as the main estimator. The model, as described by Mallinckrodt et al. (2008), utilizes the correlation between successive observations on a patient. This allows data from patients who experienced an intercurrent event to contribute to the estimation of effects at the final time point. The MMRM approach is built upon the assumption that the missing data is MAR. In other words, given the observed values of the MDS-UPDRS score, the missing data is independent of the unobserved values. We take advantage of the MAR assumption to account for the missing data due to missed intermediate visits.

9.4.6 Estimand Considerations (Time-to-Event Endpoint)

An estimand based on a time-to-event endpoint is proposed in this section because a certain progression rate of MDS-UPDRS score may be used as a threshold to define a meaningful worsening and provide sufficient information on the patient's experience (Trundell et al. 2025; Horvath et al. 2015). The sponsor might be interested in assessing a treatment effect where, for example, patients take symptomatic treatment and the experimental treatment at the same time. This is a treatment effect that can be estimated in phase II or III trials. In the following, we consider a parallel, double-blind, placebo-controlled, randomized trial.

As indicated in Sect. 9.4.2, the MDS-UPDRS is the scale traditionally used to indicate progression. Therefore, we propose an estimand based on the time needed to observe worsening in the MDS-UPDRS score. The same approach could be considered for one of the four subscales or specific items' combination as long as the progression event milestone is clinically meaningful.

The advantage of such an endpoint is that the experimental treatment effect may be accurately measured, irrespective of the potential masking effect from intensifying symptomatic background therapy, since most of the patients experience disease progression before intensifying symptomatic background therapy (Trundell et al. 2025). The target population in such a clinical trial allows the recruitment of patients who have already started symptomatic treatment.

The clinical question of interest is what the expected effect of the experimental treatment on the chances of experiencing a progression event would be after 76 weeks of treatment, compared to placebo, for patients with PD already receiving symptomatic treatment. In the following, we define the estimand, with a detailed description of its five attributes.

(a) Population
The target population includes patients with early PD who have been on a stable regimen of symptomatic treatment.
(b) Variable
The variable of interest is the time to progression, study treatment discontinuation, or death. The time-to-progression event is defined as a certain worsening in the MDS-UPDRS score from baseline.
(c) Treatment
Treatment includes experimental treatment or placebo, with symptomatic therapy as needed. Placebo is selected as the comparator arm as there are no approved disease-modifying treatments available in the market.
(d) Intercurrent Events
The intercurrent events considered for this trial are a change in symptomatic medication, treatment discontinuation, and death. Table 9.3 summarizes the proposed strategies for addressing each of the intercurrent events.

For patients who change the symptomatic treatment, the outcome after the intercurrent event is still of interest, so the upcoming progression event will be

Table 9.3 Proposed estimand strategies

Intercurrent events	Strategies	Comments
Change in symptomatic medication	Treatment policy strategy	The upcoming disease progression event is being counted irrespective of the change in symptomatic treatment
Study treatment discontinuation	Composite variable strategy	Study treatment discontinuation due to the following reasons is counted as a progression event (at the time of discontinuation): • Lack of efficacy, safety, or tolerability reason (including discontinuation due to adverse events) • Use or initiation of protocol-prohibited medication • No informative reason given
Death	Composite variable strategy	Death is being counted as a progression event

counted, irrespective of the change in symptomatic treatment, see the treatment attribute above. We selected the treatment policy strategy because a change in symptomatic treatment is not necessarily considered a meaningful progression event in early PD.

Treatment discontinuation or death are considered unfavorable events. Therefore, the composite variable strategy is used to consider them as progression events at the moment of occurrence, see the variable attribute above.

(e) Population-Level Summary

The overall treatment effect of a time-to-event analysis is measured by the estimation of the hazard ratio between the experimental treatment and the control treatment to assess the extent to which the experimental treatment slows down the disease progression by a constant factor (or percentage) relative to the control treatment at all time points and in which proportional hazards are assumed (Cox, 1972).

9.4.7 Statistical Analysis (Time-to-Event Endpoint)

The implementation of the estimand strategy in Sect. 9.4.6 is not straightforward, and the team should consider the following points during the analysis phase for the main estimator. The hazard ratio quantifies the treatment effect of the experimental treatment relative to the control as a single number under the proportional hazard assumption and, in this case, is estimated using a stratified Cox regression under the proportional hazard assumption. In practice, this assumption is often reasonable, but sensitivity analyses (e.g., assuming piecewise proportional hazard) are necessary to understand deviations from it. An aligned analysis set for the time-to-progression events needs to collect the time from randomization until a sufficient number of events for which the analysis is powered.

Different approaches can be used to handle missing data. First, if a patient misses one or two consecutive visits and if the reasons for missing data are unrelated to the trial, then we can simply ignore the missing data generated by these visits. Instead, we can focus on the measurements from subsequent visits, which will continue until the earliest occurrence of a progression event or censoring. Second, if a patient withdraws from the trial or misses more than two consecutive visits, then the patient will be censored at the time of study withdrawal. As per ICH (2019), sponsors would need to commit to attempting to ascertain a reason for missing visits, as it could be informative, and perhaps, treating certain reasons as intercurrent events.

Other key implementation elements include the date of occurrence of each event for the primary analysis and the date of the intercurrent event that should be clearly documented for analyses.

9.4.8 Summary and Discussion

This section outlines the use of two estimand approaches in early Parkinson's disease trials. For phase II trials with a continuous endpoint, the hypothetical strategy is applied to assess the effect of an experimental treatment on disease progression without symptomatic treatments, measuring the change from baseline in MDS-UPDRS score. For phase III trials with a time-to-event endpoint, a change in symptomatic medication is addressed by the treatment policy strategy to reflect clinical practice, while study treatment discontinuation and death are addressed by a composite variable strategy, as they are considered unfavorable events. Statistical analyses employ MMRM for continuous endpoints and stratified Cox regression for time-to-event endpoints, with sensitivity analyses where necessary.

9.5 Alzheimer's Disease

9.5.1 Background

Alzheimer's disease (AD) is clinically characterized by a progressive impairment in cognitive and executive abilities, which results in decreased function and gradual loss of independence (Mesterton et al. 2010). There is great interindividual variability in AD progression, and survival is dependent on many factors, including age at onset. At the early stage of AD, a slight impairment of memory, language, and visuospatial function can be observed. As AD advances, patients become progressively impaired, and the burden on caregivers significantly increases. It is well-recognized that there is a high unmet medical need in AD (Gauthier et al., 2016). Alzheimer's disease progression is typically categorized into different stages, starting from the preclinical stage without clinical manifestations to prodromal or mild cognitive impairment due to AD, followed by mild, moderate, and severe stages.

Amyloid beta (amyloid-β)-targeting therapies are based on the hypothesis that amyloid-β accumulation is the primary factor driving pathogenesis (Selkoe, 1991; Hardy & Selkoe, 2002; Selkoe & Hardy, 2016). This amyloid-β accumulation in the brain begins well before the development of clinical dementia in AD and causes a series of downstream events, leading to synaptic dysfunction, inflammation, neurodegeneration, and clinical symptoms. For these reasons, treatments that prevent, slow down, or decrease the accumulation of brain amyloid-β have been tested as therapeutic agents for AD.

For a long time, there were only symptomatic treatment options, including acetylcholinesterase inhibitors and N-methyl-d-aspartate receptor antagonists. These approved drugs are recognized to temporarily improve some clinical symptoms of AD in some patients but do not modify disease progression (Cummings et al., 2016). Recently, two different monoclonal antibody treatments, lecanemab (Van Dyck et al., 2023) and donanemab (Sims et al., 2023), targeting specific forms of amyloid beta have demonstrated a significant clinical benefit in confirmatory phase III clinical trials. Unlike symptomatic treatments, this new generation of therapeutic molecules has the potential for a disease-modifying effect. In addition to potentially disease-modifying agents targeting amyloid and tau pathways, treatments for specific symptoms are also still being actively developed, and some have recently been approved by regulatory agencies (e.g., brexpiprazole targeting agitation).

Missing data presents a significant challenge in clinical trials in AD. These trials typically target an elderly and frail population, often necessitating considerable time commitment from a care partner. In early symptomatic stages, phase III trial durations usually span up to 2 years, with dropout rates and missing data proportions ranging from 20% to 25%. Trials in preclinical stages of the disease tend to be even longer, often lasting 4 years or more. In this challenging context, the estimand framework is particularly valuable in order to facilitate a careful thought process needed to address the trial design, analysis strategy, and reporting in an appropriate and efficient manner.

9.5.2 Estimand Considerations

Both the EMA, (2018) and the FDA, (2024) provide meaningful insights into the design and analysis of clinical trials, including important aspects of the estimand to be used, see also Sect. 12.3 in Chap. 12 of this book.

Throughout this section, we will use the example of a phase III confirmatory trial conducted during the coronavirus disease (COVID-19) pandemic and before the availability of any disease-modifying treatment for AD. The objective is to evaluate a new investigational disease-modifying treatment in an early symptomatic AD population, regardless of the use or start of symptomatic treatment (see also Donohue et al. 2020).

The clinical question of interest for this trial can be formulated as assessing the impact of the investigational treatment on disease progression up to 78 weeks, without considering any significant effects of the pandemic on clinical trial operations, regardless of the use or initiation of symptomatic treatment for AD.

(a) Population
In our example, this could be patients from an amyloid-beta-positive, confirmed, mild cognitive impairment or mild AD population. Typically, the population attributes should specify the stage of the disease and any biomarker confirmation of the underlying physiological process. Different overlapping disease staging paradigms exist in the clinical community and can be used for the definition of the population attribute. Clinical trials usually apply restrictions to the recruited population, with specific inclusion and exclusion criteria. Yet the population attributes should describe the overall target population rather than specific inclusion/exclusion criteria for one trial. The recruitment of traditionally underrepresented minorities is also a critical dimension of trial design

and conduct. A clear and intentional definition of this attribute provides a strong foundation for the discussion of the generalizability of the trial results.

(b) Variable

In our example, it is a change from baseline to week 78 in the sum of boxes of the clinical dementia rating scale (CDR-SB). Typically, the primary endpoint of AD trials is based on psychometric instruments or scales. CDR-SB has been widely used as a primary endpoint in recent trials of the early symptomatic stages of the disease. Other variables have also been employed, such as the integrated Alzheimer's disease rating scale (iADRS). It is important to specify the name of the scale and the metrics, such as the total score. If different variants of the scale exist, the variable attributes should be as specific as possible. Most scales are now administered using digital equipment (tablets). However, it could be useful to specify if the variable is performed in the home setting or at the clinical site. In case of a change from baseline variable, the time point needs to be specified (e.g., week 78).

(c) Treatment

In our example, it is the study treatment or control, irrespective of the use or initiation of symptomatic treatment for AD. Generally, the dose, duration, and frequency of administration of the experimental drug are defined. If relevant, this attribute also describes any dose interruption or discontinuation prespecified to manage safety (e.g., drug interruption due to adverse events or safety events like amyloid-related imaging abnormalities or efficacy events), including drug discontinuation once a prespecified biomarker objective is attained. This attribute also specifically describes the comparator treatment in as much detail as needed to match the experimental drug. Importantly, the use of any other treatment for AD, including symptomatic treatment or rescue treatment with another disease-modifying therapy, can be described in this attribute.

(d) Intercurrent Events

Disease-modifying treatments have a different effect than symptomatic treatments. The start of a disease-modifying treatment for AD will soon become an important intercurrent event to consider for clinical trials in AD.

We present intercurrent event strategies in the context of our example, namely a trial for a disease-modifying agent in an early symptomatic AD population, run during the COVID-19 pandemic, before the availability of any disease-modifying treatments for AD. Therefore, temporary study drug interruptions due to the COVID-19 pandemic are relevant. While this intercurrent event does not apply outside of the specific context of the pandemic, it demonstrates the value of the estimand framework in adapting to unforeseen circumstances happening during the trial conduct. More details on COVID-19-related intercurrent events are discussed in Chap. 23.

Additionally, the start or change of AD symptomatic treatment can be covered in the treatment attribute but may also be listed with other intercurrent events. In clinical practice, study drug discontinuation occurs due to reasons such as a lack of efficacy, disease progression, safety concerns, or tolerability issues. These events may be managed using a treatment policy strategy. On the other hand,

Table 9.4 Proposed estimand strategies

Intercurrent events	Strategies	Comments
Study drug discontinuation due to a lack of efficacy, disease progression, safety, or tolerability	Treatment policy strategy	These intercurrent events represent events related to patients' health status or condition or the effect of intervention. These are relevant in clinical practice
Study drug discontinuation due to administrative reasons	Hypothetical strategy	These intercurrent events represent events specific to the clinical trial setting and are not relevant in clinical practice
Start of AD symptomatic treatment	Treatment policy strategy	The trial objective is to estimate the effect of treatment irrespective of whether or not patients are using AD symptomatic treatment

study drug discontinuation due to administrative reasons is addressed with a hypothetical strategy, as these events are specific to the clinical trial setting. Estimating a treatment effect as if these events had not occurred may be appropriate since these clinical trial-related events would not happen in clinical practice. Table 9.4 summarizes the intercurrent events that may occur in AD trials, including a proposal for strategies to address these intercurrent events.

(e) Population-Level Summary
In this example, the population-level summary is the difference in variable means between the treatment arms. The difference in mean change from baseline to a defined time point is the most common approach and de facto standard in AD. It has become customary in the field to report results on the scale of percent relative reduction. This could be mentioned in the estimand attribute definition or prespecified in the statistical analysis plan, such that the effect will be expressed as a relative reduction in placebo decline, defined as the difference in mean change from baseline divided by the change from baseline in the control arm.

Other summary measures may also be considered, such as the differences in the rate of progression summaries or when using a time-to-event endpoint in certain settings. In a preclinical setting, the onset of clinical symptoms is an important event. Defining a meaningful event in the symptomatic setting can be challenging, given the continuous nature and the heterogeneity in the disease trajectory.

9.5.3 Statistical Analysis

One of the main drivers to develop the estimand framework was to facilitate aligning the estimation method (estimator) with the estimand (target of estimation). In AD clinical trials with a high study discontinuation rate, it is not uncommon for intercurrent events to be followed by missing data. The proportion of intercurrent events addressed with a hypothetical strategy, whereby any data collected after the intercurrent event is not used, may also not be negligible. Assumptions about missing data should be aligned with the strategy of each of the intercurrent events, be plausibly based on the current understanding of the mechanism of action of the drug, be reasonably conservative in order to provide the most realistic treatment effect, and be in line with usual regulatory requirements. By nature, assumptions about missing data are not verifiable, and sensitivity analyses are critical to quantify their impact on trial results. The estimand framework helps differentiate between sensitivity analyses targeting the same estimand with different estimation methods or assumptions and supplementary analyses targeting different estimands. For example, a sensitivity analysis could vary parameters in missing data imputation algorithms, whereas a supplementary analysis could change the strategy for addressing an intercurrent event.

The MMRM approach has been the standard for analyzing longitudinal continuous data in Alzheimer's disease trials. It offers an unbiased estimate of the treatment effect but only under the MAR assumption for all missing data. The MAR assumption may be unplausible for certain intercurrent events and misaligned with the estimand. This can introduce bias, so other approaches should be considered. For example, the reference-based conditional mean imputation (as implemented with the `rbmi` package in `R`) was utilized to report the results of the GRADUATE trial (Bateman et al., 2023).

9.5.4 Summary and Discussion

This section explores the estimand considerations and statistical analysis for Alzheimer's disease trials, emphasizing a phase III confirmatory trial during the COVID-19 pandemic. The estimand framework helps address challenges like high dropout rates and missing data. Key attributes include defining the population with mild cognitive impairment or mild AD, the treatment regardless of symptomatic treatment use, and the primary variable as a change from baseline in the clinical dementia rating scale (CDR-SB).

Intercurrent events, such as symptomatic treatment initiation and study drug discontinuation due to a lack of efficacy, disease progression, or safety, are addressed by treatment policy strategy to reflect clinical practice. Statistical analyses like the MMRM approach assuming that the missing data is MAR may be unplausible. Alternative imputation methods, such as reference-based conditional mean imputation, are recommended.

9.6 Concluding Remarks

Clinical trials in neuroscience present significant challenges that require careful thinking at the trial design stage. There are only a few principles available across all the different indications that could guide trial design. The limitations in biological understanding in many neurological indications and the amount of missing data add to the complexity of clinical trials in neuroscience. The estimand framework, however, proves particularly valuable in such situations as it leads to thorough thinking and, often, a clearer and more transparent path forward, as illustrated in the four case studies above.

As we have seen in all four examples presented in this chapter, the heterogeneity within neuroscience is large, and there is no one-size-fits-all solution. However, when the clinical situation and the research question are well-understood, the estimand framework facilitates essential discussions that need to take place before finalizing a clinical trial design, leading to practical and reasonable solutions.

Given the amount of intercurrent events and missing data encountered in all four examples, it is not surprising that the addressing of intercurrent events is one of the most challenging problems for trial design in neuroscience. While often a treatment policy strategy turns out to be reasonable and usually acceptable to regulators, there are instances where alternative strategies are preferable. In some cases, a composite variable strategy is more appropriate, and in other cases, we suggest using a hypothetical strategy, and we discussed even a situation where—depending on the underlying research question—a principal stratum strategy is the most suitable approach.

This diversity in design challenges and their respective solutions, some of which are meaningful, while others may not be, underscores the complexity of neuroscience. It is precisely this complexity that makes neuroscience so intriguing and the application of the estimand framework so valuable.

References

Abu-Arafeh, I., Hershey, A. D., Diener, H. C., & Tassorelli, C. (2019). IHS guidelines: Guidelines of the international headache society for controlled trials of preventive treatment of migraine in children and adolescents, 1st edition. *Cephalalgia, 39*(7), 803–816. https://doi.org/10.1177/0333102419842188

Atik, A., Stewart, T., & Zhang, J. (2016). Alpha-synuclein as a biomarker for Parkinson's disease. *Brain Pathology, 26*, 410–418.

Bateman, R. J., Smith, J., Donohue, M. C., Delmar, P., Abbas, R., Salloway, S., & Doody, R. S. (2023). Two phase 3 trials of gantenerumab in early Alzheimer's disease. *New England Journal of Medicine, 389*(20), 1862–1876.

Chitnis, T., Aaen, G., & Belman, A. (2020). Improved relapse recovery in paediatric compared to adult multiple sclerosis. *Brain, 143*(9), 2733–2741. https://doi.org/10.1093/brain/awaa199

Cox, D. R. (1972). Regression models and life-tables. *Journal of the Royal Statistical Society, Series B, 34*(2), 187–220.

Cummings, J., Aisen, P. S., DuBois, B., Frölich, L., Jack, C. R., Jr., Jones, R. W., Morris, J. C., Raskin, J., Dowsett, S. A., & Scheltens, P. (2016). Drug development in Alzheimer's disease: The path to 2025. *Alzheimer's Research & Therapy, 8*, 39. https://doi.org/10.1186/s13195-016-0207-9

Diener, H.-C., Tassorelli, C., Dodick, D. W., et al. (2020). Guidelines of the international headache society for controlled trials of preventive treatment of migraine attacks in episodic migraine in adults. *Cephalalgia, 40*(10), 1026–1044. https://doi.org/10.1177/0333102420941839

Donohue, M. C., Model, F., Delmar, P., Volye, N., Liu-Seifert, H., Rafii, M. S., & Alzheimer's Disease Neuroimaging Initiative. (2020). Initiation of symptomatic medication in Alzheimer's disease clinical trials: Hypothetical versus treatment policy approach. *Alzheimer's & Dementia, 16*(5), 797–803.

EMA. (2007). *Clinical investigation of medicinal products for treatment of migraine - Scientific guideline*. EMA. https://www.ema.europa.eu/en/clinical-investigation-medicinal-products-treatment-migraine

EMA. (2018). *Guideline on the clinical investigation of medicines for the treatment of Alzheimer's disease—Scientific guideline*. EMA. https://www.ema.europa.eu/en/documents/scientific-guideline/guideline-clinical-investigation-medicines-treatment-alzheimers-disease-revision-2_en.pdf

European Parkinson's disease association (EPDA) (2017). Rating scales. Available at http://www.epda.eu.com/about-parkinsons/symptoms/rating-scales/

Evers, S., Afra, J., Frese, A., Goadsby, P. J., Linde, M., May, A., & Sándor, P. S. (2009). EFNS guideline on the drug treatment of migraine--revised report of an EFNS task force. *European Journal of Neurology, 968-81*. https://doi.org/10.1111/j.1468-1331.2009.02748.x

Fahn S (2008) Clinical aspects of Parkinson disease. In: Nass R, Przedborsky R (editors): Parkinson's disease: Molecular and therapeutic insights from model systems. 1st edidion Elsevir; 3–8.

FDA. (2018). *Migraine: Developing Drugs for Acute Treatment—Guidance for*. https://www.fda.gov/media/89829/download

FDA. (2024). *Early Alzheimer's disease: Developing drugs for treatment guidance for industry*. https://www.fda.gov/media/110903/download

Gauthier, G. S., Feldman, H. H., Schneider, L. S., Wilcock, G. K., Frisoni, G. B., Hardlund, J. H., Moebius, H. J., Bentham, P., Kook, K. A., Wischik, D. J., Schelter, B. O., Davis, C. S., Staff, R. T., Bracoud, L., Shamsi, K., Storey, J. M. D., Harrington, C. R., & Wischik, C. M. (2016). Efficacy and safety of tau-aggregation inhibitor therapy in patients with mild or moderate Alzheimer's disease: A randomised, controlled, double-blind, parallel-arm, phase 3 trial. *Lancet, 388*(10062), 2873–2884. https://doi.org/10.1016/S0140-6736(16)31275-2

GBD. (2016). Parkinson's disease collaborators. Global, regional, and national burden of Parkinson's disease, 1990-2016: A systematic analysis for the global burden of disease study 2016. *Lancet Neurology, 17*(11), 939–953. https://doi.org/10.1016/S1474-4422(18)30295-3

Goetz, C. G., Tilley, B. C., Shaftman, S. R., et al. (2008). Movement Disorder Society-sponsored revision of the unified Parkinson's disease rating scale (MDS-UPDRS): Scale presentation and clinimetric testing results. *Movement Disorders, 23*(15), 2129–2170.

Hardy, J., & Selkoe, D. J. (2002). The amyloid hypothesis of Alzheimer's disease: Progress and problems on the road to therapeutics. *Science, 297*(5580), 353–356. https://doi.org/10.1126/science.1072994

He, J., Ford, H. C., Carroll, J., Douglas, C., Gonzales, E., Ding, S., Fearnley, I. M., & Walker, J. E. (2018). Assembly of the membrane domain of ATP synthase in human mitochondria. *Proceedings of the National Academy of Sciences of the United States of America, 115*(12), 2988–2993.

Headache Classification Committee of the International Headache Society. (2018). *Cephalalgia, 38*(1), 1–211. https://doi.org/10.1177/0333102417738202

Holden, S. K., Finseth, T., Sillau, S. H., & Berman, B. D. (2018). Progression of MDS-UPDRS scores over five years in De novo Parkinson disease from the Parkinson's progression markers Initiative cohort. *Movement Disorders Clinical Practice, 5*, 47–53. https://doi.org/10.1002/mdc3.12553

Horvath, K., Aschermann, Z., Kovacs, M., et al. (2015). Minimal clinically important difference on the motor examination part of MDS-UPDRS. *Parkinsonism & Related Disorders, 21*(12), 1421–1426.

ICH. (2019). *E9 (R1) addendum on estimands and sensitivity analysis in clinical trials to the guideline on statistical principles for clinical trials*. www.ich.org

Kappos, L., Bar-Or, A., Cree, B. A., Fox, R. J., Giovannoni, G., Gold, R., et al. (2018). Siponimod versus placebo in secondary progressive multiple sclerosis (EXPAND): A double-blind, randomised, phase 3 study. *The Lancet, 391*(10127), 1263–1273.

Katsarava, Z., Buse, D. C., Manack, A. N., Richard, B., & Lipton, R. B. (2012). Defining the differences between episodic migraine and chronic migraine. *Current Pain and Headache Reports, 16*(1), 86–92. https://doi.org/10.1007/s11916-011-0233-z

Kurtzke, J. F. (1983). Rating neurologic impairment in multiple sclerosis: An expanded disability status scale (EDSS). *Neurology, 33*(11), 1444–1452. https://doi.org/10.1212/wnl.33.11.1444

Lublin, F. D., Häring, D. A., Ganjgahi, H., Ocampo, A., Hatami, F., Čuklina, J., Aarden, P., Dahlke, F., Arnold, D., Wiendl, H., Chitnis, T., Nichols, T. E., Kieseier, B. C., & Bermel, R. A. (2022). How multiple sclerosis patients acquire disability. *Brain, 145*(9), 3147–3161.

Luquin, M. R., Kulivsky, J., Martinez-Martin, P., et al. (2017). Consensus on the definition of advanced Parkinson's disease: A neurologists based Delphi study (CEPA study). *Parkinsons dis, 4047392.*

Magnusson, B. P., Schmidli, H., Rouyrre, N., & Scharfstein, D. O. (2019). Bayesian inference for a principal stratum estimand to assess the treatment effect in a subgroup characterized by postrandomization event occurrence. *Statistics in Medicine, 38*(23), 4761–4771.

Mallinckrodt, C. H., Lane, P. W., Schnell, D. J., Peng, J., & Mancuso, J. P. (2008). Recommendations for the primary analysis of continuous endpoints in longitudinal clinical trials. *Drug Information Journal, 42*(4), 303–319. https://doi.org/10.1177/009286150804200402

Mészáros, L., Lasch, F., Delafont, B., Guizzaro, L. (2023). *Strategies for addressing intercurrent events in CNS trials*. https://ssrn.com/abstract=4516200

Mesterton, J., Wimo, A., By, A., et al. (2010). Cross sectional observational study on the societal costs of Alzheimer's disease. *Current Alzheimer Research, 7*, 358–367.

Noci, A., Wolbers, W., Abt, M., Baayen, C., Burger, H. U., Jin, M. R., & W.Z. (2022). A comparison of estimand and estimation strategies for clinical trials in early Parkinson's disease. *Statistics in Biopharmaceutical Research, 15*, 491. https://doi.org/10.1080/19466315.2022.2116476

Parkinson's Disease Foundation. (2019).

Parkinson's Disease Foundation. (2023).

Pinter, B., Diem-Zangerl, A., Wenning, G. K., Scherfler, C., Oberaigner, W., Seppi, K., & Poewe, W. (2015). Mortality in Parkinson's disease: A 38-year follow-up study. *Movement Disorders, 30*(2), 266–269. https://doi.org/10.1002/mds.26060. Epub 2014 Dec 1.

Poewe, W., & Wenning, G. (2002). The differential diagnosis of Parkinson's disease. *European Journal of Neurology, 3*, 23–30.

Poewe, W., Seppi, K., Tanner, C. M., Halliday, G. M., Brundin, P., Volkmann, J., Schrag, A. E., & Lang, A. E. (2017). Parkinson disease. *Nature Reviews Disease Primers, 3*, 17013.

Polverejan, E., O'Kelly, M., Hefting, N., Norton, J. D., Lim, P., & Walton, M. K. (2023). Defining clinical trial Estimands: A practical guide for study teams with examples based on a psychiatric disorder. *Therapeutic Innovation & Regulatory Science, 57*, 911. https://doi.org/10.1007/s43441-023-00524-2

Postuma, R. B., Berg, D., Adler, C. H., et al. (2016). The new definition and diagnosis criteria of Parkinson's disease. *Lancet Neurology, 15*, 546–548.

Selkoe, D. J. (1991). The molecular pathology of Alzheimer's disease. *Neuron, 6*(4), 487–498. https://doi.org/10.1016/0896-6273(91)90052-2

Selkoe, D. J., & Hardy, J. (2016). The amyloid hypothesis of Alzheimer's disease at 25 years. *EMBO Molecular Medicine, 8*(6), 595–608. https://doi.org/10.15252/emmm.201606210

Silberstein, S. D., Holland, S., Freitag, F., Dodick, D. W., Argoff, C., & Ashman, E. (2012). Quality standards Subcommittee of the American Academy of neurology and the American headache society. Evidence-based guideline update: Pharmacologic treatment for episodic migraine prevention in adults: Report of the quality standards Subcommittee of the American Academy of neurology and the American headache society. *Neurology, 78*(17), 1337–1345. https://doi.org/10.1212/WNL.0b013e3182535d20. Erratum in: Neurology 2013 Feb 26;80(9):871. PMID: 22529202; PMCID: PMC3335452.

Sims, J. R., Zimmer, J. A., Evans, C. D., Lu, M., Ardayfio, P., Sparks, J., & Kaul, S. (2023). Donanemab in early symptomatic Alzheimer disease: The TRAILBLAZER-ALZ 2 randomized clinical trial. *JAMA, 330*(6), 512–527.

Tassorelli, C., Diener, H. C., Dodick, D. W., Silberstein, S. D., Lipton, R. B., Ashina, M., Becker, W. J., Ferrari, M. D., Goadsby, P. J., Pozo-Rosich, P., & Wang, S. J. (2018). International headache society clinical trials standing committee. Guidelines of the international headache society for controlled trials of preventive treatment of chronic migraine in adults. *Cephalalgia, 38*(5), 815–832. https://doi.org/10.1177/0333102418758283

Trundell, D., Davies, E. W., Barrett, L., et al. (2025). Estimation of and clinical consensus on the meaningful motor progression threshold on MDS-UPDRS part III. *Journal of Parkinson's Disease, 15*, 97–110.

Van Dyck, C. H., Swanson, C. J., Aisen, P., Bateman, R. J., Chen, C., Gee, M., & Iwatsubo, T. (2023). Lecanemab in early Alzheimer's disease. *New England Journal of Medicine, 388*(1), 9–21.

Walton, C., King, R., & Rechtman, L. (2020). Rising prevalence of multiple sclerosis worldwide: Insights from the atlas of MS, third edition. *Multiple Sclerosis Journal, 26*, 1816–1821.

Wang, Y., Tu, W., Kim, Y., et al. (2023). (2023). Statistical methods for handling missing data to align with treatment policy strategy. *Pharmaceutical Statistics, 22*(4), 650–670. https://doi.org/10.1002/pst.2299

Wolbers, M., Noci, A., Delmar, P., Gower-Page, C., Yiu, S., & Bartlett, J. W. (2022). Standard and reference-based conditional mean imputation. *Pharmaceutical Statistics, 21*(6), 1246–1257.

Chapter 10
Applying the Estimand Framework: Case Studies in Cardiovascular, Respiratory, and Infectious Diseases and Vaccines

Alice Wang, Cui Xiong, Rong Fu, Zhiwei Jiang, Folke Folkvaljon, Zelie Bailes, Dawn Edwards, Wenting Li, and Peter Mesenbrink

Abstract The estimand framework has been widely applied in drug development to define trial objectives and establish clear estimands across various therapeutic areas. Unique challenges and specific considerations may arise in practice across different therapeutic areas. This chapter illustrates the practical implementation of the estimand framework in cardiovascular, respiratory, and infectious diseases and preventive vaccines through case studies in chronic heart failure (HF), asthma, coronavirus disease (COVID-19), and rabies vaccine, respectively. Each case study

A. Wang (✉)
Biometrics, R&D, AstraZeneca, Shanghai, China
e-mail: alice.wang2@astrazeneca.com

C. Xiong
Biostatistics, GlaxoSmithKline, Shanghai, China
e-mail: cui.2.xiong@gsk.com

R. Fu
Biostatistics and Research Decision Sciences, MSD R&D (China) Co., Ltd., Beijing, China
e-mail: rong.fu1@merck.com

Z. Jiang
KeyTech, Beijing, China
e-mail: zhi.wei.jiang@ktstat.com

F. Folkvaljon
HTA Statistics, BioPharmaceuticals, AstraZeneca, Barcelona, Spain
e-mail: folke.folkvaljon@astrazeneca.com

Z. Bailes · D. Edwards
Biostatistics, GlaxoSmithKline, London, UK
e-mail: zelie.a.bailes@gsk.com; Dawn.M.Webber@gsk.com

W. Li
Biostatistics, dMed Biopharmaceutical Co., Ltd, Shanghai, China
e-mail: wenting.li@caidya.com

P. Mesenbrink
Advanced Quantitative Sciences, Novartis Pharmaceuticals Corporation, East Hanover, USA
e-mail: peter_g.mesenbrink@novartis.com

J. Wei et al. (eds.), *Estimands in Clinical Trials*, Springer Series in Pharmaceutical Statistics, https://doi.org/10.1007/978-3-032-02192-2_10

discusses the development of the primary estimand, strategies for addressing the intercurrent events, and the rationale behind these choices, along with the associated analysis methods. Additionally, it explores alternative estimands and relevant supplementary analyses. The thinking process illustrated in these case studies offers broad insights that are applicable to other fields.

10.1 Introduction

The previous chapters in Part 2 illustrated the implementation of the estimand framework in therapeutic areas such as oncology, hematology, immunology, inflammation, and neuroscience. In this chapter, we focus on its practical application in other therapeutic areas, including chronic heart failure (HF) (Sect. 10.2), asthma (Sect. 10.3), coronavirus disease (COVID-19) (Sect. 10.4), and preventive vaccine trials (Sect. 10.5).

Each case study begins with a description of the trial objective and design, followed by the primary estimand and its attributes. Subsequently, we elaborate on the strategies and rationale for addressing the intercurrent events and explain the corresponding analysis methods.

The case studies in this chapter are not intended to provide standard or unified estimand considerations in these specific therapeutic areas. Alternative primary estimands and strategies for handling intercurrent events may be employed in other contexts within these therapeutic areas. Nevertheless, we believe that the thinking process illustrated through these estimand case studies will be broadly applicable.

10.2 Chronic Heart Failure

10.2.1 Background

Heart failure (HF) is a complex clinical syndrome caused by structural and/or functional abnormalities of the heart. It is characterized by dyspnea, fatigue, and pulmonary congestion and/or peripheral edema due to fluid retention. HF is one of the leading causes of mortality, hospitalization, and suboptimal quality of life. Even with the best possible treatment, the five-year survival rate for HF patients is worse than for most cancers (Braunwald, 2015). Patients with signs and symptoms of HF are diagnosed and often categorized into one of three categories based on the left-ventricular ejection fraction (LVEF) measurements: HF with reduced LVEF (HFrEF, $\leq$40%), HF with mildly reduced LVEF (HFmrEF, 41–49%), or HF with preserved LVEF (HFpEF, $\geq$50%) (McDonagh et al., 2021; McDonagh et al., 2023).

Previous studies have shown that treatment with diuretics, angiotensin-converting enzyme inhibitors, angiotensin II receptor blockers, angiotensin II receptor blocker neprilysin inhibitors, mineralocorticoid receptor antagonists, and beta-blockers for HFrEF can improve symptoms and hemodynamics, as well as reduce hospitalizations for HF and mortality (Iwaz et al., 2016). Data from cardiovascular outcome trials of sodium-glucose cotransporter-2 (SGLT-2) inhibitors (empagliflozin and canagliflozin) indicate that treatment with SGLT-2 inhibitors can reduce the risk of cardiovascular death and hospitalization due to HF in patients with type 2 diabetes overall, and in patients with type 2 diabetes and concomitant HF (Zinman et al., 2015; Ferreira et al., 2016; Fitchett et al., 2016; Neal et al., 2017; Rådholm et al., 2018).

In clinical trials evaluating the effect of treatment in HF patients, the commonly used composite primary endpoint includes events of cardiovascular death and hospitalization due to HF. Other important endpoints include changes in HF symptoms, degree of physical limitation, and exercise capacity.

10.2.2 Trial Objective and Design

DETERMINE-reduced (ClinicalTrials.gov identifier: NCT03877237 , n.d.) is an international, multicenter, parallel-group, randomized, double-blind, placebo-controlled, phase III trial in HFrEF patients (with or without type 2 diabetes), evaluating the effect of dapagliflozin 10 mg versus placebo, given once daily, in addition to background local standard-of-care (SOC) therapy, on changes in HF symptoms, physical limitation, and exercise capacity (McMurray et al., 2023).

HFrEF patients who meet all of the inclusion and none of the exclusion criteria are randomly assigned in a 1:1 ratio to receive either once-daily dapagliflozin 10 mg or a matching placebo. Patients receive the study drug until week 16, after which patients receive SOC therapy at the discretion of the investigator. All patients receive local standard background therapy for HFrEF and comorbidities (including treatment for hypertension, ischemic heart disease, atrial fibrillation, diabetes, and hyperlipidemia). All patients are prohibited from using open-label SGLT-2 inhibitors during the trial. If treatment with an SGLT-2 inhibitor alone or in combination is deemed essential, the study drug must be discontinued before that treatment is started.

Through metabolic-independent mechanisms, SGLT-2 inhibitors can improve abnormalities such as increased intraglomerular pressure, hypertension, proteinuria, and fluid/sodium overload. Therefore, it is expected that patients with heart failure and reduced renal function can benefit from the initiation of treatment with dapagliflozin, regardless of treatment discontinuation, subsequent treatment after discontinuation of study treatment, and the use of concomitant treatments.

Efficacy and safety assessments are performed at screening, randomization, week 8, week 16, and at the early withdrawal visit or early treatment discontinuation visit. Patients who temporarily or permanently discontinue the study drug continue to be followed up and assessed according to the protocol at the scheduled visits, and relevant data are collected until the end of the trial.

Three separate scores/outcomes are used to evaluate the degree of HF symptoms, physical limitation, and exercise capacity, all of which are clinically important for HF patients and are, therefore, used in this trial:

1. Change in total symptom score on the Kansas City Cardiomyopathy Questionnaire (KCCQ-TSS) from baseline to week 16
2. Change in physical limitations score on the Kansas City Cardiomyopathy Questionnaire (KCCQ-PLS) from baseline to week 16
3. Change in six-minute walk distance (6MWD) from baseline to week 16

Among these three endpoints, KCCQ is a patient-reported outcome instrument developed specifically for chronic HF patients. The scores of KCCQ-TSS and KCCQ-PLS can effectively and reliably evaluate HF symptoms and the degree of physical limitation, respectively, with good responsiveness. 6MWD is a standard method to evaluate the submaximal exercise capacity in response to treatment in patients with severe heart or lung disease.

10.2.3 Estimand Considerations

The trial aims to compare dapagliflozin with a placebo in patients with HFrEF. The primary objective is to demonstrate the superiority of the experimental arm over the control arm in reducing symptoms and physical limitations associated with HF and improving exercise capacity in terms of median difference for each variable. Patients who die are assigned the worst outcome. The treatment effect of primary interest is regardless of the discontinuation of study treatment, subsequent treatment after discontinuation of study treatment, and the use of concomitant treatments. In the following, we describe the estimands corresponding to each of the three endpoints, KCCQ-TSS, KCCQ-PLS, and 6MWD, with a detailed description of the five attributes.

(a) Population: HFrEF patients who meet the trial's inclusion and exclusion criteria.
(b) Variables: Composite outcome of separate scores (KCCQ-TSS, KCCQ-PLS, and 6MWD) and death, where death is treated as the worst outcome (see the population-level summary below for more details).
(c) Treatment: Initiation of daily dapagliflozin 10 mg or placebo on top of local SOC therapy for HFrEF and comorbidities, regardless of treatment discontinuation, subsequent treatment after treatment discontinuation, and the use of concomitant treatment.
(d) Intercurrent events and strategies are described in Table 10.1. A composite variable strategy is used for death as an intercurrent event; see the variable attribute above. A treatment policy strategy is used for the other three intercurrent events (discontinuation of study treatment, subsequent treatment after discontinuation of study treatment, and the use of concomitant treatments); see the treatment attribute above.

Table 10.1 Proposed estimand strategies

Intercurrent events	Strategies	Comments
Discontinuation of study treatment	Treatment policy strategy	Discontinuation of study treatment reflects the clinical practice, as described in the treatment attribute
Use of concomitant treatments	Treatment policy strategy	The use of concomitant treatment reflects the clinical practice, as described in the treatment attribute
Subsequent treatment after discontinuation of study treatment	Treatment policy strategy	The use of subsequent treatment after discontinuation of study treatment reflects the clinical practice, as described in the treatment attribute
Death	Composite variable strategy	Death is treated as the worst possible outcome, as described in the variable attribute

(e) Population-level summary: The Hodges–Lehmann median difference between the two arms is used for each variable. The worst rank is assigned to patients who died for the pairwise comparisons in the primary analysis, regardless of the time from randomization to death. The time from randomization to death is considered when assigning ranks to the patients who died in one of the supplementary analyses. This is done to address and evaluate the impact of potential treatment differences in mortality time on the assessment of the primary efficacy endpoints. The Hodges–Lehmann median difference is not sensitive to outliers and can, therefore, accommodate deaths without imputing explicit (implausible) values for patients who died. This approach also accommodates the expected non-normal distribution of changes from baseline in KCCQ-TSS and KCCQ-PLS, caused by the floor (0 points) and ceiling (100 points) of these values, together with the noncentral distribution at baseline.

10.2.4 Statistical Analysis

10.2.4.1 Analysis Set

The full analysis set includes all randomized patients, irrespective of their protocol adherence, addition or modification of background rescue medications, switches to alternative medications, or continued participation in the trial.

10.2.4.2 Primary Analysis

The primary objective of this trial is to confirm the superiority of dapagliflozin over placebo in any of the primary endpoints (KCCQ-TSS, KCCQ-PLS, and 6MWD). A rank analysis of covariance model is employed to test the differences between the treatment arms in changes in KCCQ-TSS, KCCQ-PLS, and 6MWD, respectively, from baseline at week 16 (Koch et al., 1998). The difference between the treatment arms in each variable is estimated using the Hodges–Lehmann method, based on the median of all pairwise differences in changes in each variable (Hodges & Lehmann, 1963). Multiple imputation based on the placebo arm is used to impute the missing values due to reasons other than death before ranking, the patients who died before week 16 are assigned the worst outcome, and ordering among deaths is based on the last value while alive (the lower the last observed value of change from baseline before death, the lower/worse the rank). A gatekeeping procedure (Dmitrienko et al., 2011) is used to control the overall type I error rate at level 0.05 (two-sided).

10.2.4.3 Sensitivity Analysis

To examine the robustness of the primary analysis results regarding missing data handling, a tipping point sensitivity analysis is planned. For patients who have missing data for changes in KCCQ-TSS, KCCQ-PLS, and 6MWD from baseline at week 16, missing data are first replaced using the multiple imputation procedure described above. The imputed post-baseline values in the active arm are then subsequently shifted toward a null hypothesis (i.e., subtracting a certain value up to 100 meters for 6MWD and up to 40 points for KCCQ-TSS and KCCQ-PLS, respectively) until the significance of the model estimates is overturned to identify the point at which the conclusion changes.

10.2.4.4 Supplementary Analysis

To examine the impact of the addressing of deaths in the composite variable strategy and the robustness of the primary analysis results regarding death, the following supplementary analyses are planned:

- The time from randomization to death is considered when assigning ranks to the patients who died, with a shorter time corresponding to a lower/worse rank. Other missing data handling methods and analysis methods are the same as those used in the primary analysis.
- Patients who died before week 16 are excluded from the analysis. The missing values are imputed in the same way as in the primary analysis. An analysis of covariance model is conducted with non-ranked values. The mean difference of each variable between the treatment arms is estimated.

10.2.5 Summary and Discussion

We conclude this section with a few additional considerations on the estimand choice above. In this case study, a treatment policy strategy is implemented for most of the intercurrent events in the primary estimands because they are believed to reflect clinical practice and need to be considered in the evaluation of the treatment effect. A hypothetical strategy may be considered to address these intercurrent events as a supplementary analysis to evaluate a treatment effect as if the intercurrent events would not occur.

A composite variable strategy is used for death as an intercurrent event. Other strategies, such as treatment policy, hypothetical or principal stratum approaches. These three strategies/approaches are in parallel and the exact terms are used in the ICH E9(R1) guideline: treatment policy strategy, hypothetical strategy, or principal stratum strategy. to address the intercurrent event of death, seem to have limited clinical utility and less value to clinicians, patients, and regulators. As a result, these strategies are not implemented in this case study.

The Hodges–Lehmann median difference of the changes in each variable between the two arms is used for a population-level summary of each primary estimand. Alternatively, a trimmed mean difference between the treatment arms may be considered as a population-level summary (Permutt & Li, 2017). However, this is not preferred for our case study, as it will not accommodate the composite variable strategy to address death as an intercurrent event, i.e., assigning worse ranks to patients who died prior to week 16.

10.3 Asthma

10.3.1 Background

Asthma is a common chronic airway disease, imposing a significant burden on families, healthcare systems, and the workplace. It is characterized by airway inflammation, increased airway responsiveness, and bronchoconstriction (GINA, 2019). The goal of asthma treatment is to achieve and maintain asthma control, enabling patients to avoid symptoms and flare-ups and lead productive lives with near-normal lung function.

Despite the availability of treatments and published guidelines, patients may have asthma that is inadequately controlled. The prevalence of inadequately controlled asthma varies based on the definition used for control. In a sample of asthmatics visiting their healthcare provider for any reason, 58% of adult asthmatics were estimated to have uncontrolled asthma based on the asthma control test (ACT), defined as an ACT score less than or equal to 19 (ClinicalTrials.gov identifier: NCT02924688 , n.d.).

The Global Initiative for Asthma guideline (GINA, 2019) recommends a long-acting muscarinic antagonist (LAMA) as an add-on treatment option for adults with asthma who are currently taking medium-to-high-dose inhaled corticosteroid (ICS)/ long-acting beta2 agonist (LABA) treatment and have a history of exacerbations. Exacerbation is an important endpoint to reflect the effect of treatment in asthma patients; however, improving lung function and symptom control are also important in determining which patients could benefit from a step-up therapy.

10.3.2 Trial Objective and Design

The phase III trial named CAPTAIN (ClinicalTrials.gov identifier: NCT02924688 , n.d.; Lee et al., 2021) aims to evaluate a once-daily closed triple therapy consisting of an ICS/LAMA/LABA combination [fluticasone furoate (FF)/umeclidinium (UMEC)/vilanterol (VI)] administered via a single ELLIPTA® dry powder inhaler. The goal is to provide a new treatment option for the management of asthma by improving lung function and symptom control over established combination therapies.

This randomized, double-blind, active-controlled, global multicenter trial consists of six parallel treatment arms to evaluate the safety and efficacy of FF/UMEC/VI (100/31.25/25, 100/62.5/25, 200/31.25/25, and 200/62.5/25 micrograms [mcg]) versus FF/VI (100/25 and 200/25 mcg), given once daily in the morning. By comparing a closed triple therapy to a standard-of-care ICS/LABA combination therapy, this trial provides important information to prescribers regarding the benefit of stepping up to closed triple therapy for patients who are uncontrolled on ICS/ LABA therapy.

The primary efficacy endpoint is trough forced expiratory volume in 1 s (FEV1) at the end of the 24-week treatment period. FEV1 is a measure of lung function and is defined as the maximal volume of air that can be forcefully exhaled in 1 s. Trough FEV1 on treatment is defined as the highest FEV1 value obtained prior to the morning dose of the investigational product. Trough FEV1 can efficiently evaluate the effects on lung function, which is the primary objective of this trial and is aligned with regulatory agencies. In addition, endpoints relevant to exacerbation and symptom control are also included as secondary endpoints to further assess the benefits of a step-up therapy for the patients.

The trial requires approximately 2250 randomized patients, with 375 patients allocated to each of the six double-blind treatment arms. It consists of five phases: prescreening (visit 0), screening/run-in, recruitment/stabilization, randomization/ treatment, and follow-up. All patients who meet the predefined eligibility criteria following the run-in and stabilization period are randomized to one of the six treatment arms. The duration of the treatment period is variable, with a minimum of

24 weeks and a maximum of 52 weeks. Patients are to have up to six on-treatment clinic visits scheduled at visits 3, 4, 5, 6, 7, and 8 (end of trial) at weeks 0, 4, 12, 24, 36, and 52, respectively. A follow-up visit is to be conducted approximately 7 days after the end of the treatment period or, if applicable, after the early withdrawal visit. Patients who prematurely discontinue treatment are encouraged to remain in the trial.

10.3.3 Estimand Considerations

The trial compares FF/UMEC/VI with FF/VI in patients with inadequately controlled asthma. The primary objective is to demonstrate the superiority of adding UMEC at two dosage strengths, 62.5 mcg and 31.25 mcg, in a single inhaler to FF/VI on change from baseline in trough FEV1 at the end of the 24-week treatment period. The primary comparison of interest is the treatment effect, regardless of the intercurrent events, including the discontinuation of study treatment, use of rescue medication, temporary treatment interruption, and treatment switch. This trial was planned before the estimand framework was published, but the principles of the primary analyses are aligned with the ICH E9 (R1) guideline (ICH 2019). Based on the original analyses defined in the statistical analysis plan, the primary estimand and its five attributes can be interpreted as follows:

(a) Population: Patients with inadequately controlled asthma despite requiring treatment with ICS/LABA.
(b) Variable: Change from baseline in trough FEV1 at week 24.
(c) Treatment: FF/UMEC/VI (100/62.5/25 mcg; 200/62.5/25 mcg; 100/31.25/25 mcg; 200/31.25/25 mcg) or FF/VI (100/25 mcg; 200/25 mcg), regardless of the discontinuation of study treatment, use of rescue medication, temporary treatment interruption, and treatment switch.
(d) Intercurrent events and strategies are described in Table 10.2.
(e) Population-level summary: The primary treatment comparisons are based on the differences in mean change from baseline in trough FEV1 at week 24 for FF/UMEC/VI versus FF/VI.

Table 10.2 Proposed estimand strategies

Intercurrent events	Handling strategies	Comments
Treatment discontinuation	Treatment policy strategy	This estimand is intended to represent what may happen when the treatment is used in clinical practice, as described in the treatment attribute
Use of rescue medication	Treatment policy strategy	
Temporary treatment interruption	Treatment policy strategy	
Treatment switch	Treatment policy strategy	

10.3.4 Statistical Analysis

10.3.4.1 Analysis Set

The analysis set is defined as all randomized patients, excluding those who are randomized in error. A patient who is recorded as a screen failure, run-in failure, or stabilization failure, but is randomized and does not receive a dose of trial treatment, is considered to be randomized in error.

10.3.4.2 Primary Analysis

A mixed-model repeated measures (MMRM) analysis is performed in the primary analysis with covariates sex, region, visit, pre-study ICS dosage at screening, age, and baseline value for clinic FEV1. Since the primary clinical question of interest is the treatment effect regardless of treatment discontinuation and other intercurrent events, all FEV1 data collected following discontinuation of randomized treatment for patients who remain in the trial are included in the primary analyses. More discussions about the statistical analysis of continuous endpoints can be found in Chap. 15.

The MMRM analysis assumes that missing data are missing at random (MAR), where missingness is assumed to depend on observed data, conditional on covariates and measurement history. No imputation of missing data is planned; instead, the missing data are addressed via MMRM. Sensitivity analyses are performed to explore the robustness of statistical inference when this assumption is violated.

10.3.4.3 Sensitivity Analysis

The missing data in the primary analysis are assumed to be MAR. Deviation from this assumption may affect the primary analysis result, so sensitivity analyses, including tipping point analysis and jump-to-reference imputation, are performed using alternative assumptions to assess the robustness of the primary analysis results.

The tipping point analysis explores the potential effect of missing data on the reliability of the results by using different assumptions regarding the primary endpoint outcome in patients who withdraw from the trial early. For patients who withdraw from the trial earlier than week 24, missing data are first imputed under the assumption of MAR and then adjusted by adding a shift before analyzing the imputed datasets and combining the results. This shift is varied separately for FF/UMEC/VI and FF/VI and specified in advance, representing a change in trough FEV1. If the observed treatment effect from the primary analysis is x, the shift to be investigated will range from $-3x$ to $+x$ milliliter for both active and placebo arms, in increments of $0.5x$ milliliter. For the missing data, the relevant shifts (positive and/or negative) are added to the imputed FEV1 using multiple imputation under MAR for each respective treatment arm. This analysis allows for the determination of the tipping point of the values for missing data that would cause a change in the statistical significance of the result of the treatment comparison.

Jump-to-reference imputation assumes that patients with posttreatment missing data in the test arms (FF/UMEC/VI) would have provided data similar to those in the reference arm (FF/VI). This approach represents the situation where the patients' expected mean change from baseline in trough FEV1 is shifted to that of the reference arm (FF/VI with the same FF dose), regardless of the UMEC dose in their randomized treatment. Posttreatment missing data in the reference arms (FF/VI 100/25 or 200/25 mcg) are imputed under MAR.

10.3.4.4 Supplementary Analysis

A supplementary analysis based on on-treatment data is performed, which excludes the data collected post withdrawal from treatment. The purpose of this is to enable comparison of the results with those of previous trials, which did not collect post-treatment data. All other intercurrent events are still addressed via treatment policy (i.e., rescue medication and treatment interruptions are ignored). For this supplementary analysis, only on-treatment FEV1 data collected prior to and at week 24 are analyzed, using MMRM with the same covariates as the primary analysis. Posttreatment data are not utilized in the analysis, and imputation is not made for any missing data.

10.3.5 Summary and Discussion

Before the ICH E9 (R1) guideline was released, many trials did not specify the intercurrent events or collect data after the discontinuation of study treatment. In this case study, the sponsor aligned with regulators that this trial was of interest in assessing the treatment effect regardless of intercurrent events and confirmed that the data collected after intercurrent events retain value for assessing treatment effect. Therefore, the treatment policy was used as the strategy for the primary estimand. Conversely, to enable comparison with previous trials that did not collect data after treatment discontinuation, a supplementary analysis based only on on-treatment data was used for the intercurrent event of premature treatment discontinuation, and an MMRM model was performed. This analysis was planned before the estimand framework was in place; however, it could be interpreted as a hypothetical strategy where patients would not discontinue treatment. This also provided a comparison with the primary estimand of the treatment policy to confirm the impact of intercurrent events on the assessment of treatment effect.

10.4 COVID-19

10.4.1 *Background*

The COVID-19 outbreak, caused by the severe acute respiratory syndrome coronavirus 2 (SARS-CoV-2), started in December 2019 and escalated into a global pandemic. The virus is mainly transmitted through respiratory droplets and contact, and infected individuals may be asymptomatic (WHO, 2023). Symptomatic individuals may experience fever, fatigue, cough, shortness of breath, and loss of taste and smell, typically appearing 1–14 days post-incubation. While most symptomatic patients exhibit mild-to-moderate symptoms, hospitalization may be necessary for those with severe symptoms, requiring supportive care, and/or with a higher risk factor of complications. In view of the global COVID-19 crisis, regulatory agencies rapidly issued a series of guidelines and policies to accelerate drug development for both hospitalized and nonhospitalized patients, among which the FDA, (2023) provided recommendations for defining estimands in clinical trials evaluating COVID-19 treatment (see also Sect. 13.4 in Chap. 13 of this book). This section presents a case study, JWT629A12301, illustrating the application of the estimand framework to a COVID-19 clinical trial in hospitalized patients (ClinicalTrials.gov identifier: NCT04358081 , n.d.).

10.4.2 *Trial Objective and Design*

This case study is on a multicenter, randomized, double-blind, three-arm, placebo-controlled phase III clinical trial. The trial evaluated the safety and efficacy of hydroxychloroquine (HCQ) monotherapy or in combination with azithromycin (AZI) in hospitalized adult patients with moderate-to-severe COVID-19. No drugs had been approved or received emergency use authorization for the treatment of hospitalized COVID-19 patients during the design stage of this trial. Available clinical data at that time suggested that HCQ (monotherapy or in combination with AZI) may provide benefits for patients with moderate-to-severe COVID-19. It was, therefore, selected as the treatment of interest. In addition, standard supportive care for COVID-19 was added to reflect actual clinical practice.

On day 1, patients were randomly assigned in equal proportions to one of three treatment arms: HCQ monotherapy, HCQ in combination with AZI, or placebo. Treatment was administered from days 1 to 10, followed by a posttreatment observation period from days 11 to 40. For patients who were discharged from the hospital before the end of the treatment period, treatment continued at home if their corrected QT interval using Fridericia's formula at discharge was less than or equal to 480 milliseconds; otherwise, treatment was terminated at discharge. Patients who terminated study treatment early were still required to continue follow-up and assessment per the planned visit, unless they withdrew their informed consent.

Throughout the trial, all patients received the best standard supportive care for COVID-19 according to local treatment guidelines. Depending on the disease severity, supportive care included oxygen supplementation, antibiotic prophylaxis, concomitant medications for comorbidities, ventilator support, or intensive care management after disease progression. Rescue therapies beyond the standard supportive care were potentially administered to patients with worsening conditions at the investigator's discretion.

Since the target population included hospitalized patients, a composite variable of discharge and survival was chosen as the criterion for clinical response. An improvement in clinical response was considered a relevant measure to assess the treatment effect of COVID-19 drugs. The definition of clinical response varied, depending on the patients' premorbid oxygen requirement.

10.4.3 Estimand Considerations

The objective of this trial is to compare HCQ monotherapy or HCQ + AZI combination therapy with placebo in hospitalized patients with moderate-to-severe COVID-19 who are receiving standard supportive care. The primary objective is to demonstrate the superiority of HCQ monotherapy or HCQ + AZI combination therapy compared with placebo in improving the clinical response by day 15 after randomization. The treatment effect of primary interest is regardless of the discontinuation of study treatment or rescue therapies. In the following, we define the estimand, with a detailed description of its five attributes.

(a) Population: Adults (at least 18 years of age) who are confirmed to be infected with SARS-COV-2 by polymerase chain reaction or rapid test within 4 days prior to randomization and are currently hospitalized or required hospitalization due to COVID-19.
(b) Variable: Clinical response by day 15 after randomization. For patients with a premorbid oxygen requirement, it is defined as discharge (or readiness for discharge) or survival without the need for mechanical ventilation. For patients without a premorbid oxygen requirement, it is defined as discharge (or ready for discharge) or survival without the need for mechanical ventilation or supplemental oxygen over the past 24 h. The readiness for discharge is determined by assessing their normal body temperature, respiratory rate, and stable oxygen saturation while breathing ambient air or requiring less than or equal to two liters of supplemental oxygen.
(c) Treatment: HCQ monotherapy, HCQ + AZI combination therapy, or placebo, added to concomitant standard supportive care for moderate-to-severe COVID-19, regardless of the discontinuation of study treatment or rescue therapies.
(d) Intercurrent events and strategies are specified in Table 10.3. Rescue therapies were allowed in the trial to reflect clinical practice. Likewise, the occurrence of

Table 10.3 Proposed estimand strategies

Intercurrent events	Strategies	Comments
Rescue therapies	Treatment policy strategy	Clinical practice allows for rescue therapies, as described in the treatment attribute
Discontinuation of study treatment	Treatment policy strategy	Discontinuation of study treatment may occur in clinical practice, as described in the treatment attribute

discontinuation of study treatment was considered possible clinical practice. A treatment policy strategy was, therefore, used to address both intercurrent events because the clinical question of interest was to evaluate the treatment effect regardless of rescue therapy and treatment discontinuation; see the treatment attribute above. Patients were followed up after the occurrence of either of these intercurrent events.

(e) Population-level summary: Odds ratio comparing the experimental arm (HCQ monotherapy or HCQ + AZI combination therapy) to the placebo arm.

10.4.4 Statistical Analysis

10.4.4.1 Analysis Set

The analysis includes all randomized patients except those with erroneous randomization.

10.4.4.2 Primary Analysis

The objective is to demonstrate the superiority of HCQ monotherapy (or the HCQ + AZI combination therapy) compared to placebo in achieving a clinical response by day 15. The treatment effect is measured using the odds ratio. Accordingly, a logistic regression model is fitted to estimate the odds ratio for achieving a clinical response (HCQ monotherapy versus placebo and HCQ + AZI combination therapy versus placebo, respectively). The model includes the treatment arm as the independent variable and oxygen supplementation at randomization as a covariate variable. Patients are to be included in the primary analysis, regardless of whether they take rescue therapies or discontinue treatment.

Since this trial involves hospitalized patients, it is anticipated that their clinical outcomes will be carefully collected, minimizing the possibility of missing data in the primary analysis. Consequently, no sensitivity analysis regarding missing data is planned.

10.4.5 Summary and Discussion

This case study illustrates the estimand framework for a clinical trial of a COVID-19 drug in hospitalized patients, see also FDA, (2023) guidelines for further considerations on how to address intercurrent events in clinical trials of COVID-19 drugs (see Sect. 13.4 in Chap. 13). For trials involving hospitalized patients, the FDA, (2023) suggests using the composite strategy for death and the treatment policy strategy for other intercurrent events. Specifically, in this case study, the definition of the clinical response endpoint is a composite of survival and clinical improvement, which is in accordance with the recommended strategy for death.

Although the acute crisis of COVID-19 has passed, the significant challenges it posed to the conduct of clinical trials and the interpretation of trial results motivate us to learn from this experience. It is worth considering how to effectively manage similar situations within the estimand framework in the future. The impact of the pandemic on estimand attributes such as population, treatment, variable, and intercurrent events, as well as on data collection and analysis, has compromised the trial's ability to accurately assess the treatment effect in a non-pandemic setting (Degtyarev et al., 2020; Yassi et al., 2021).

The pandemic altered the characteristics of the recruited patients, especially regarding their medical conditions and disease severity. It is crucial to thoroughly assess and address the representativeness of the recruited population relative to the original target population.

Maintaining adherence to the assigned treatment during the pandemic posed significant challenges, with a higher frequency of interruptions, delays, or modifications to treatment regimens due to the strain on the healthcare system or changes in standard of care. Any alterations in treatment conditions should be carefully considered, particularly in determining whether the intended treatment effect should account for those disruptions due to the pandemic (i.e., focusing on the non-pandemic clinical practice) or incorporate them as part of the medical practice and treatment conditions. Different strategies for relevant intercurrent events, which may be selected based on the frequency and causes of these intercurrent events, can address different clinical questions of interest. Prespecifying them would help prevent biased estimations and misinterpretation of the treatment effect. We refer to Chap. 23 in this book for more details.

The COVID-19 pandemic has also impacted the clinical endpoint variable in various ways. For example, due to the high mortality and morbidity associated with COVID-19, there have been potential changes in overall survival due to interruptions in treatment and alterations in disease progression pathways. Furthermore, COVID-19-related events, such as illness or hospitalizations, may significantly impact the occurrence of intercurrent events, rendering subsequent trial outcome measurements unsuitable for treatment effect assessment within the defined estimand framework. This also highlights the importance of carefully defining the variable that is most clinically relevant to the treatment effect.

The estimand framework is a valuable tool for addressing the complexities introduced by a pandemic like COVID-19, ensuring that the treatment effect is clearly defined and that the collected data are appropriate for providing a valid estimate.

10.5 Preventive Vaccine

10.5.1 Background

Preventive vaccines are crucial for safeguarding public health as they help prevent the occurrence of infectious diseases or alleviate the severity of the disease caused by viruses, bacteria, or other pathogens. The gold standard design for evaluating the efficacy and safety of experimental vaccines is the randomized, controlled efficacy trial, where a vaccine's efficacy is claimed based on the reduction in disease incidence in vaccinated subjects compared to unvaccinated subjects. For example, the vaccine efficacy of COVID-19 vaccines, human papillomavirus (HPV) vaccines, and herpes zoster vaccines has been evaluated using this approach in randomized, placebo-controlled efficacy trials. However, when the disease incidence is low, an efficacy trial may require a large sample size and a long follow-up period to accumulate disease cases, or it may even be infeasible. Alternatively, for diseases where the predictive relationship between an immune response and vaccine efficacy has been established (i.e., an immune response has been verified as an immune correlate of protection), immunogenicity trials can replace efficacy trials (e.g., rabies vaccine and polio vaccine). In that case, a non-inferiority design on immunogenicity endpoints is usually used to demonstrate the experimental vaccine's efficacy. However, if there are no scientifically accepted immune responses that are reasonably likely to predict vaccine efficacy, an efficacy trial is generally required for a new vaccine.

The lot-to-lot consistency trial is a critical and unique component of the clinical development of preventive vaccines. This trial serves to demonstrate manufacturing consistency by proving the equivalence of immunogenicity across three consecutive lots of the experimental vaccine. To achieve this, the trial is designed to compare post-vaccination antibody titers between each pair of the three lots, in terms of the prespecified equivalence criteria. The successful completion of this trial is essential to ensure that each manufacturing lot of the vaccine induces a similar level of immune response, thus providing equivalent protection against the targeted disease.

In addition, ensuring the safety of preventive vaccines is also important in clinical evaluation, especially because they are typically administered to a healthy population. To this end, a vaccine trial is sometimes designed with a primary objective to evaluate safety with a statistical hypothesis. For example, determining whether there is an increased risk of intussusception following rotavirus vaccination is an important safety question surrounding rotavirus vaccines.

This section aims to illustrate the estimand framework introduced by the ICH E9 (R1) guideline in preventive vaccine trial settings.

10.5.2 Estimand Considerations

In this section, we discuss some of the general considerations of estimands in preventive vaccines. These considerations may reflect different clinical questions of interest, and the specific definition of an estimand needs to fit the purpose of the trial objective (Fu et al., 2023; Nauta, 2024).

(a) Population
Preventive vaccines are generally administered to healthy individuals. In immunogenicity trials, the population can comprise either only seronegative individuals (e.g., for rabies vaccines) or all individuals, regardless of their serostatus (e.g., for influenza vaccines), based on the targeted infectious disease. Factors to consider when defining the population include the proportion of naturally infected or immunized individuals and the expected efficacy of the vaccine across different subpopulations (EMA, 2023).
In efficacy trials, a naïve population comprising seronegative individuals who have no ongoing infection with the targeted pathogen is often the target population of interest. For example, in a COVID-19 vaccine trial, the primary objective was to assess vaccine efficacy in a population that was seronegative at baseline and had no evidence of COVID-19 up to 14 days after the second dose (Kaabi et al., 2021; Jiang et al., 2021).

(b) Variable
In immunogenicity trials, primary variables typically include seroconversion and antibody titer or concentration at a post-vaccination time point. It is important to specify the time point of measurement when defining the variable. For example, in a rabies vaccine trial, the primary variables included antibody titer at 14 days following the first dose, seroconversion at 14 days following the first dose, and seroconversion at 14 days following the last dose.
In efficacy trials, the clinical outcome of interest is usually the occurrence of confirmed disease. The variable used to assess the vaccine efficacy may include the occurrence of the disease in a specified period. When the clinical objective is focused on efficacy post full vaccination, the disease surveillance period (i.e., the period during which subjects are monitored for the development of the disease endpoint of interest) starts after the completion of the vaccination rather than right after randomization. This timing allows for full immunization to stimulate sufficient immunity. For example, in a COVID-19 vaccine trial, the primary variable was the occurrence of COVID-19, confirmed by reverse transcription polymerase chain reaction occurring 14 days post dose 2 (Kaabi et al., 2021).

(c) Treatment
In either immunogenicity or efficacy trials, the treatment typically consists of the experimental vaccine and the comparative product. Depending on the objective of the trial, it may also be specified by dosing regimens, dosing intervals, route of administration (e.g., intramuscular versus subcutaneous), or concomitant use of other vaccines. For example, in a COVID-19 vaccine trial, the

treatment was the SARS-CoV-2 vaccine versus an aluminum hydroxide-only control at a two-dose regimen, with the second dose administered 21 days after the first dose.

(d) Intercurrent Events and Strategies
Table 10.4 provides common intercurrent events that may occur in vaccine trials, along with the strategies that could be adopted to address them. Discussions on the implementation of the principal stratum strategy in vaccine trials are also provided.

In preventive vaccine trials, the primary clinical question of interest is typically to assess the efficacy after full vaccination. For instance, in a COVID-19 vaccine efficacy trial, the primary objective was to demonstrate that the vaccine reduced the incidence of COVID-19 of any severity occurring at least 14 days after full vaccination compared to placebo, while assessing efficacy after the first dose was a secondary objective (Kaabi et al., 2021; Jiang et al., 2021). In a rabies vaccine lot-to-lot consistency trial, the primary objective was to demonstrate the equivalence of antibody titers 14 days after full vaccination (see Sect. 10.5.3).

To address the intercurrent event of not completing the vaccine regimen (e.g., due to loss to follow-up, withdrawal of informed consent, or adverse events) in vaccine trials, the principal stratum strategy can be employed to define a population consisting of subjects who would complete the vaccine regimen regardless of treatment assignment (i.e., always completers). The principal stratum strategy is discussed in detail in Chap. 19. However, it may be necessary to consider different assumptions when estimating the principal stratum estimand to address the discontinuation of vaccination due to different reasons.

The occurrence of the intercurrent event of not completing the vaccine regimen due to loss to follow-up or withdrawal of informed consent can be assumed to be at random and not dependent on treatment assignment. Therefore, an

Table 10.4 Common intercurrent events and strategies in vaccine trials

Intercurrent events	Strategies	Comments
Not completing the vaccine regimen (e.g., due to loss to follow-up, withdrawal of informed consent, or adverse events)	Principal stratum strategy	Applied to both efficacy and immunogenicity trials
Acquisition of the disease being targeted prior to the disease endpoint case surveillance period	Principal stratum strategy	Applied to efficacy trials
Experiencing events that could affect the efficacy assessments (e.g., the use of concomitant vaccines or medications) prior to the disease endpoint case surveillance period	Principal stratum strategy	Applied to efficacy trials
Receipt of a similar vaccine product during the disease endpoint case surveillance period	While on treatment strategy	Applied to efficacy trials
Experiencing events that could affect the immunogenicity assessments (e.g., the use of concomitant vaccines or medications)	Hypothetical strategy	Applied to immunogenicity trials

analysis population, including trial participants who completed their assigned vaccine regimen, provides an unbiased estimate of the corresponding principal stratum estimand in terms of the subjects' potential status of occurrence of the intercurrent event under both treatment arms (Lou et al., 2019).

The occurrence of the intercurrent event of not completing the vaccine regimen due to adverse events can be assumed to satisfy the assumption of monotonicity in placebo-controlled vaccine trials. This means that if such an event occurs under the placebo arm, it will also occur under the vaccine arm (Gilbert et al., 2013). As shown by Lou et al. (2019), an analysis set simply excluding participants who discontinued the vaccination due to adverse events may lead to selection bias in estimation. It is recommended to perform descriptive analyses of baseline characteristics between the treatment arms to assess the balance in the analysis set and conduct sensitivity analyses to evaluate the causal inference on the primary estimand.

The principal stratum strategy is also useful in efficacy trials to address intercurrent events, such as acquisition of the disease being targeted prior to the disease endpoint case surveillance period or experiencing events (e.g., the use of concomitant vaccines or medications) that could impact the efficacy assessments in this period. This strategy defines the target population as subjects who would not experience these events, regardless of treatment assignments (i.e., always compliers). As discussed above, an unbiased estimation of a principal stratum estimand generally requires additional assumptions, which, however, cannot be verified by observed data. An analysis by excluding subjects who have experienced these intercurrent events may introduce bias in the estimation. However, it is worth noting that in large-scale vaccine trials, the proportion of subjects who have experienced these intercurrent events is usually too small to significantly affect the robustness of the estimate of the primary estimand, especially when the incidence of the targeted disease is low, such as in HPV vaccine trials, rotavirus vaccine trials, and hand-foot-mouth disease vaccine trials (Joura et al., 2015; Li et al., 2014; Ruiz-Palacios et al., 2006). However, if a breakout occurs before the surveillance period, the number of subjects who acquire the disease prior to the start of the efficacy endpoint surveillance period could be significant, and sensitivity analyses could be performed to explore the robustness of the estimate of the primary estimand.

(e) Population-Level Summary

In immunogenicity trials, the population-level summary for treatment comparison regarding the antibody titer or concentration variable is the ratio of geometric mean titers (GMT) or geometric mean concentrations. For the variable of seroconversion, the population-level summary for treatment comparison is usually the difference in seroconversion rates. In efficacy trials, vaccine efficacy is calculated as the percentage reduction in the risk of disease when comparing the experimental vaccine to the control, and is used as the population-level summary. The quantification of the risk of disease depends on the variable, such as the person-year incidence rate when the variable is the occurrence of the disease or the hazard rate when the variable is the time to the disease onset.

10.5.3 *Case Study*

10.5.3.1 Trial Objective and Design

We consider a randomized, double-blind, equivalence trial to evaluate the lot-to-lot consistency among three consecutive lots of a rabies vaccine. A total of 594 healthy subjects aged 10–60 years are randomized in a 1:1:1 ratio to receive one of the three lots of the rabies vaccine in a five-dose regimen (days 0, 3, 7, 14, and 28). Blood samples are collected for immunogenicity evaluation prior to dose 1, 14 days post dose 1, and 14 days post dose 5.

The primary objective of the trial is to demonstrate the equivalence of anti-rabies virus antibody titers at 14 days post dose 5 between each pair of lots in baseline seronegative subjects. The lot-to-lot consistency is to be claimed if the 95% confidence intervals of the GMT ratios of anti-rabies virus antibody titers at 14 days post dose 5 between each pair of lots fall within the range of 2/3–3/2.

10.5.3.2 Estimand Considerations

The trial aims to compare each pair of three consecutive lots of rabies vaccine in healthy subjects aged 10–60 years, who are seronegative at baseline and who would have completed all five doses regardless of treatment assignment. The primary objective is to demonstrate the clinical equivalence between each pair of the vaccine lots in terms of anti-rabies antibody titers at 14 days post dose 5 (assessed via the ratio of GMTs), in the absence of concomitant vaccines or medications within 14 days of vaccination that can affect the immune response.

This trial was planned and conducted before the release of the ICH E9 (R1) guideline. Based on the original trial objective and corresponding analyses and estimand considerations in Sect. 10.5.2, the primary estimand and its five attributes of this trial can, therefore, be formulated retrospectively as follows. The primary analysis is aligned with this estimand.

(a) Population: Healthy subjects aged 10–60 years, who are seronegative at baseline and who would have completed all five doses regardless of treatment assignment. The seronegative subjects are the sensitive population to detect potential differences in immunogenicity data, which are preferred in lot-to-lot consistency trials from a clinical perspective. The primary population, defined by the principal stratum who would complete all five doses, is therefore of interest for the clinical question to assess the vaccine-induced immune response after completion of the full series of vaccinations.
(b) Variable: Anti-rabies virus antibody titers at 14 days after dose 5.
(c) Treatment: Rabies vaccine from three consecutive manufacturing lots administered in a five-dose regimen on days 0, 3, 7, 14, and 28, if concomitant vaccines or medications would not be available within 14 days of vaccination.

(d) Intercurrent events and strategies are described in Table 10.5. Besides the intercurrent event of not completing the full vaccine regimen, which is addressed by the principal stratum strategy (incorporated in the definition of population), this trial also considers the impact of using concomitant vaccines or medications within 14 days of full vaccination that can affect the immune response. A hypothetical strategy is utilized to address this intercurrent event, as subsequent immune responses measured after this event may be confounded and unsuitable for assessing the immunogenicity induced by the rabies vaccine. The clinical question of interest is to compare the antibody titers of each pair without this intercurrent event. Therefore, the hypothetical strategy is implemented to allow for the assessment of the treatment effect in a scenario where this intercurrent event would not have occurred, as described in the treatment attribute above.
(e) Population-level summary: The ratio of GMTs between each pair of lots.

10.5.3.3 Statistical Analysis

10.5.3.3.1 Analysis Set

According to the definition of the population in the primary estimand, the clinical interest is on the immunogenicity in the principal stratum of baseline seronegative subjects, who would complete all five doses following the 0-, 3-, 7-, 14-, and 28-day immunization schedule, regardless of treatment assignment. In this trial, the treatment across arms is the same rabies vaccine but from three different manufacturing lots. It is, therefore, reasonable to assume that there is no difference in terms of adverse reactions to the vaccine across the three arms and that the intercurrent event of not completing the vaccine regimen due to adverse events is not related to the treatment arm. Also, the intercurrent event of not completing the

Table 10.5 Proposed estimand strategies

Intercurrent events	Strategies	Comments
Not completing the vaccine regimen (e.g., due to loss to follow-up, withdrawal of informed consent, or adverse events)	Principal stratum strategy	This strategy defines the population in a subset of subjects who would not have this intercurrent event regardless of treatment assignment
Use of concomitant vaccines or medications within 14 days of full vaccination that could affect the immune response	Hypothetical strategy	This intercurrent event confounds subsequent immunogenicity data, and any measured values afterward are not appropriate to be used for equivalence assessment. Under this strategy, equivalence is assessed in a hypothetical scenario that this intercurrent event would not have occurred

vaccine regimen due to loss to follow-up or withdrawal of informed consent is considered to be at random. Under these assumptions, the subset of subjects who complete all five doses is considered to be unbiased to the principal stratum. Therefore, an analysis set, which includes all randomized subjects who are sero-negative at baseline and complete all five doses, is used for the primary analysis of the primary estimand.

10.5.3.3.2 Primary Analysis

The primary analysis employs an analysis of variance model based on the analysis set defined in Sect. 10.5.3.3.1. The model includes the log-transformed post-vaccination antibody titer as the dependent variable, treatment as the fixed effect, and log-transformed pre-vaccination antibody titer as a covariate. From the model, the least square-adjusted GMT in each arm and the GMT ratio between each pair of lots, together with their corresponding 95% confidence intervals, are estimated. Note that the estimate from subjects who complete the vaccine regimen is unbiased to the principal stratum estimand only under the assumed conditions. Therefore, conducting sensitivity analyses to assess the robustness of the primary analysis results in light of deviations from these assumptions may be necessary. The necessity of these sensitivity analyses also depends on the proportion of subjects who do not complete the vaccine regimen.

As an implementation of the hypothetical strategy, the last observation carried forward method is employed to impute the missing data in the primary analysis. To assess the robustness of the primary analysis, a tipping point analysis is also conducted under the assumption of missing not at random. Note that the last observation carried forward method, as described in Sect. 22.2 of Chap. 22, may not be a conservative approach in equivalence trials. Alternative imputation methods, such as multiple imputation, can be considered to improve assay sensitivity.

10.5.4 Summary and Discussion

This case represents a typical immunogenicity vaccine trial, and the estimand framework is illustrated. The primary population of medical interest in vaccine trials usually comprises subjects who have completed the full vaccine regimen. This is different from other therapeutic areas where patients who have taken at least one dose are the target population of interest. Considering whether or not completing the assigned vaccine regimen is observed post-randomization, the principal stratum strategy is an appropriate approach to define the target population, based on their potential compliance status with the vaccination. However, since it is generally unknown about the subjects' membership to the principal stratum, specific assumptions are needed to make a valid estimate of the treatment effect within a principal stratum. In this case, sensitivity analyses may also be necessary to evaluate the robustness of the primary results if the given assumptions are violated. Similar considerations also apply to efficacy trials, for which common intercurrent events and the corresponding strategies are discussed in Table 10.4.

10.6 Concluding Remarks

In conclusion, this chapter has illustrated the challenges and considerations involved when implementing the estimand framework in various therapeutic areas. As demonstrated by the case studies, it is critical to define clear trial objectives first and then establish meaningful estimands.

Depending on the trial objectives, different primary endpoints/variables may be used in the same disease setting. For instance, as illustrated in Sect. 10.5.2, in the preventive vaccine area, the primary variable in an immunogenicity clinical trial is different from that in an efficacy clinical trial. In the field of chronic heart failure, time to the first occurrence of any event in the composite of cardiovascular death, hospitalization for heart failure, or an urgent heart failure visit can serve as the primary efficacy variable. Similarly, in the asthma disease setting, the annual asthma exacerbation rate can be used as the primary efficacy variable. Consequently, the corresponding estimands need to be defined differently to ensure accurate assessment and interpretation of the treatment outcomes. We encourage readers to refer to the relevant chapters in Part IV of this book for discussions on statistical analysis under the estimand framework (Chap. 16 for binary endpoints and Chap. 18 for time-to-event endpoints).

As shown in the case studies, the treatment policy strategy is quite common for addressing intercurrent events like treatment discontinuation, the use of concomitant or rescue treatment, and treatment switch to reflect clinical practice in chronic disease clinical trials. Nonetheless, it is imperative to explore additional strategies for intercurrent events and supplementary analyses to ensure the robustness and reliability of the treatment effect assessment. Most importantly, initiating early discussions and achieving alignment between trial sponsors and regulatory agencies are essential to guarantee the scientific robustness and regulatory success of the clinical trials.

References

Braunwald, E. (2015). The war against heart failure: The lancet lecture. *The Lancet, 385*, 812–824.

Degtyarev, E., Rufibach, K., Shentu, Y., Yung, G., Casey, M., Industry Working Group on Estimands in Oncology, et al. (2020). Assessing the impact of COVID-19 on the clinical trial objective and analysis of oncology clinical trials-application of the estimand framework. *Statistics in Biopharmaceutical Research, 12*, 427–437.

Dmitrienko, A., Millen, B. A., Brechenmacher, T., & Paux, G. (2011). Development of gatekeeping strategies in confirmatory clinical trials. *Biometrical Journal, 53*, 875–893.

EMA. (2023). *Guideline on clinical evaluation of vaccines (draft)*. https://www.ema.europa.eu/en/documents/scientific-guideline/guideline-clinical-evaluation-vaccines-revision-1_en.pdf

FDA. (2023). *COVID-19: Developing drugs and biological products for treatment or prevention*. https://www.fda.gov/

Ferreira, J. P., Duarte, K., Graves, T. L., Zile, M. R., Abraham, W. T., et al. (2016). Natriuretic peptides, 6-min walk test, and quality-of-life questionnaires as clinically meaningful endpoints in HF trials. *Journal of the American College of Cardiology, 68*, 2690–2707.

Fitchett, D., Zinman, B., Wanner, C., Lachin, J. M., Hantel, S., et al. (2016). Heart failure outcomes with empagliflozin in patients with type 2 diabetes at high cardiovascular risk: Results of the EMPA-REG OUTCOME® trial. *European Heart Journal, 37*, 1526–1534.

Fu, R., Li, H., Wang, X., Shou, Q., & Wang, W. W. B. (2023). Application of estimand framework in ICH E9 (R1) to vaccine trials. *Journal of Biopharmaceutical Statistics, 33*, 502–513.

Gilbert, P. B., Shepherd, B. E., & Hudgens, M. G. (2013). Sensitivity analysis of per-protocol time-to-event treatment efficacy in randomized clinical trials. *Journal of the American Statistical Association, 108*, 1. https://doi.org/10.1080/01621459.2013.786649

GINA. (2019). *Global strategy for asthma management and prevention*. http://www.ginasthma.org/

Hodges, J. L., & Lehmann, E. L. (1963). Estimates of location based on rank tests. *The Annals of Mathematical Statistics, 34*, 598–611.

Iwaz, J. A., Le, E., Aramin, H., Romero, D., Iqbal, N., et al. (2016). New targets in the drug treatment of heart failure. *Drugs, 79*, 187–201.

Jiang, Z., Wang, X., & Xia, J. (2021). Considerations on the clinical development of COVID-19 vaccine from trial design perspectives. *Human Vaccines & Immunotherapeutics, 17*, 656–660.

Joura, E. A., Giuliano, A. R., Iversen, O. E., Bouchard, C., Mao, C., et al. (2015). A 9-valent HPV vaccine against infection and intraepithelial neoplasia in women. *The New England Journal of Medicine, 372*, 711–723.

Kaabi, N. A., Zhang, Y., Xia, S., Yang, Y., Aqhtani, M. A., et al. (2021). Effect of 2 inactivated SARS-CoV-2 vaccines on symptomatic COVID-19 infection in adults: A randomized clinical trial. *The Journal of the American Medical Association, 326*, 35–45.

Koch, G. G., Tangen, C. M., Jung, J. W., & Amara, I. A. (1998). Issues for covariance analysis of dichotomous and ordered categorical data from randomized clinical trials and non-parametric strategies for addressing them. *Statistics in Medicine, 17*, 1863–1892.

Lee, L. A., Bailes, Z., Barnes, N., Boulet, L. P., Edwards, D., et al. (2021). Efficacy and safety of once-daily single-inhaler triple therapy (FF/UMEC/VI) versus FF/VI in patients with inadequately controlled asthma (CAPTAIN): A double-blind, randomised, phase 3A trial. *The Lancet Respiratory Medicine, 9*, 69–84.

Li, R., Liu, L., Mo, Z., Wang, X., Xia, J., et al. (2014). An inactivated enterovirus 71 vaccine in healthy children. *The New England Journal of Medicine, 370*, 829–837.

Lou, Y., Jones, M. P., & Sun, W. (2019). Assessing the ratio of means as a causal estimand in clinical endpoint bioequivalence studies in the presence of intercurrent events. *Statistics in Medicine, 38*, 5214–5235.

McDonagh, T. A., Metra, M., Adamo, M., ESC Scientific Document Group, et al. (2021). ESC guidelines for the diagnosis and treatment of acute and chronic heart failure: Developed by the task force for the diagnosis and treatment of acute and chronic heart failure of the European Society of Cardiology (ESC) with the special contribution of the heart failure association (HFA) of the ESC. *European Heart Journal, 36*, 3599–3726. https://doi.org/10.1093/eurheartj/ehab368

McDonagh, T. A., Metra, M., Adamo, M., ESC Scientific Document Group, et al. (2023). Focused update of the 2021 ESC guidelines for the diagnosis and treatment of acute and chronic heart failure: Developed by the task force for the diagnosis and treatment of acute and chronic heart failure of the European Society of Cardiology (ESC) with the special contribution of the heart failure association (HFA) of the ESC. *European Heart Journal, 44*, 3627–3639.

McMurray, J. J. V., Docherty, K. F., de Boer, R. A., Hammarstedt, A., Kitzman, D. W., et al. (2023). Effect of dapagliflozin versus placebo on symptoms and 6-minute walk distance in patients with heart failure: The DETERMINE randomized clinical trials. *Circulation, 149*, 825–838.

Nauta, J. (2024). Estimand for non-inferiority influenza vaccine immunogenicity trials. *Vaccine, 42*, 840–843.

NCT02924688. (n.d.) *Study protocol*. Retrieved December 31, 2023, from https://classic.clinicaltrials.gov/ProvidedDocs/88/NCT02924688/Prot_000.pdf

NCT03877237. (n.d.). *DETERMINE-reduced study protocol and statistical analysis plan*. Retrieved December 31, 2023, from https://clinicaltrials.gov/ct2/show/NCT03877237

NCT04358081. (n.d.). *Study protocol*. Retrieved September 9, 2023, from https://classic.clinicaltrials.gov/ProvidedDocs/81/NCT04358081/Prot_000.pdf

Neal, B., Perkovic, V., Mahaffey, K. W., de Zeeuw, D., Fulcher, G., for the CANVAS Program Collaborative Group, et al. (2017). Canagliflozin and cardiovascular and renal events in type 2 diabetes. *The New England Journal of Medicine, 377*, 644–657.

Permutt, T., & Li, F. (2017). Trimmed means for symptom trials with dropouts. *Pharmaceutical Statistics, 16*, 20–28.

Rådholm, K., Figtree, G., Perkovic, V., Solomon, S. D., Mahaffey, K. W., et al. (2018). Canagliflozin and heart failure in type 2 diabetes mellitus: Results from the CANVAS program. *Circulation, 138*, 458–468.

Ruiz-Palacios, G. M., Pérez-Schael, I., Velázquez, F. R., Abate, H., Breuer, T., et al. (2006). Safety and efficacy of an attenuated vaccine against severe rotavirus gastroenteritis. *The New England Journal of Medicine, 354*, 11–22.

World Health Organization (WHO). (2023). *Coronavirus disease (COVID-19) pandemic*. https://www.who.int/emergencies/diseases/novel-coronavirus-2019?adgroupsurvey=%7badgroupsurvey%7d&gclid=EAIaIQobChMI78reqcCugAMVPCqDAx2EjgOoEAAYASAAEgJ3_PD_BwE

Yassi, N., Hayward, K. S., Campbell, B. C. V., & Churilov, L. (2021). Use of the estimand framework to manage the disruptive effects of COVID-19 on stroke clinical trials. *Stroke, 52*, 3739–3747.

Zinman, B., Wanner, C., Lachin, J. M., Fitchett, D., Bluhmki, E., et al. (2015). Empagliflozin, cardiovascular outcomes, and mortality in type 2 diabetes. *The New England Journal of Medicine, 373*, 2117–2128.

Part III
Regulatory Guidelines and Their Relationship to the Estimand Framework

This part of the book provides a detailed overview of regulatory guidelines related to the use of the estimand framework in clinical trials. It begins with a comprehensive description of guidelines issued by the International Council for Harmonisation (ICH), including ICH E8(R1), ICH M11, and ICH E20. Subsequent chapters review disease-specific guidance documents released by national or regional regulatory agencies, starting with guidelines from the European Medicines Agency (EMA) on conditions such as diabetes mellitus, Alzheimer's disease, chronic noninfectious liver diseases, chronic heart failure, and gout. It then turns to the US Food and Drug Administration (FDA), highlighting the incorporation of estimand principles in guidelines for the treatment of acute myeloid leukemia, chronic rhinosinusitis with nasal polyps, COVID-19, and eosinophilic esophagitis. Finally, this part concludes with a review of guidelines from the China National Medical Products Administration (NMPA), including documents addressing Crohn's disease, ulcerative colitis, real-world evidence, and pediatric extrapolation.

Chapter 11
ICH Guidelines and Their Relationship to the Estimand Framework

Cui Xiong, Frank Bretz, Jiawei Wei, Byron Jones, Christine Fletcher, William W. Wang, Jun Wang, Luyan Dai, Jielai Xia, and Jianhong Pan

Abstract The International Council for Harmonisation (ICH) develops guidelines to standardize pharmaceutical development, strengthen global regulatory practices, and enhance the reliability of clinical trials. Among these, the ICH E9(R1) guide-

---

C. Xiong (✉)
Biostatistics, GlaxoSmithKline, Shanghai, China
e-mail: cui.2.xiong@gsk.com

F. Bretz
Advanced Methodology and Data Sciences, Novartis, Basel, Switzerland
e-mail: frank.bretz@novartis.com

J. Wei
Advanced Methodology and Data Sciences, Novartis Institutes for Biomedical Research Co., Shanghai, China
e-mail: jiawei.wei@novartis.com

B. Jones
Patient Engagement Data Science, Novartis Pharma AG, Basel, Switzerland
e-mail: byron.jones_ext@novartis.com

C. Fletcher
Biostatistics, GlaxoSmithKline, Stevenage, UK
e-mail: chrissie.a.fletcher@gsk.com

W. W. Wang
Biostatistics and Research Decision Sciences (BARDS), Merck & Co., Inc, Rahway, NJ, USA
e-mail: William_wang@merck.com

J. Wang · J. Pan
Office of Statistics and Clinial Pharmacology, Center for Drug Evaluation, National Medical Products Administration, Beijing, China
e-mail: wangj@cde.org.cn; panjh@cde.org.cn

L. Dai
Graceful Plume Consulting, Shanghai, China
e-mail: luyan.dai@g-plume.com

J. Xia
Xijing Hospital, Xian, China
e-mail: xiajielai@fmmu.edu.cn

J. Wei et al. (eds.), *Estimands in Clinical Trials*, Springer Series in Pharmaceutical Statistics, https://doi.org/10.1007/978-3-032-02192-2_11

line, published in 2019, provides a structured framework for aligning clinical trial objectives, design, data collection, and analysis approaches. Given its broad relevance, the ICH E9(R1) guideline is closely related to other ICH guidelines. This chapter focuses on the relationship between the estimand framework in the ICH E9(R1) guideline and other ICH guidelines, including ICH E8(R1), ICH M11, and ICH E20, along with earlier ICH guidelines predating the formal introduction of the estimand framework The discussion highlights how these guidelines either align with the principles of the estimand framework or may be influenced by the ICH E9(R1) guideline during their implementation. Understanding these interconnections can help harmonize global practices, refine the scientific and statistical rigor of clinical trials, improve trial transparency and reliability, and ensure high-quality, evidence-based regulatory decisions.

11.1 Introduction

The International Council for Harmonisation (ICH) of Technical Requirements for Pharmaceuticals for Human Use was established in 1990 as a collaborative effort between regulatory authorities and the pharmaceutical industry of the United States, Europe, and Japan. Since then, ICH has expanded its membership over the years to include regulatory authorities and pharmaceutical associations from many other regions and countries.

The primary goal of ICH is to promote global harmonization in the development, registration, and post-approval processes of pharmaceutical products. By fostering international collaboration and mutual acceptance of scientific and technical standards, ICH aims to ensure that safe, effective, and high-quality medicines are developed, registered, and maintained in the most resource-efficient manner while meeting high standards.

Over the years, ICH has produced a range of significant guidelines and documents that have become instrumental in guiding the pharmaceutical industry's practices and regulatory decision-making. ICH operates through four main categories of guidelines: Efficacy (E), Safety (S), Quality (Q), and Multidisciplinary (M).

- Efficacy guidelines focus on the design, conduct, safety, and reporting of clinical trials. It also covers novel types of medicines derived from biotechnological processes and the use of pharmacogenetic/genomic techniques to produce better targeted medicines.
- Safety guidelines help uncover potential risks like carcinogenicity, genotoxicity, and reprotoxicity. A recent breakthrough has been a nonclinical testing strategy for assessing the QT interval prolongation liability: the single most important cause of drug withdrawals in recent years.
- Quality guidelines include the conduct of stability studies, defining relevant thresholds for impurity testing and a more flexible approach to pharmaceutical quality based on Good Manufacturing Practice risk management.

- Multidisciplinary guidelines address topics that do not fit uniquely into one of the Quality, Safety, and Efficacy categories. They include the ICH medical terminology Medical Dictionary for Regulatory Activities (MedDRA), the Common Technical Document, and the development of the Electronic Standards for the Transfer of Regulatory Information.

The formal ICH procedure is a stepwise process consisting of five steps (ICH, 2023). This procedure is followed for the harmonization of all new ICH topics and is initiated with the endorsement by the ICH assembly of a concept paper and business plan. An Expert Working Group (EWG) is subsequently established. The EWG works to develop a draft guideline and take it through the various steps of the procedure, which culminate in Step 5 and the implementation of a harmonized guideline in the ICH regions.

- Step 1: The EWG works on a consensus draft of the technical document, based on the objectives set out in the concept paper.
- Step 2: When consensus on the Step 1 expert technical document is reached and adopted by the ICH assembly, the ICH regulatory members will take the actions they deem necessary to develop the draft guideline.
- Step 3: Occurring in three distinct stages, this includes regulatory consultation, discussion, and the finalization of the Step 3 expert draft guideline.
- Step 4: The Step 4 final document is adopted by the ICH regulatory members of the ICH assembly as an ICH harmonized guideline.
- Step 5: The regulatory implementation is carried out according to the same national/regional procedures that apply to other regional regulatory guidelines and requirements in the ICH regions.

The success of ICH can be attributed to several factors. First, the organization's unique collaborative model brings together regulatory authorities and industry representatives from different regions, fostering the exchange of expertise, perspectives, and experiences. Second, ICH's commitment to transparency and openness in the guideline development process has enhanced trust and credibility among stakeholders, contributing to the widespread adoption of ICH guidelines by regulatory agencies worldwide. Third, ICH's ability to adapt and address emerging challenges in the pharmaceutical industry, such as advances in science and technology, has kept its guidelines relevant and up-to-date. Last, the voluntary nature of ICH guidelines allows countries to implement them based on their specific needs and regulations, further facilitating their adoption across various regulatory frameworks.

In this chapter, we review recent ICH guidelines that refer to the estimand framework, as introduced by ICH (2019a, 2019b), which by itself is an ICH guideline in the form of an addendum to the ICH E9 guideline (ICH, 1998). Section 11.2 discusses considerations that are closely related to the estimand framework, as part of the ICH E8(R1) guideline on general considerations for clinical trials. Section 11.3 summarizes key estimand considerations for the clinical electronic structured harmonised protocol (CeSHarP) introduced by the draft ICH M11 guideline. Section 11.4 discusses how the estimand framework applies to adaptive clinical trials according to the forthcoming draft ICH E20 guideline. Other ICH guidelines that refer to concepts related to the estimand framework are briefly discussed in Section 11.5. Where applicable, we provide, in each section, an introduction to the guideline, its key estimand considerations, and a brief summary.

11.2 ICH E8(R1) on General Considerations for Clinical Studies

11.2.1 Introduction

In July 1997, the ICH officially released the ICH E8 guideline on general considerations for clinical studies (ICH, 1997). Its revision, ICH E8(R1), was adopted by the regulatory members of the ICH assembly under Step 4 in October 2021 (ICH, 2021); it provides guidance on the clinical development life cycle, including designing quality into clinical trials, considering the broad range of clinical trial designs and data sources used.

One of the key purposes of this guideline is to emphasize that clinical trials should be designed, planned, conducted, analyzed, and reported according to sound scientific principles to achieve their objectives. The primary objective of any clinical trial should be clearly and explicitly stated and reflect the scientific questions that the trial needs to answer.

The ICH E8(R1) guideline states that the development plan should cover the entire product life cycle, including different stages of drug development. Trials should be strictly designed around achieving trial objectives and carefully consider design elements, such as the selection of trial populations, response variables, corresponding analysis methods, possible intercurrent events, and strategies to address them, while also minimizing biases as much as possible. This should be done using the principles of quality-by-design. Building quality into the design is a key recommendation of the ICH E8(R1) guideline.

As described in the ICH E8(R1) guideline, there is now a wide range of trial designs and data sources to choose from, including those with and without randomization. The purpose of a clinical trial will affect the selection of trial design and data sources, thereby affecting regulatory decisions and clinical practice. Clear objectives will help specify the trial design, and conversely, the process of specifying the design may help further clarify the objectives. At the planning stage, the objectives may need to be modified if substantial practical considerations and limitations or other risks to critical-to-quality factors are identified. The trial objectives are further refined through the specification of estimands. Estimands, as discussed in the ICH E9(R1) guideline, provide a precise description of the treatment effects that reflect the clinical questions posed by the trial objectives (ICH, 2019a, 2019b). An estimand summarizes at a population level what the outcomes would be in the same patients under the different treatment conditions being compared.

11.2.2 Considerations for Estimands

The ICH E8(R1) guideline discusses several important quality factors in clinical trials, including the population; treatment; response variables; methods for reducing bias, such as randomization; and statistical analysis. These factors are aligned with the basic principles of the ICH E9(R1) guideline.

- Population
  The trial population should be selected to support the trial objective and reflect the target population. The inclusion and exclusion criteria for the trial population should be clearly defined.
- Variable (or Endpoint)
  Variables (or endpoints) are attributes of interest that may be affected by the drug. Variables may originate from pharmacokinetics, pharmacodynamics, efficacy, and/or safety or focus on the use of the drug, for example, the adherence to risk minimization measures after approval. The trial endpoints are the response variables used to evaluate the drug effects.
- Treatment
  The treatment(s), including the control arm(s), should be clearly and specifically described. Treatment may be an individual treatment (different doses or regimens), combinations of treatments, or no treatments and may also include background therapy. The definition of treatment should align with the trial's purpose.
- Methods to Reduce Bias: Consideration of Intercurrent Events
  Potential sources of bias that may affect the reliability of the results should be scientifically controlled in the trial design. As mentioned in the ICH E8(R1) guideline, randomization can effectively minimize the possibility of selection bias in treatment allocation, but it cannot prevent bias generated by other confounding factors that occur during the trial after randomization. Events that occur after randomization, particularly intercurrent events, may affect the validity and interpretation of comparisons between the treatment arms. Intercurrent events may also lead to changes in follow-up patterns between the treatment arms. For example, patients in different arms may terminate the trial at different rates due to adverse events or a lack of efficacy. Careful consideration of intercurrent events during the trial process, evaluating their impact on the results, will help clarify important factors that affect the quality of the trial, such as minimizing trial withdrawal and collecting data after treatment discontinuation as much as possible (if applicable). When defining the treatment effect (estimand), consideration of the occurrence and addressing of intercurrent events is particularly important.
- Statistical Analysis
  The statistical analysis of clinical trials should enable the trial to address its trial objectives. The protocol should provide a detailed definition of the estimands for the primary and secondary objectives and a summary of the planned statistical analyses. The protocol should also prespecify sensitivity analyses for each estimand to evaluate the impact of assumptions made in the primary and secondary

analyses on the trial results. The statistical analysis plan should provide more detailed descriptions of the statistical analysis of the primary and secondary endpoints of the trial and can provide further details of the corresponding estimands.

11.2.3 Summary and Discussion

Taken together, the basic principles of the ICH E8(R1) and ICH E9(R1) guidelines emphasize the importance of clearly defining the trial objectives, which should lead to the choice of corresponding estimands. It should be noted that these basic principles apply to research at all stages, such as pre- and post-approval studies, as well as to different types of trials, such as interventional and observational trials. Throughout the product life cycle (i.e., different stages of drug development), research plans should be defined as early as possible, and clinical scientific questions that need to be answered and the corresponding research objectives should be determined early on. Communication with regulatory authorities should be conducted in a timely manner to achieve consensus throughout the drug development stages. Additionally, estimands and planned statistical analyses should be agreed upon when trials are being designed.

11.3 ICH M11 on Clinical Electronic Structured Harmonised Protocol

11.3.1 Introduction

In March 2025, the ICH signed off the ICH M11 guideline on clinical electronic structured harmonised protocol (CeSHarP) (ICH, 2025a) as a Step 2 document to be issued by the ICH regulatory members for a second public consultation, thereby subject to change due to public comments. The ICH M11 guideline is a new harmonized guideline on clinical protocols that specifies comprehensive organization with standardized content (including both required and optional components).

The purpose of the guideline is to describe the general protocol design principles and approach used to develop the separate associated documents, the ICH M11 clinical electronic structured harmonised protocol template (template), and the technical specification of the template that are acceptable to all regulatory authorities of the ICH regions. The template and technical specification are applicable to interventional clinical trials of medicinal products across all phases and therapeutic areas of clinical research. In this section, we will focus on the protocol template.

A clinical protocol describes the processes and procedures directing the conduct and analysis of a clinical trial of medicinal product(s) in humans. To date, no internationally adopted harmonized standard has been established for the format and content of the clinical protocol to support consistency across sponsors and health authority review across regions and for the electronic exchange of protocol information.

The protocol template was designed based on general principles that would support a harmonized standard protocol to facilitate consistency and efficiency in the development, amendment, review, conduct, and closeout of a clinical trial and the exchange of protocol information. The use of the clinical trial protocol template aids the sponsor or sponsor investigator in the development of a protocol that is complete, free from ambiguity, well-organized, and aligned with the quality-by-design principles, as set forth in other ICH guidelines. By conveying information consistently and in the same location across clinical trial protocols, the protocol template is intended to provide value to all parties that include sponsors, investigators, clinical site personnel, trial patients, ethics committees, and regulators.

11.3.2 Considerations for Estimands

The template presents the format and structure of the protocol, including the table of contents, common headers, and contents. It must clearly support the development of a final protocol that meets the needs of its diverse audience, which includes investigators, site staff, regulatory reviewers, and sponsor personnel. The template aligns with the estimand framework and requires relevant estimand discussions in, but not limited to, the following sections.

11.3.2.1 Section 3 on "Trial Objectives and Associated Estimands"

This section should precisely define each trial objective and refine each trial objective into a precise clinical question of interest by defining the associated estimand. For all trials, each primary trial objective should be precisely stated by providing a "meaningful and concise description of the treatment effect of interest using natural, nontechnical language for clear understanding of sponsors, investigators, clinical site personnel, trial participants, ethics committees, and regulators."

When constructing an estimand for trials intended to estimate a treatment effect or test a hypothesis related to a treatment effect, all estimand attributes need to be described, including the treatment, the endpoint (or variable), the population of patients targeted by the clinical question of interest, other intercurrent events (if applicable), and a population-level summary. As stated in ICH (2025a), precise specifications of treatment, population, and variables are likely to address many of the key intercurrent events. Other key intercurrent events not already addressed in the clinical question of interest by the aforementioned attributes should be described with their associated strategies.

11.3.2.2 Section 4 on "Trial Design," Especially Section 4.2.1 on "Rationale for Estimand(s)"

It is important to provide a rationale for the estimand(s) described in Sect. 3 on "Trial Objectives and Associated Estimands." This should include a rationale that the selected endpoint(s) are clinically relevant and provide a reliable and valid measurement of the intended intervention effect. It should also include a rationale for the selected strategies for addressing intercurrent events.

11.3.2.3 Section 7 on "Participant Discontinuation of Trial Intervention and Discontinuation or Withdrawal from Trial"

This section must align with the intercurrent events introduced in Sect. 3 on "Trial Objectives and Associated Estimands" and the treatment described in Sect. 6 on "Trial Intervention and Concomitant Therapy."

11.3.2.4 Section 10 on "Statistical Considerations," Especially Section 10.4 and Section 10.5

Section 10.4 on "Analyses Associated with the Primary Objective(s)" introduces the statistical analysis plan and provides an overview of the subsequent subsections that will provide the details. It entails explaining the methods of estimation (analytic approach) in alignment with the defined estimands. Sensitivity analyses and how their assumptions changed from the assumptions of the main statistical analysis should also be described. Moreover, supplementary analysis should be described, if applicable.

It is important to ensure that the statistical hypothesis/model/analysis (and the corresponding assumptions) align with the primary estimand(s).

For each intercurrent event related to the primary estimand(s), a clear explanation should be provided on how the data will be addressed during the statistical analysis in accordance with the primary estimand. Addressing the intercurrent events through the statistical analysis should be aligned with the specific estimand strategies being employed.

Furthermore, this section should outline the approach for dealing with missing data. When the estimand framework is employed, reference should be made to the E9(R1) guideline.

Section 10.5 on "Analysis Associated with the Secondary Objective(s)" focuses on estimands for secondary objectives. Here, the statistical analysis, addressing of intercurrent events, handling of missing data, sensitivity analysis, and supplementary analysis corresponding to each secondary estimand should be described.

Finally, Section 10.11 on "Sample Size Determination" emphasizes that the sample size calculation should be aligned with the primary estimand and the primary analysis; otherwise, a justification is needed.

11.3.3 Summary and Discussion

A harmonized clinical protocol template and technical specification for electronic exchange of protocol information will enhance the ability of sponsors, regulators, investigators, and other stakeholders to initiate, review, and conduct clinical research, resulting in more efficient drug development and delivery of medicines to patients. The protocol template also provides a harmonized standard for estimand definition and related discussions in terms of format and content to support consistency across sponsors. Additionally, it is crucial that estimands and analysis approaches are aligned to inform an adequate sample size.

The recommendations in this section are also aligned with the ICH E6(R3) guideline on good clinical practice, which offers recommendations on the various aspects of a clinical trial that should be included in a protocol (ICH, 2025b). Importantly, ICH (2025b) emphasizes the need to document estimands in the protocol section on "Trial Objectives and Purpose," thereby providing a clear description of the scientific objectives and the purpose of the trial.

11.4 ICH E20 on Adaptive Clinical Trials

11.4.1 Introduction

In June 2018, the ICH assembly endorsed a new topic, E20 on adaptive clinical trials. As described in the ICH E20 Concept Paper (ICH, 2019a, 2019b), there is an increasing interest in using adaptive clinical trials in modern drug development. The potential advantages of adaptive designs include limiting patient exposure to unsafe or ineffective treatments, saving trial resources, and accelerating the development process while ensuring that the adaptive clinical trials can provide the evidence for regulatory decision-making. However, there are uncertainties due to the lack of common principles for the design, conduct, analysis, and interpretation of adaptive clinical trials and the lack of common expectations for the documentation to support regulatory review. Hence, it is critical to develop a harmonized guideline to eliminate some of the limiting factors and ensure appropriate use of the potentially efficient designs in the global development of effective treatments.

An EWG was subsequently convened and held its first meeting at the end of 2019. Since then, it has been working on the development of a global harmonized regulatory guideline on the design, conduct, analysis, and interpretation of adaptive clinical trials. The goal is to provide a transparent and harmonized set of principles for the regulatory review of these studies in a global drug development program. A Step 2 document was released in 2025 for public consultation (ICH, 2025c).

The principles contained in ICH (2025c) provide a framework to evaluate and discuss innovative approaches to clinical trial design throughout the development process. For the purpose of this guideline, an adaptive design is defined as a clinical trial design that allows for prospectively planned modifications to one or more aspects of the trial based on an interim analysis of accumulating data from patients in the trial. The term "prospectively planned" means that the potential trial adaptations are planned and described in the clinical trial protocol prior to the initiation of the trial. The scope of this guideline does not include trials with unplanned modifications to the design based on external information or accumulating data within the trial.

11.4.2 Considerations for Estimands

As discussed in Sect. 11.2, adequate planning is important for all clinical trials to ensure that the design, conduct, and analysis are appropriate and that the results are reliable and interpretable. Proper trial planning distinguishes between the target of estimation (trial objective and estimand) and the analysis method. The statistical analysis of clinical trial data should be aligned with the estimands that reflect the trial objectives and ensure reliable estimates. The principal features of trial design, conduct, and statistical analysis should be described in the protocol. These include the primary estimand(s) of interest and corresponding primary analysis method(s), as well as other estimands and analysis methods important for regulatory decision-making and labeling of the product information. Further details may be provided, where necessary, in additional documents, such as the statistical analysis plan.

Adaptive designs for confirmatory trials allow for prospectively planned modifications to one or more aspects of the trial design based on an interim analysis, which should be carefully planned and properly documented. Careful planning includes following the general estimand framework from the ICH E9(R1) guideline. This is particularly true for adaptive designs, which include the selection of an estimand in an interim analysis as part of the adaptation step. Examples of such estimand selection designs include two-stage treatment selection or enrichment designs, where a treatment or a specific patient population is selected at the interim analysis. In both examples, an estimand would be selected from within a prespecified set after the first stage to continue in the trial for final inference at its conclusion. For such estimand selection designs, all candidate estimands should be properly prespecified at the planning stage of the trial. Along with the estimand(s) of interest, other aspects of trial planning should be specified prior to trial initiation, including the anticipated number and timing of interim analyses, the rationale and type of adaptation, the anticipated rule governing the adaptation decision, the statistical methods for the interim and final analyses, and procedures to maintain trial integrity.

For a given estimand, an aligned method of analysis should be implemented that allows a reliable interpretation of the analysis results at trial end. The evaluation of efficacy often involves a primary estimand of interest and a corresponding primary analysis method, with specific criteria for determining whether there is evidence of a treatment effect. The standard approach in confirmatory trials to limit erroneous conclusions of efficacy is to select the design and analysis approach such that the type I error rate with respect to the primary estimand of interest is controlled at a prespecified significance level. Some adaptive designs use Bayesian methods that involve the selection of decision criteria for the primary analysis in terms of the posterior distribution for the estimand of interest (e.g., a threshold on the posterior probability for efficacy). The thresholds should be selected such that the success criteria are clinically meaningful, and the operating characteristics of the design are appropriate. Trial protocols should include decision criteria for all primary and secondary estimands intended to be included in product labeling if the product is approved, along with a rationale for the choice of criteria, which may be different across these estimands. In addition, for a given clinical trial estimand, an aligned method of analysis should be implemented that limits the bias and variability of estimates to ensure reliable interpretation at trial end. Sensitivity analyses to assess the robustness of the conclusions to deviations from the underlying assumptions of the estimator are also important.

11.4.3 Summary and Discussion

In settings amenable to the use of an adaptive design, the added flexibility can lead to a variety of advantages. The decision to use or not use specific adaptive elements in a clinical trial, however, will often depend on many factors. It is critical to understand the extent to which the adaptive elements being considered add uncertainty about the ability of the trial to adhere to the key principles discussed in the ICH E20 guideline and, therefore, produce reliable and interpretable information. Having a clear understanding of the objectives of an adaptive trial design, i.e., its estimand(s), as well as the reliability of estimates and decisions related to those objectives, will help ensure that the trials are fit for purpose within the overall development program. Many types of adaptations concern the selection of an estimand at an interim analysis, such as treatment or population selection designs, and all candidate estimands should be properly prespecified at the planning stage of the trial. For further considerations and examples, we refer to Sect. 22.3 in this book.

11.5 ICH Guidelines Released Before ICH E9(R1)

11.5.1 Introduction

Several ICH guidelines published after the release of the ICH E9(R1) guideline either refer to estimands or align with the principles described therein. However, if we take into consideration the ICH guidelines finalized before the estimand framework was introduced, some will be impacted by the ICH E9(R1) guideline, while others have used concepts and language that are already aligned with the ICH E9(R1) guideline. For example, the ICH E2A guideline on clinical safety data management (ICH, 1994) provides requirements of expedited reporting, which should now reflect the estimand thinking introduced by the ICH E9(R1) guideline when describing and interpreting safety results. For example, if an estimand is to assess the treatment effect regardless of treatment discontinuation, then the clinical safety data after that should be collected and analyzed.

This section describes three other ICH guidelines that were released before the ICH E9(R1) guideline and are indirectly related to the estimand framework. Other ICH guidelines that will refer to the estimand framework will undoubtedly be developed in the future. One recent example is the ICH E11A guideline on pediatric extrapolation (ICH, 2024), which was released in its final form after this chapter had been accepted for publication.

11.5.2 ICH E3, E10, and E17

11.5.2.1 ICH E3

The ICH E3 guideline on the structure and content of clinical study reports, released in 1995, is a key ICH guideline (ICH, 1995). This guideline describes a comprehensive, integrated clinical study report for individual trials involving any therapeutic, prophylactic, or diagnostic agent (referred to as a drug or treatment) conducted in patients. In this report, clinical and statistical descriptions, presentations, and analyses are integrated into a single document. The impact of the ICH E9(R1) guideline on the ICH E3 guideline concerns the estimands for clinical trials designed before, whose results are reported after the release of the estimand framework. This encompasses, but is not limited to, the following aspects:

- Trial objectives
- Trial design, including the choice of control arm
- Treatment
- Efficacy and safety variables
- Trial population
- Statistical analyses

For example, the primary treatment effect of interest and relevant intercurrent events, which may impact the interpretation of the trial results, should be reflected in trial objectives. While the ICH E3 guideline is broadly aligned with the five estimand attributes (population, treatment condition, variables, intercurrent events, and summary measure), these attributes need to be explicitly addressed in clinical study reports to be aligned with the ICH E9(R1) guideline. This is particularly important for the description of intercurrent events, relevant estimand strategies, missing data assumptions, and sensitivity analyses. These elements should be well-defined in the statistical analysis section of a clinical study report. Results from the main, sensitivity, and supplementary analyses should be systematically reported in the clinical study report, specifying whether each analysis was prespecified, introduced while the trial was still blinded, or performed post hoc.

11.5.2.2 ICH E10

The ICH E10 guideline on the choice of control groups in clinical trials was released in 2000 (ICH, 2000). The purpose of this guideline is to describe the general principles involved in selecting a control group for clinical trials intended to demonstrate the efficacy of a treatment and discuss related trial design and conduct issues. The purpose of control groups is to allow discrimination of patient outcomes (for example, changes in symptoms, signs, or other morbidity) caused by an experimental treatment from outcomes caused by other factors, such as the natural progression of the disease. Consequently, the choice of the control group will be reflected in one of the estimand attributes introduced by the ICH E9(R1) guideline, specifically the treatment condition of interest.

Note that the ICH E10 guideline already anticipates causal treatment effects, in the sense that a control group experience helps infer "what would have happened to patients if they had not received the test treatment or if they had received a different treatment known to be effective" (ICH, 2000). Although the ICH E9(R1) guideline does not explicitly use the phrase "causal," it was conceived with causal treatment effects in mind. It addresses central questions for drug development and licensing, stressing the need to "establish the existence, and to estimate the magnitude, of treatment effects: how the outcome of treatment compares to what would have happened to the same subjects under alternative treatment (i.e., had they not received the treatment, or had they received a different treatment)." Therefore, both the ICH E10 and ICH E9(R1) guidelines are well-aligned and should be read in conjunction regarding the appropriate choice of the control group as part of the treatment attribute introduced with the estimand framework.

11.5.2.3 ICH E17

The ICH E17 guideline on the general principles for the planning and design of multiregional clinical trials, released in 2017, aims to increase the acceptability in global regulatory submissions (ICH, 2017). Although it was released prior to the ICH E9(R1) guideline and does not directly include the estimand concept, the requirements outlined in this guideline are aligned with the estimand framework. For instance, the ICH E17 guideline mentions that in planning a multiregional clinical trial, the primary analysis strategy should carefully consider the (1) population, (2) variables of primary interest, (3) relevant intrinsic and extrinsic factors in multiregional settings, and (4) population-level summary required to describe the treatment effect. For most multiregional clinical trials, the primary analysis will correspond to a test of the hypothesis about the treatment effect and the estimation of that effect, taking into account data from all regions and subpopulations included in the trial. This is aligned with the ICH E9(R1) guideline, even while it was still at its draft stage. Any multiregional clinical trial should include considerations about intercurrent events, which can be different between different regions (e.g., the background therapies might depend on the region, thus potentially impacting the frequency and patterns of intercurrent events).

The ICH E17 guideline also mentioned that if agreement about a single (primary) endpoint cannot be reached by the regulatory authorities due to well-justified scientific or regulatory reasons, a single protocol should be developed with endpoint-related subsections tailored to meet the respective requirements of the regulatory authorities. Therefore, if in a multiregional clinical trial, regulatory requirements for the primary estimand strategy or analysis methods differ due to well-justified scientific or regulatory reasons, the strategies planned to satisfy the different requirements should be described in the trial protocol.

Even though the ICH E17 guideline does not explicitly mention the estimand framework, applying this framework can further enhance the design and analysis of multiregional clinical trials. For example, in the consistency evaluation across regions, one can examine the consistency of each attribute of the primary or secondary estimand. The similarity of population description across regions, the compliance rate of treatment regimen across regions, the validated collection of trial endpoints, and the level of intercurrent events (e.g., the use of rescue medication) can also help elucidate the consistency of treatment effect summary metrics.

11.6 Summary

The advent of the ICH E9(R1) guideline marked a pivotal moment in the evolution of clinical research, leading to a paradigm shift in the way we conceptualize and plan clinical trials. It has changed the way of framing or designing clinical trials, including considerations for trial conduct, data collection, and planned statistical analyses. While key principles underpinning clinical research have not changed, the ICH E9(R1) guideline proposes a structured framework to strengthen the dialogue between disciplines and stakeholders involved in the formulation of clinical trial objectives, design, conduct, analysis, and interpretation, as well as the treatment effect(s) of interest that a clinical trial should address. Several ICH guidelines issued after the release of the ICH E9(R1) guideline either reference estimands or adhere to the principles outlined in it. Conversely, guidelines that were finalized prior to the introduction of the estimand framework may be affected by the ICH E9(R1) guideline. Although the ICH E9(R1) guideline introduced the estimand framework as a structured approach to describe treatment effects of interest, it is important to recognize that this does not render older guidelines obsolete. Rather, it serves as an evolutionary framework that builds upon the solid foundation laid out by, for example, the ICH E3, ICH E10, and ICH E17 guidelines. As a result, clinical trial sponsors must navigate the intricate landscape of regulatory guidelines to ensure a comprehensive approach to estimands. Early engagement with regulatory authorities about their requirements is important, and it is highly recommended to have early discussions with them and obtain their agreement on the proposed estimands.

References

ICH. (1994). *ICH E2A Clinical safety data management: definitions and standards for expedited reporting*. www.ich.org
ICH. (1995). *ICH E3 Structure and content of clinical study reports*. www.ich.org
ICH. (1997). *ICH E8 General considerations for clinical studies*. www.ich.org
ICH. (1998). *ICH E9 Statistical principles in clinical trials*. Step 4 document. www.ich.org
ICH. (2000). *ICH E10 Choice of control group in clinical trials*. www.ich.org
ICH. (2017). *ICH E17 General principles for planning and design of multi-regional clinical trials*. www.ich.org
ICH. (2019a). *ICH E9(R1) addendum on estimands and sensitivity analysis in clinical trials to the guideline on statistical principles for clinical trials*. Step 4 document. www.ich.org
ICH. (2019b). *Final Concept Paper ICH E20 Adaptive clinical trials*. www.ich.org
ICH. (2021). *ICH E8(R1) General considerations for clinical studies*. Step 4 document. www.ich.org
ICH. (2023). *Standard operating procedure of the ICH working groups*. Version 13.0. https://admin.ich.org/sites/default/files/inline-files/SOP_Approved_v13-0_2023_0512.pdf
ICH. (2024). *ICH E11A Paediatric extrapolation*. Step 4 document available at www.ich.org
ICH. (2025a). *ICH M11 Clinical electronic structured harmonized protocol*. Step 2 document. www.ich.org
ICH. (2025b). *ICH E6(R3) Good clinical practice (GCP)*. Step 4 document. www.ich.org
ICH. (2025c). *ICH E20 Adaptive clinical trials*. Step 2 document available at www.ich.org

Chapter 12
EMA Guidelines and Their Relationship to the Estimand Framework

Jiawei Wei, Frank Bretz, Cui Xiong, Zhiyue Huang, Xiaoling Wei, Alice Wang, Xin Zhang, Luyan Dai, Mouna Akacha, and Chunquan Ou

Abstract The European Medicines Agency (EMA) adopted the International Council for Harmonization (ICH) E9(R1) guideline on estimands and sensitivity analysis in clinical trials in early 2020. The ICH E9(R1) guideline has significantly

J. Wei (✉)
Advanced Methodology and Data Sciences, Novartis Institutes for Biomedical Research Co., Shanghai, China
e-mail: jiawei.wei@novartis.com

F. Bretz · M. Akacha
Advanced Methodology and Data Sciences, Novartis Pharma AG, Basel, Switzerland
e-mail: frank.bretz@novartis.com; mouna.akacha@novartis.com

C. Xiong
Biostatistics, GSK, Shanghai, China
e-mail: cui.2.xiong@gsk.com

Z. Huang
Quantitive Science and Evidence Generation, Astellas Pharma Inc., Shanghai, China
e-mail: zhiyue.huang@astellas.com

X. Wei
Advanced Quantitative Sciences, Novartis Institutes for Biomedical Research Co., Shanghai, China
e-mail: xiaoling.wei@novartis.com

A. Wang
Biometrics, R&D, AstraZeneca, Shanghai, China
e-mail: Alice.wang2@astrazeneca.com

X. Zhang
Global Biometrics & Data Management, Pfizer Inc., Shanghai, China
e-mail: xin.zhang6@pfizer.com

L. Dai
Graceful Plume Consulting, Shanghai, China
e-mail: luyan.dai@g-plume.com

C. Ou
Biostatistics, Southern Medical University, Guangzhou, China
e-mail: ocq@smu.edu.cn

J. Wei et al. (eds.), *Estimands in Clinical Trials*, Springer Series in Pharmaceutical Statistics, https://doi.org/10.1007/978-3-032-02192-2_12

influenced the design and analysis of confirmatory studies by providing a structured framework for addressing intercurrent events. Since its adoption, there has been a shift in how sponsors approach clinical trials for a wide range of therapeutic areas. This chapter discusses the EMA's implementation of the estimand framework across various guideline documents, including treatments for diabetes mellitus, Alzheimer's disease, chronic noninfectious liver diseases, gout, trials with recurrent event endpoints, and registry-based studies. In most of these guidelines, common intercurrent events in specific disease areas and estimand strategies were discussed, which inform trial design, data collection, and choice of analysis method.

12.1 Introduction

The European Medicines Agency (EMA) adopted in early 2020 the ICH E9(R1) guideline on estimands and sensitivity analysis in clinical trials (ICH, 2019), which came into effect July 30, 2020. Since then, sponsors conducting confirmatory studies have been embracing this new framework, and it can even be applied to other settings beyond confirmatory trials. Mészáros et al. (2023) recently surveyed the estimand strategies proposed by applicants and endorsed by regulators within the European jurisdiction. More specifically, they identified strategies for addressing intercurrent events in confirmatory central nervous system (CNS) trials and searched scientific advice letters issued by the EMA between 2017 and 2022. The authors concluded that for different occurring intercurrent events in confirmatory CNS trials, different strategies are of regulatory interest, depending on the trial objective, underlying disease properties, disease prevalence, as well as the frequency and timing of intercurrent events and their relatedness to the disease. Cro et al. (2022) also conducted a survey to evaluate how often the precise research question being addressed about an intervention (the estimand) is stated or can be determined from reported methods in phase 2–4 randomized trials. The authors concluded that the precise research question being investigated in most trials is unclear, mainly because of a lack of clarity on the approach to addressing intercurrent events. In addition, Mitroiu et al. (2020) systematically evaluated what estimands, especially what strategies for intercurrent events, are advised in EMA disease guidelines, used in sponsors' trials, and additionally requested by the EMA in assessment dossiers.

At the same time, the estimand framework found its way to some extent into various guideline documents released by the EMA, although elements and attributes of the estimand framework were present, to some extent, in guidelines long before ICH (2019). In this chapter, we focus on selected documents issued by the EMA since it adopted the addendum that have embraced the estimand framework. Section 12.2 discusses considerations of estimands in the guideline on clinical investigation of medicinal products in the treatment or prevention of diabetes mellitus. Section 12.3 provides considerations of estimands for the clinical investigation of medicines for the treatment of Alzheimer's disease. Section 12.4 summarizes the regulatory requirements for the development of medicinal products for chronic noninfectious liver diseases. Section 12.5 discusses the use of the estimand framework for treatment effect measures when using recurrent event endpoints. The use of estimands in the treatment of gout and in registry-based studies is briefly discussed in Sections 12.6 and 12.7, respectively. Where applicable, we provide in each section an introduction to the guideline, disease background, and relevant considerations for the estimands and statistical analyses.

The list of guidelines presented in this chapter is not exhaustive; it aims to offer a snapshot at this stage. For example, EMA (2018a) refers to the estimand framework when discussing the adjustment for crossover in estimating effects in oncology trials. Likewise, estimand considerations are also available for the development of new medicinal products for the treatment of Crohn's disease (EMA, 2018b) and ulcerative colitis (EMA, 2018c), depression (EMA, 2023c), among others. EMA (2020b, 2022) acknowledges that, in view of the COVID-19 pandemic and the war in Ukraine, the emergence of new unforeseen disruptive events may require the revision of the prespecified estimand and/or the addition of estimands may be warranted (see Chap. 23 in this book for more details). More recently, EMA (2023a) provides guidance to assessors of the summary of product characteristics (SmPC) in centralized procedures, and the EMA Day 80 assessment report—clinical template—was updated by incorporating the estimand framework (EMA, 2024). Moreover, applicants and marketing authorization holders are expected to consider this document when preparing an SmPC for review, e.g., in the context of a marketing authorization application or an extension of indication. As indicated in EMA (2023b), the implementation of the estimand framework outlined in ICH (2019) will result in language and concepts in many European guidelines being updated in the future.

12.2 Diabetes Mellitus

12.2.1 Introduction to Guideline Principles

In 2002, the EMA released the guideline on clinical investigation of medicinal products in the treatment or prevention of diabetes mellitus (EMA, 2002), which detailed the EMA's regulatory position on the development of new drugs for the treatment or prevention of diabetes. The guideline was initially revised in 2012, and a second version was published in 2023 (EMA, 2023d). This version significantly enriched the safety section with respect to cardiovascular events. Furthermore, it brought updates to various aspects such as treatment effects on diabetes complications, requirements for first-line indications, and so forth. As one of the key components for clinical trials, the principles of estimands for diabetes mellitus are also discussed in this version. In this section, we briefly summarize the common considerations for the estimands in randomized controlled trials of treatment for diabetes mellitus, as suggested in the guideline.

12.2.2 Disease Background

Diabetes mellitus is a metabolic disorder characterized by the presence of hyperglycemia due to defective insulin secretion, insulin action, or both. The chronic hyperglycemia of diabetes mellitus is associated with significant long-term sequelae, particularly damage, dysfunction, and failure of various organs, such as the kidneys, eyes, nerves, heart, and blood vessels.

Type I diabetes is the result of pancreatic beta-cell destruction and is prone to acute complications, such as ketoacidosis. In type I diabetes, the main goal is optimal blood glucose control to be achieved by optimal insulin replacement therapy, extensive education, and disease management. Type II diabetes is a complex disorder that involves various degrees of decreased beta-cell function, peripheral insulin resistance, and abnormal hepatic glucose metabolism. Glucose control in type II diabetes deteriorates progressively over time, and, after failure of diet and exercise alone, patients need, on average, a new intervention with glucose-lowering agents every 3–4 years to obtain/retain good control.

Studies have shown that normalization or near-normalization of blood glucose levels (evaluated by changes in glycated hemoglobin A1c (HbA1c)) in patients with type I and type II diabetes can significantly reduce the risk of microvascular complications such as retinopathy, nephropathy, and neuropathy.

12.2.3 Considerations for Estimands

This guideline suggests that the primary estimand should estimate a treatment effect based on the change in HbA1c from baseline to the end-of-trial (or other predefined time for assessment of the effect) between the experimental treatment and a control treatment. It is important to be precise with respect to the trial objectives. In particular, intercurrent events will occur after treatment initiation that affect either the interpretation or the existence of the measurements associated with the clinical question of interest. For example, a certain proportion of patients may not adhere to randomized treatment (e.g., due to intolerance, lack of efficacy) and require rescue medication or a change of background medication. It is important to consider these events prospectively and to address them when defining a treatment effect of interest. Specification of strategies to address these intercurrent events to precisely define a treatment effect of interest should then, in turn, inform trial design, data collection, and choice of estimation.

(a) Population
    The patients recruited into clinical trials must be representative of the target population in terms of demography, ethnic background, comorbidities (including cardiovascular disease), and type, duration, and severity of diabetes.

(b) Variable
Treatment of patients with type II diabetes should be based on a holistic approach to improve blood glucose levels and reduce the risk of both micro- and macrovascular complications. Even though the primary objective of the confirmatory studies with the glucose-lowering agent is to demonstrate a favorable effect on blood glucose control, it is also important to consider the effects of the test agent on other CV risk factors. Specific efficacy endpoints include:

1. Glycated hemoglobin (HbA1c) is the most widely accepted measure of overall, long-term blood glucose control in patients with diabetes. It reflects the mean glucose concentration over the past 2–3 months. Reduction of HbA1c is known to reduce the long-term risk of development of microvascular complications. Therefore, HbA1c is an appropriate primary endpoint to support a claim based on glycemic control.
2. Change in fasting plasma glucose (FPG) is an acceptable secondary efficacy endpoint. Changes in average plasma glucose recorded at regular intervals (mean of at least seven measurements: before and after each of three meals and at bedtime) or the area under the curve of glucose are also acceptable endpoints. Nocturnal hypoglycemia may also be a relevant endpoint.
3. Improvement of insulin sensitivity and beta-cell function is currently not validated as surrogate markers for the reduction of micro- and macrovascular complications but can be assessed as secondary endpoints.

(c) Treatment
The treatment arm will be experimental drugs for the treatment or delay of diabetes onset and prevention. Placebo-controlled trials are accepted when added to an established background therapy, which represents the standard of care in the studied population; however, at least one active-controlled trial (e.g., non-inferiority of the new agent to an established active comparator) is recommended to be submitted with the marketing authorization application.

(d) Intercurrent Events and Strategies
The primary target of estimation should estimate a treatment effect based on the change in HbA1c from baseline to the end-of-trial (or other predefined time for assessment of the effect) between the experimental treatment and a control treatment. The actual adherence to treatment should be reflected in the target of estimation. Specifically, the guideline highlights "patients are not expected to benefit once treatment is discontinued (e.g., due to adverse events), the treatment effect should be estimated based on observed or modelled data reflecting adherence to treatment as observed in the clinical trial," which can be interpreted as using the "treatment policy" strategy that the clinical outcome data of the variable/endpoint data after treatment discontinuation will be used for assessment, and the missing data (e.g., due to discontinuation from the trial) can be imputed based on modeled data reflecting adherence to treatment. Other important intercurrent events to consider are the changes to, or introduction of, other medications that will influence HbA1c values, including the use of protocol-defined rescue medication. The impact of additional medication complicates the evaluation of the effect of the test product compared to placebo or

Table 12.1 Intercurrent events and estimand strategies for different efficacy endpoints

Efficacy endpoints	Intercurrent events	Strategies
HbA1c	Treatment discontinuation	Treatment policy strategy
	Rescue therapy	Hypothetical strategy
	Use of other medications that will influence HbA1c values	Hypothetical strategy
FPG	Treatment discontinuation	Treatment policy strategy
	Rescue therapy	Hypothetical strategy
	Use of other medications that will influence HbA1c values	Hypothetical strategy
Insulin parameters	Rescue therapy	Composite variable strategy
	Meaningful increase in concomitant treatment	Composite variable strategy

active control. Therefore, the treatment effect can be estimated under the assumption that rescue medication, or use of other medications that will influence HbA1c values, was not introduced (hypothetical scenario), provided that a reliable estimate of that effect can be obtained.

When evaluating the treatment effect on FPG, the strategy for addressing intercurrent events can be the same as that for the primary endpoint of HbA1c.

For insulin parameters, patients with a meaningful increase in concomitant treatment or use of rescue medication would be classified as nonresponders, and it shall be reflected in the endpoint definition, such as "achieving an improvement in insulin parameters without any meaningful increase in concomitant treatment or use of rescue medication."

Based on these discussions in the guideline, the intercurrent event and relevant estimand strategies can be interpreted as presented in Table 12.1.

12.2.4 Statistical Analysis

The analytical approach, including the handling of missing data, should be aligned with the agreed estimand. For example, for the primary estimand of endpoint HbA1c, data obtained after discontinuation of treatment are of interest, and the missing data (e.g., due to trial discontinuation) after early withdrawal from treatment might be imputed, which should reflect the adherence to treatment as observed in the clinical trial. In addition, the data collected after initiation of rescue medication are not of interest (they reflect the effect of the additional or rescue medication itself); statistical modeling would be required. Modeling based on data collected in the control arm might be an acceptable approach to reflect unobserved data after discontinuation from treatment and a scenario in which additional medication was not introduced. Please note this is suggested for this case, and for illustration purposes, the reader is advised to consider their own statistical analysis for their trial.

12.2.5 Summary and Discussion

This guideline intends to address the EMA position on the topics of clinical development of new products in the treatment or delay in onset/prevention of diabetes. Although this guideline does not discuss the estimand strategies directly, it provides general principles on clinical questions of interest and estimation of treatment effect, as well as intercurrent events we need to consider in the clinical trials, which are fully aligned with the estimand framework.

In addition, the estimand considerations may be different with different health authorities; therefore, early interaction between sponsors and regulators would help achieve alignment on trial objectives and clinical questions of interest, with corresponding estimands. A motivating example is in a clinical trial for dapagliflozin that was conducted before the ICH E9(R1) guideline mentioned in Chap. 1; the FDA pointed out that the preferred analysis method was to use data after the patients had taken rescue treatment. Clearly, there are differences in the definition of the primary estimand between this case study and the guideline of EMA (2023d) on the development of new diabetes drugs. This further indicates that early interaction with regulatory authorities about the estimate and interpretation of treatment effects to reach a consensus on clinical questions to be answered as early as possible is paramount.

12.3 Alzheimer's Disease

12.3.1 Introduction to Guideline Principles

In 2018, the EMA released the guideline on clinical investigation of medicines for the treatment of Alzheimer's disease (EMA, 2018d). This guideline covers the impact of new Alzheimer's disease diagnostic criteria, including early and even asymptomatic stages of the disease. The guideline discussed the consideration points in the development, design, and analysis of trials at different disease stages. This guideline was one of the first few using the estimand framework language. In this section, we briefly summarize the common considerations for the estimands in randomized controlled trials of drugs for treating Alzheimer's disease as proposed in the guideline. The summary of considerations for estimands in Alzheimer's disease trials can be seen in Table 12.2.

Table 12.2 Intercurrent events and estimand strategies corresponding to different populations and outcomes

Population	Outcomes	Intercurrent events	Strategies	Comments
Severe Alzheimer's disease patient population	Function and global clinical assessment	Treatment discontinuation	Treatment policy strategy	Patients will not benefit after treatment, and treatment compliance is considered
		Change initial concomitant medication	Hypothetical strategy	Only effect of the investigational treatment is of interest
		Death	NA	Depends on the interest in patients' survival in the trial objective
Mild to moderate Alzheimer's disease patient population	Cognition as a primary endpoint could also be co-primary with function or global clinical assessment	Treatment discontinuation	Treatment policy strategy	Patients will not benefit after treatment and treatment compliance is considered
		Change initial concomitant medication	Hypothetical strategy	Only effect of the investigational treatment is of interest
MCI to preclinical Alzheimer's disease patient population	Composite endpoint including cognitive and functional scores	Initiate symptomatic treatment with a non-study treatment	Hypothetical strategy	Only effect of the investigational treatment is of interest
			Composite variable strategy	The occurrence of the intercurrent event is considered as disease progression
		Initiate symptomatic treatment with a non-investigational treatment	Hypothetical strategy	Only effect of the investigational treatment is of interest
			Composite variable strategy	The occurrence of the intercurrent event is considered a disease progression

12.3.2 Disease Background

Alzheimer's disease is characterized by memory impairment as the most common initial symptom, followed by impairments in other cognitive domains, behavioral and psychiatric symptoms, and functional decline, causing a significant burden to families and society. Commonly used diagnostic criteria for Alzheimer's disease include the International Working Group (IWG) criteria and the National Institute on Aging-Alzheimer's Association (NIA-AA) criteria. Both sets of criteria divide Alzheimer's disease into three stages based on disease progression: preclinical Alzheimer's disease, mild cognitive impairment (MCI) due to Alzheimer's disease, or prodromal Alzheimer's disease.

12.3.3 Considerations for Estimands

This guideline discusses the considerations for estimands in terms of population, variable, treatment, intercurrent events and strategies, and population-level summary.

(a) Population
The clinical trial population for Alzheimer's disease studies is typically divided based on disease progression. Both NIA-AA and IWG diagnostic criteria recognize the existence of a preclinical stage of Alzheimer's disease and accept the diagnosis of Alzheimer's disease with or without the use of biomarkers before the onset of dementia. Both criteria also include atypical (IWG) or non-amnestic (NIA-AA) Alzheimer's disease. However, there are differences between the two diagnostic criteria in terms of the conceptualization of Alzheimer's disease, the use of terminology, and the consideration of biomarkers in the diagnosis. Of particular note is that the preclinical Alzheimer's disease population defined by IWG criteria differs significantly from the MCI population defined by NIA-AA criteria. It is still unclear which criterion has the best sensitivity and specificity in a clinical setting. From a regulatory perspective, the following factors should be considered:

1. The preclinical population is defined as asymptomatic individuals with Alzheimer's disease pathology determined by biomarkers (e.g., Aβ and Tau).
2. There should be an open attitude toward diagnostic criteria, especially for the determination of MCI or prodromal populations, but efforts should be made to ensure that the population or homogeneous patient group with a determined rate of Alzheimer's disease dementia progression is detected.
3. Enrichment strategies are recommended to identify and characterize high-risk patients who will develop clinical symptoms during the trial.

(b) Variable

- Alzheimer's Disease Population
  For patients with Alzheimer's disease, treatment effects can be demonstrated in three areas: cognition, function, and clinical global assessments. In mild to moderate Alzheimer's disease, clinically significant cognitive improvement can be used to demonstrate treatment effect. However, the clinical significance of cognitive improvement needs to be confirmed by functional or clinical global assessment. Therefore, functional or clinical global assessment can be used as a co-primary endpoint with cognition. In severe Alzheimer's disease, function and clinical global assessments are more appropriate as primary clinical endpoints, as cognitive improvement may not be sufficient to demonstrate treatment effect.
- MCI or Prodromal Population
  Due to the limitations of existing detection tools, it is difficult to use cognitive and functional scores or clinical global assessments in clinical trials for patients with MCI or prodromal populations. Although composite endpoints including cognitive and functional scores are more appropriate as primary endpoints, treatment effect in each area should still be considered.
- Preclinical Alzheimer's Disease Population
  Currently, there are no standard endpoints to measure treatment effect in preclinical Alzheimer's disease populations. Diagnosis of dementia based on critical score rating and significant cognitive decline, or change, can be used as primary endpoints for primary and secondary prevention trials. In addition, new tools that monitor small neurocognitive changes or the time to onset of cognitive impairment can be used for supplementary analysis. Time-to-event can also be used as a supplementary endpoint to support the relevance of the selected endpoint, but the definition of the event needs to be clinically significant. At the same time, when using time-to-event as the endpoint, attention needs to be paid to the length of the clinical trial and the dropout rate.

(c) Treatment
There are two types of treatment for Alzheimer's disease: symptomatic treatment and disease-modifying treatment. The former can temporarily improve cognition but cannot slow disease progression, while the latter targets the pathological mechanisms of Alzheimer's disease and delays disease progression. In the selection of control treatment, because there are some symptomatic treatments for mild to moderate and severe Alzheimer's disease, if the investigational treatment belongs to symptomatic treatment, an active control should be set. At the same time, due to different population selection and placebo effects, it is still recommended to add a placebo arm outside the active control arm. In the mild cognitive impairment or preclinical Alzheimer's disease population, as there is no approved symptomatic treatment, a placebo can be used as a control treatment. Per the guideline, a placebo can also be used as a clinical trial control in Alzheimer's disease populations at any stage, given that no disease-modifying treatment was approved at the time of guideline release. However, it is

worthwhile to note that, depending on local medical practice, active controls are generally favored for ethical and practical considerations and readily interpretable trial results per ICH E10 (ICH, 2020).

(d) Intercurrent Events and Strategies
Intercurrent events include but are not limited to treatment discontinuation, dose modification, use of non-study treatments (including rescue treatment in the protocol), behavioral therapy, events unrelated to treatment but related to endpoints, and death. Generally speaking, unless there is a legitimate reason, treatment compliance should be reflected in the estimand (i.e., "treatment policy strategy" should be applicable to such intercurrent events). The consideration of other intercurrent events and their strategy may be influenced by different factors, but ultimately, the clinical questions of interest are on the target population.

- Alzheimer's Disease Population
Treatment discontinuation or changes in initial concomitant medication are common intercurrent events in the moderate-to-severe Alzheimer's disease population. As we believe that patients will not continue to benefit after stopping treatment and focus on the effectiveness of treatment under actual compliance, we adopt a treatment policy strategy for treatment discontinuation. However, sometimes patients change their initial concomitant medication with or without the investigational treatment, and the change in concomitant medication may affect the treatment outcomes. In this case, to study the pure treatment effect (excluding the impact of changes in concomitant medication on the investigational treatment efficacy), we can use a hypothetical strategy.
  Severe Alzheimer's disease patients often die during the trial, and death may affect the interpretation of the treatment efficacy. There is no recommended intercurrent event strategy to address death, although options are limited. The final strategy for dealing with death will depend on whether we are interested in the treatment effect on survival time. A composite variable strategy, in which death is defined as a composite of the treatment outcomes, could be adopted to reflect the treatment effect on survival time. It can be viewed as implementing the intention-to-treat principle in some cases where the original measurement of the variable might not exist or might not be meaningful, but where the intercurrent event itself meaningfully describes the patient's outcome, such as when the patient dies. On the other hand, the "while alive" strategy could also be considered if the treatment effect on patients while they are alive is of interest.
- MCI or Preclinical Alzheimer's Disease Population
The MCI or preclinical Alzheimer's disease population does not receive standard background treatment from the beginning of the trial, so starting non-study symptomatic treatment is considered an intercurrent event. To obtain the pure treatment effect (excluding the impact of symptomatic treatment on the investigational treatment effect), we can use a hypothetical strategy. Another strategy is a composite variable strategy. We can include this

intercurrent event as part of the study endpoint. For example, if a patient is treated by a non-investigational symptomatic anti-AD treatment, he or she will be considered a nonresponder to the investigational treatment, and the intercurrent event is reflected in the definition of endpoint.

(d) Population-Level Summary
For scale endpoints, we usually use the difference in mean change from baseline between arms as the population-level summary for the treatment effect. For disease-modifying therapies, the difference in time slope between arms can be considered, but the validity should be noted, such as the change from baseline in scale endpoints being a linear function of time. Population-level summaries from time-to-event analyses, such as hazard ratio or event-free rate ratio, are also commonly used to describe the disease-modifying effect of treatment on disease progression.

12.3.4 Summary and Discussion

This guideline provides an example of how different stages of a disease (Alzheimer's disease population, mild, moderate, and MCI to preclinical) and treatment (symptomatic or disease-modifying treatment) could impact the estimand considerations and trial designs.

12.4 Chronic Noninfectious Liver Diseases

12.4.1 Introduction to Guideline Principles

In 2018, EMA released a draft reflection paper on regulatory requirements for the development of medicinal products for chronic noninfectious liver diseases (primary biliary cholangitis (PBC), primary sclerosing cholangitis (PSC), NASH) (EMA, 2018e), which provided a high-level description of the requirements for drug development in noninfectious liver diseases. The reflection paper provides a framework for estimands for three different noninfectious liver diseases (NASH, PBC, and PSC) and is anticipated to be of some reference value for other chronic liver diseases. In this section, we briefly summarize the considerations for the estimands in randomized controlled trials of medicines for treating chronic noninfectious liver diseases as proposed in the reflection paper.

12.4.2 Nonalcoholic Steatohepatitis

12.4.2.1 Disease Background

Nonalcoholic steatohepatitis (NASH) is considered a progressive phenotype of nonalcoholic fatty liver disease and is the most prevalent chronic liver disease worldwide. The progression of this disease is related to the development of liver cell stress, subsequent inflammation, and fibrosis, with the potential development of cirrhosis and end-stage liver disease. The diagnosis of NASH is based on exclusion criteria (involving the exclusion of relevant alcohol intake and infectious and noninfectious liver disease) and positive confirmation of the features by liver biopsy and histology (including features of steatosis, hepatocellular ballooning, lobular inflammation, and fibrosis).

12.4.2.2 Considerations for Estimands

This guideline discusses the considerations for estimands for NASH in terms of population, variable, treatment, intercurrent events and strategies, and population-level summary.

(a) Population
The patient population should represent the target population, especially in terms of demographic characteristics and comorbidities. The diagnosis of NASH is a positive diagnosis based on liver biopsy, which excludes other related diseases.

(b) Variable
The long-term endpoint of NASH clinical trials includes a composite endpoint of all-cause mortality, liver transplantation, and the manifestation of decompensation (variceal bleeding, ascites, encephalopathy, etc.). For patients with fibrosis stages 2 and 3, the recommended long-term endpoint is a composite endpoint consisting of all-cause mortality, decompensation of liver disease (with a complete listing), as well as (histological) diagnosis of liver cirrhosis and model for end-stage liver disease (MELD) score above the threshold of 14. However, considering the feasibility of long-term studies and the unmet medical needs of NASH, early efficacy assessments are also necessary. Acceptable short-term endpoints (intermediate endpoints) consist of two composite endpoints:

1. The resolution of NASH with the presence of any grade of steatosis, no ballooning, and only minimal (grade 1) lobular inflammation, and at the same time, no worsening of the stage of fibrosis.
2. The improvement of fibrosis by at least 1 stage without any worsening of NASH (no worsening of ballooning and lobular inflammation; a 1-grade change in steatosis may be acceptable).

For patients who have already developed cirrhosis, a long-term endpoint that includes a composite endpoint of all-cause mortality and liver decompensation events may be considered. When using this long-term endpoint, the trial population should be enriched with patients with advanced cirrhosis. For non-decompensated patients, a short-term endpoint that may be considered is the reversal of cirrhosis (e.g., defined as "improvement of liver cirrhosis to non-cirrhotic liver disease (1 or more point improvement in fibrosis stage)"). In the case of late-stage liver cirrhosis patients, an acceptable short-term endpoint is the occurrence of decompensation events since the prognosis for patients with decompensated cirrhosis is markedly worse than those with compensated cirrhosis. Other potential short-term endpoints (such as lowering of MELD score below a certain threshold or of the hepatic portal venous gas below 10 mm Hg) may also be considered based on specific reasons.

(c) Treatment
Currently, there is no standard drug therapy for NASH, and placebo control is acceptable.

(d) Intercurrent Events and Strategies
Expected intercurrent events are events related to the clinical question of interest, such as treatment discontinuation and use of additional medication. The use of rescue medication may not be relevant for the time being since there is no specific treatment available for NASH, but it may become relevant in the future. Changes in background medication (including excessive lifestyle changes with weight loss or uptake of relevant alcohol intake) may affect treatment outcomes and may need to be considered. A treatment policy strategy is recommended for managing intercurrent events.

(e) Population-Level Summary
For response or composite endpoints, treatment risk difference or odds ratio can also be considered as a population-level summary in general.

12.4.3 Primary Biliary Cholangitis

12.4.3.1 Disease Background

Primary biliary cholangitis (PBC) is a chronic liver disease characterized by slow progressive autoimmune cholestasis. The pathogenesis of the disease is not fully understood. Its characteristics are cholestasis and the presence of specific antibodies. Histologically, it is accompanied by chronic granulomatous and lymphocytic small bile duct cholangitis. The disease course is progressive and may eventually lead to the presence of cirrhosis and end-stage liver disease.

12.4.3.2 Considerations for Estimands

This guideline discusses the considerations for estimands for PBC in terms of population, variable, treatment, intercurrent events and strategies, and population-level summary.

(a) Population
The selection of the patient population depends on the intended place in therapy of the investigational agent. First-line treatment trials can include both newly diagnosed and/or untreated patients, as well as patients already treated with ursodeoxycholic acid (UDCA). Add-on therapy to UDCA requires the inclusion of patients with an insufficient response to UDCA and may also include patients intolerant to standard UDCA therapy.

(b) Variable
In this population, it is almost impossible to evaluate all potential long-term outcomes. Considerable endpoints can be a composite endpoint including relevant serum biomarkers, alkaline phosphatase (ALP), and (total) bilirubin. Reduction in total bilirubin and ALP (including percentage decrease and proportion below certain thresholds) has previously been used as a primary endpoint in trials and has been accepted. In PBC, these endpoints are considered acceptable short-term efficacy outcomes. Additional long-term outcomes are required to support new compounds. Advocacy for strict definitions of response, with the ALP criterion being at least ALP < 1.5x Upper Limit of Normal (ULN) with at least a 40% decrease, and total bilirubin ≤ULN, should be considered. Additional criteria regarding transaminases, gamma-glutamyl-transferase, and/or Mayo score may be considered. Long-term outcome data, such as histological manifestation of cirrhosis, decompensation of cirrhosis, MELD score above a certain threshold, liver transplantation, and death, should be the basis for long-term follow-up efficacy evaluations, as the validity of these short-term endpoints has not been fully established.

(c) Treatment
For first-line drug trials, in addition to direct comparison with UDCA, placebo arms for determining sensitivity may be considered. For add-on therapy to UDCA trials, treatments are UDCA plus drug versus UDCA plus placebo.

(d) Intercurrent Events and Strategies
Potential intercurrent events include lack of adherence to treatment and the intake of rescue medication. The use of rescue therapy should be considered a treatment failure (corresponding to composite strategies). For other intercurrent events, treatment policy strategies may be considered. Refer to Table 12.3 for details.

(e) Population-Level Summary
For response or composite endpoints, treatment risk difference or odds ratio can also be considered as a population-level summary in general.

Table 12.3 Intercurrent events and estimand strategies

Intercurrent events	Strategy
Lack of adherence to treatment (including treatment discontinuation, treatment interruption, and/or other incompliance events)	Treatment policy strategy
Use of rescue medication	Composite variable strategy
Other intercurrent event	Treatment policy strategy

12.4.4 *Primary Sclerosing Cholangitis*

12.4.4.1 Disease Background

Primary sclerosing cholangitis (PSC) is a rare, chronic, heterogeneous, and idiopathic inflammatory disease characterized by the development of intra- and/or extrahepatic stricturing of bile ducts and the development of fibrosis. The natural history of PSC includes the development of complications (e.g., bacterial cholangitis), progression of fibrosis to cirrhosis, and ultimately end-stage liver disease with decompensation, liver transplantation, or death. Diagnosis is generally based on serum markers of potential cholestasis and the presence of stricturing cholangiopathy, usually diagnosed by magnetic resonance cholangiopancreatography. Final confirmation of the diagnosis also requires exclusion of associated secondary cholangitis, particularly Immunoglobulin G4-related disease.

12.4.4.2 Considerations for Estimands

This guideline discusses the considerations for estimands for PSC in terms of population, variable, treatment, intercurrent events and strategies, and population-level summary.

(a) Population
The diagnosis of PSC mainly relies on elevated ALP and abnormal cholangiography. A minimal threshold for ALP and transaminases elevations should be defined. The availability of a liver biopsy consistent with PSC is a compulsory requirement. The selection of PSC patients should allow for the occurrence of related complications in the patient population. If patients have a dominant stricture at the time of inclusion, their serum biomarkers should not have a history of fluctuation records, and there should not be relevant cholestasis. The presence of cholangial and gallbladder carcinoma, as well as colon carcinoma, should be excluded. Typically, patients with active inflammatory bowel disease should not be included. The presence of decompensation symptoms should also be an exclusion criterion, but cirrhotic patients without signs and/or symptoms of decompensation can be included.

(b) Variable
Using short-term endpoints to demonstrate efficacy at early time points and then confirming long-term benefits on long-term endpoints is an acceptable option. The combined use of histological evaluation and ALP changes is currently considered an acceptable short-term endpoint. Histological evaluation is best based on the newer staging system, according to Nakamura. ALP changes can be considered for response type evaluation: reduction of ALP to 1.3xULN, or a combination of the reduction to 1.5–1.3xULN with at least a 40% reduction from baseline. Long-term endpoints can consider composite endpoints including (histological diagnosis) cirrhosis, MELD score higher than 14, decompensation events (such as encephalopathy, variceal bleeding, and ascites), liver transplantation, and death.

(c) Treatment
Currently, there are no licensed treatments for PSC, and placebo-controlled trials are acceptable.

(d) Intercurrent Events and Strategies
Considerable intercurrent events include lack of adherence to treatment and the occurrence of malignancy. A treatment policy strategy can be considered for both.

(e) Population-Level Summary
For response or composite endpoints, treatment risk difference or odds ratio can also be considered as a population-level summary in general.

12.4.5 Symptomatic Treatment Trials (PBC and PSC)

If treatment is targeted at disease-specific symptoms, measuring disease-specific symptoms should be part of the primary evaluation, and the development of such tools to measure patient-reported outcomes is encouraged. A treatment policy strategy can be considered for addressing intercurrent events.

12.4.6 Summary and Discussion

Chronic, noninfectious liver diseases are a medical field of high unmet medical needs. The specifics of the diseases create major challenges for the development of new medicinal products. The guidance provides a framework for estimands for three different noninfectious liver diseases (NASH, PBC, and PSC) with a high-level description of the requirements for drug development in the field. To be noted, for all three disease entities, the regulatory experience with the licensing of new medicinal products is limited. Therefore, the guidance aims at a preliminary definition of development strategies only, which, in the case of several successful marketing authorization applications occurring in the future, will have to be refined.

12.5 Chronic Diseases with Recurrent Event Endpoints

12.5.1 Introduction to Guideline Principles

In 2020, the European Medicines Agency (EMA) published the qualification opinion of clinically interpretable treatment effect measures based on recurrent event endpoints that allow for efficient statistical analyses (EMA, 2020c). This document provides guidance on the definition of estimands in clinical trials for various chronic diseases using recurrent events as endpoints, including multiple sclerosis, pulmonary disease exacerbation and asthma, migraine headache attacks, hypoglycemic events in diabetes, epilepsy, and chronic heart failure. In this section, we briefly summarize the considerations for the estimands in randomized controlled trials with recurrent event endpoints, focusing on chronic heart failure disease, as proposed in the guideline.

12.5.2 Disease Background

Chronic heart failure refers to the persistent state of heart failure. Due to abnormalities in cardiac structure or function, patients with chronic heart failure require repeated hospitalizations and have a higher risk of cardiovascular death than the general population. The general goals of heart failure treatment are not only to improve symptoms and quality of life but also to delay and prevent the development of myocardial remodeling and reduce hospitalization and mortality caused by heart failure.

12.5.3 Considerations for Estimands

In clinical trials for chronic heart failure, the primary endpoint is typically the time to the first composite event of cardiovascular death or first hospitalization, whichever occurs first. This composite endpoint is more specific than time to death alone and avoids some competing risks and multiplicity issues by using only one rather than two endpoints (i.e., time to cardiovascular death and time to first hospitalization). However, while these events reflect clinically meaningful information, this composite endpoint disregards all recurrent hospitalizations that occur after the first hospitalization and does not account for death after the first hospitalization. Additionally, improvements in medical care can simultaneously decrease hospitalization rates and mortality rates. Therefore, the sample size required for these classic disease-related mortality and morbidity trials is usually large, making it increasingly challenging to conduct trials with sufficient statistical power. Including all recurrent hospitalization and death information can better describe the burden of disease and ultimately construct more clinically meaningful treatment effect measures and higher statistical power. However, because hospitalization and death share some common risk factors, there are significant challenges in determining the estimand for recurrent hospitalization in chronic heart failure.

12.5.3.1 Scenarios without Terminal Event (or with Low Terminal Event Rate)

For scenarios without a terminal event or with a low terminal event rate, EMA (2020c) only considers the intercurrent event treatment discontinuation. Two estimands are proposed: one based on a hypothetical strategy (if the patient continues to receive treatment) and the other based on a treatment policy strategy (regardless of whether the patient continues to receive treatment). EMA (2020c) does not aim to address which estimand is more acceptable for regulatory decision-making. However, the general concern regarding the hypothetical strategy applied to treatment discontinuation should be noted, where it is not understood why a patient who discontinued in the trial, for example, because of a severe toxicity, would have continued with the medication outside the trial. In earlier phase trials, where the purpose is not to gain regulatory approval, the strategy is easier to understand.

12.5.3.2 Scenarios with Terminal Event

In scenarios with a terminal event, such as cardiovascular death and non-cardiovascular death, the estimation of recurrent heart failure hospitalizations is complicated by the presence of death, as patients will not experience hospitalization after death. Therefore, the EMA (2020c) guideline document focuses on treatment discontinuation, cardiovascular death, and non-cardiovascular death as intercurrent events and proposes the following two estimands.

Estimand 1

(a) Population: atients with chronic heart failure defined by inclusion/exclusion criteria.
(b) Variable: Number of heart failure hospitalizations before death or trial termination (at T years).
(c) Treatment: Treatment arm vs. control arm.
(d) Intercurrent Events and Strategies: See Table 12.4.
(e) Population-Level Summary: The ratio of the expected number of heart failure hospitalizations per unit time alive in the treatment arm to that in the control arm.

Estimand 2

(a) Population: Patients with chronic heart failure defined by inclusion/exclusion criteria.

Table 12.4 Intercurrent events and estimand strategies

Intercurrent events	Strategies
Treatment discontinuation	Treatment policy strategy
Cardiovascular death	While alive strategy
Non-cardiovascular death	While alive strategy

Table 12.5 Intercurrent events and estimand strategies

Intercurrent events	Strategies
Treatment discontinuation	Treatment policy strategy
Cardiovascular death	Composite variable strategy
Non-cardiovascular death	While alive strategy

(b) Variable: Number of unfavorable events, including heart failure hospitalizations and cardiovascular deaths, before death or trial termination (T years).
(c) Treatment: Treatment arm vs. control arm.
(d) Intercurrent Events and Strategies: See Table 12.5.
(e) Population-Level Summary: The ratio of expected unfavorable event rates per unit time alive in the treatment arm to those in the control arm.

Estimand 1 targets the following question that patients may have regarding treatment effect: "How many heart failure hospitalizations can I expect to have in the next T years, relative to how long I can expect to live in the next T years, regardless of any treatment discontinuation?" Estimand 2 targets the following question that patients may have regarding treatment effect: "How many unfavorable events, including heart failure hospitalizations and cardiovascular death, can I expect to have in the next T years, relative to how long I can expect to live in the next T years, regardless of any treatment discontinuation?"

EMA (2020c) has evaluated these two endpoints, and first of all, both endpoints are based on an *exposure-weighted method* that calculates the weighted average of the event rates for each patient, with the weights being the proportion of the follow-up time contributed by that patient; that is, patients who were followed up for longer are given more weight in the analysis. In Estimand 1, this method means that the size of the treatment effect on recurrent heart failure hospitalizations depends on the treatment's effect on cardiovascular death (the earlier the cardiovascular death, the fewer hospitalizations), leading to difficulties in clinical interpretation. Therefore, Estimand 1 is only applicable to situations where the death rate is not high or where the death rate is similar in both arms. For Estimand 2, there is no clear clinical interpretation for the composite endpoint of hospitalization and cardiovascular death (because cardiovascular death and heart failure hospitalization have the same weight). Ideally, trial data should be analyzed for both aspects of the treatment effect on recurrent heart failure hospitalization and cardiovascular death. EMA (2020c) also proposes another population-level summary method called *patient-weighted rate*, which is the average of the rates observed for each patient, with each patient being given equal weight, regardless of exposure. EMA (2020c) discusses both methods and points out that the exposure-weighted rate seems to be of some relevance to the population. For example, if a hospital was estimating the admission rates they should expect for heart failure, the exposure-based method might provide useful information in terms of events per year that they might see. However, for a patient considering what annual rate they as an individual might expect while they are alive, the patient-weighted rate would be the most informative, as every individual patient studied would have an equal chance of representing them; there is no more chance that they would be like one of the patients with long follow-up. Therefore, the equal-weighted method seems to be more relevant when describing the treatment's effect on specific patients.

12.5.4 Summary and Discussion

Chronic diseases are often characterized by the repeated occurrence of events like relapses in relapsing-remitting multiple sclerosis or hospitalizations in chronic heart failure. Treatments for such diseases are then expected to impact the first as well as subsequent recurrent events. Hence, their effect is best characterized by using a recurrent event endpoint rather than a time-to-first-event endpoint. For chronic diseases, where deaths during a clinical trial are more common, the situation is far more complex. Although the clinical meaningfulness of recurrent heart failure hospitalizations has been recognized in the recent Committee for Medicinal Products for Human Use (CHMP) guideline on the clinical investigation of medicinal products for the treatment of chronic heart failure (CHMP, 2017), it is acknowledged that experience in this setting is limited. There are two main challenges. First, the definition of a clinically interpretable treatment effect measure needs attention, especially when there is a terminal event such as in chronic heart failure trials, since the size of the treatment effect on recurrent heart failure hospitalizations depends on the treatment's effect on cardiovascular death. This guideline discusses two estimands for the scenarios with a terminal event. Second, finding suitable analysis methods (estimators) that target the estimand of interest is challenging. Extensive simulations in this guideline show that estimators including a recurrent event endpoint are typically more efficient than a Cox model based on a time-to-first-event endpoint. The CHMP also suggests further exploring analysis methods that deliver separate estimates that appropriately summarize the expected effect of the treatment on the (annual event rate for the) recurrent event while alive and the effect on the terminal event for confirmatory decision-making.

From both a clinical and a statistical efficiency perspective, a better understanding of those patient characteristics that determine differences in the frequency of rehospitalizations for worsening heart failure would be of interest and could be used for adjustment in statistical models, ultimately leading to a reduction in variability and an increase in efficiency.

12.6 Gout

In 2019, the EMA published the guideline on clinical investigation of medicinal products for the treatment of gout (EMA, 2019), which provides general guidance on the development of medical products (primarily urate-lowering and anti-inflammatory therapies) for the treatment of gout.

Gout is a common disorder caused by hyperuricemia and the formation of monosodium urate crystal deposits, which may induce an inflammatory reaction when accumulating in joints, tendons, and the surrounding soft tissues. Gout may manifest as intermittent acute gouty arthritis (i.e., flares) with symptom-free periods between attacks. In severe cases, chronic tophaceous gouty arthropathy may occur, characterized by inflamed tophi at multiple joints and bone erosions, where patients are not symptom-free in between flares. Gout may progress to renal damage and kidney stone formation.

The standard of care treatment of gout is urate-lowering therapy (ULT). However, it may lead to gout flares as a sudden drop in serum uric acid levels induced by ULT may trigger a host defense to dissolve crystals. Therefore, standardized prophylactic therapy should be used concurrently in the short term to prevent flares.

In the section on confirmatory trials in urate-lowering therapies of this guideline, it is specified that the statistical analysis plan must address how to address intercurrent events, such as the dropout due to flares shortly after the introduction of ULT or after the withdrawal of concurrent flare prophylaxis treatment, or differential adherence to the investigational treatment. Flare is an event of concern in ULT, and the dropout due to flares should be addressed appropriately in the trials. However, it is not specified in the guideline what strategies, as proposed in the ICH E9(R1) guideline, should be used to address the intercurrent events of interest accordingly.

12.7 Registry-Based Studies

In 2021, the EMA released the guideline on registry-based studies (EMA, 2021), which provides recommendations on key methodological aspects that are specific to the use of patient registries by marketing authorization applicants and holders to conduct registry-based studies. Registry-based studies use databases or patient populations of one or more patient registries to investigate a research question, with or without randomization allocation. The trial design should follow the requirements of the ICH E9(R1) guideline on estimands and sensitivity analysis in clinical trials. Data collection and analysis should be aligned with the estimand(s) of interest, with adequate estimation and testing methods. Sensitivity analysis should be planned to explore the robustness of the estimates on the primary estimand under potential deviations from underlying assumptions and data limitations.

The registry population is the source of the patient population for the registry-based study. The choice of the trial population should be based on the trial objectives, which could be the entire population of the registry center or only a subset defined by predetermined characteristics.

When registry-based studies involve secondary use of data, the trial protocol should specify the events of interest already collected by the registry center and discuss the risks of bias and unmeasured confounding. A detailed and complete search strategy, coding list, or adjudication should be used for the precise definition of variables, including both outcomes of interest and baseline covariates.

The estimation of sample size should be described and justified in the protocol. The feasibility of achieving the required sample size within the registry for the trial should be evaluated based on realistic assumptions. Effect and sample size should be considered based on the primary estimand, intercurrent events, missing data, and whether they need to be imputed.

Missing data may lead to bias and confounding. The approaches for handling missing data should be detailed in the trial protocol and statistical analysis plan. Justifications should be provided for the assumptions related to approaches for handling missing data used in statistical analysis, such as their distribution, causes, and timing. The ICH E9 (R1) guideline, EMA Guideline on Missing Data in Confirmatory Clinical Trials (EMA, 2010), and European Network of Centers for Pharmacoepidemiology and Pharmacovigilance (ENCePP) Guide on Methodological Standards in Pharmacoepidemiology (ENCePP, 2023) provide guidance on how to handle missing data.

12.8 Concluding Remarks

The ICH E9(R1) guideline was published in 2019 and subsequently adopted by EMA. Since then, it has been implemented with various degrees of specification and detail in some disease guidelines. This chapter presented selected documents issued by the EMA in the past years that have embraced the estimand framework, including guidelines on diabetes mellitus, Alzheimer's disease, chronic noninfectious liver diseases, gout, trials with recurrent event endpoint and registry-based studies. In most of these guidelines, common intercurrent events in specific disease areas and estimand strategies were discussed, which would inform trial design, data collection, and choice of analysis method. According to the Accelerating Clinical Trials EU Methodology Workshop by the EMA, methodology guidelines will be developed or updated to incorporate the E9 (R1) framework, and more clinical guidelines will be updated to reflect recommendations specific to that disease. Early engagement with regulatory authorities about their treatment effects of interest and alignment on planned analysis methods is highly recommended, especially in disease areas that have not yet incorporated the estimand framework. Sharing case studies may help with the process of updating more disease guidelines.

References

CHMP. (2017). *Guideline on clinical investigation of medicinal products for the treatment of chronic heart failure*. https://www.ema.europa.eu/

Cro, S., Kahan, B. C., Rehal, S., Chis Ster, A., Carpenter, J. R., White, I. R., & Cornelius, V. R. (2022). Evaluating how clear the questions being investigated in randomised trials are: Systematic review of estimands. *BMJ (Clinical research ed.), 378*, e070146. https://doi.org/10.1136/bmj-2022-070146

EMA. (2002). *Note for guideline on clinical investigation of medicinal products in the treatment or prevention of diabetes mellitus*. https://www.ema.europa.eu/

EMA. (2010). *Guideline on Missing Data in Confirmatory Clinical Trials*. https://www.ema.europa.eu/

EMA. (2018a). *Question and answer on adjustment for cross-over in estimating effects in oncology trials*. https://www.ema.europa.eu/

EMA. (2018b). *Guideline on the development of new medicinal products for the treatment of Crohn's Disease*. https://www.ema.europa.eu/

EMA. (2018c). *Guideline on the development of new medicinal products for the treatment of Ulcerative Colitis*. https://www.ema.europa.eu/

EMA. (2018d). *Guideline on the clinical investigation of medicines for the treatment of Alzheimer's disease*. https://www.ema.europa.eu/

EMA. (2018e). *Reflection paper on regulatory requirements for the development of medicinal products for chronic non-infectious liver diseases* (PBC, PSC, NASH). https://www.ema.europa.eu/

EMA. (2019). *Guideline on clinical investigation of medicinal products for the treatment of gout*. https://www.ema.europa.eu/

EMA. (2020b). *Points to consider on implications of Coronavirus disease (COVID-19) on methodological aspects of ongoing clinical trials*. https://www.ema.europa.eu/

EMA. (2020c). *Qualification opinion of clinically interpretable treatment effect measures based on recurrent event endpoints that allow for efficient statistical analyses*. https://www.ema.europa.eu/

EMA. (2021). *Guideline on registry-based studies*. https://www.ema.europa.eu/

EMA. (2022). *Points to consider on the impact of the war in Ukraine on methodological aspects of ongoing clinical trials*. https://www.ema.europa.eu/

EMA (2023a). *Assessment of SmPC section 5.1 (draft)*. EMA/CHMP/566497/2023 available at https://www.ema.europa.eu/

EMA. (2023b). *Draft revised consolidated 3-year work plan for the methodology working party (MWP)*. EMA/CHMP/478317/2023. https://www.ema.europa.eu/

EMA. (2023c). *Guideline on clinical investigation of medicinal products in 4 the treatment of depression*. https://www.ema.europa.eu/

EMA. (2023d). *Guideline on clinical investigation of medicinal products in the treatment or prevention of diabetes mellitus*. https://www.ema.europa.eu/

EMA. (2024). *Day 80 assessment report—Clinical template with guidance—Rev.04.24 Revamp*. https://www.ema.europa.eu/

ENCePP. (2023). *ENCePP Guide on Methodological Standards in Pharmacoepidemiology (Revision 11)*. EMA/95098/2010. Methodological Guide—European Union

ICH. (2019). *ICH E9 (R1) addendum on estimands and sensitivity analysis in clinical trials to the guideline on statistical principles for clinical trials*. Step 4 document. https://ich.org/

ICH. (2020). *ICH E10 Choice of control group in clinical trials*. Step 5 document. https://ich.org/

Mészáros, L., Lasch, F., Delafont, B., Guizzaro, L. (2023). *Strategies for addressing intercurrent events in CNS trials*. https://ssrn.com/abstract=4516200

Mitroiu, M., Oude Rengerink, K., Teerenstra, S., et al. (2020). A narrative review of estimands in drug development and regulatory evaluation: Old wine in new barrels? *Trials, 21*, 671. https://doi.org/10.1186/s13063-020-04546-1

Chapter 13
FDA Guidelines and Their Relationship to the Estimand Framework

Wenting Li, Sheinchung Chow, Xue Yang, Qiong Du, Alice Wang, Na Yang, and Liwen Liang

Abstract The Food and Drug Administration (FDA) adopted the ICH E9(R1) guideline on estimands and sensitivity analysis in clinical trials in 2021. The ICH E9(R1) guideline has substantially reshaped the planning and evaluation of confirmatory studies by offering the estimand framework for addressing intercurrent events. Its implementation has led to more transparency about the targeted treatment effects in clinical trials across therapeutic areas. This chapter discusses the FDA's implementation of the estimand framework across various guideline documents, including treatments for acute myeloid leukemia, chronic rhinosinusitis with nasal polyps, COVID-19, and eosinophilic esophagitis. In these guidelines, the five esti-

W. Li (✉)
Biostatistics, dMed Biopharmaceutical Co., Ltd, Shanghai, China
e-mail: wenting.li@caidya.com

S. Chow
Biostatistics and Bioinformatics, Duke University School of Medicine, North, USA
e-mail: sheinchung.chow@duke.edu

X. Yang
Statistics and Decision Sciences, Johnson & Johnson Innovative Medicine, R&D, Shanghai, China
e-mail: xyang36@its.jnj.com

Q. Du
China Biometrics, ClinChoice Enterprise Management (Shanghai) Co., Ltd., Shanghai, China
e-mail: qiong.du@clinchoice.com

A. Wang
Biometrics, AstraZeneca Global R&D (China) Co., Ltd., Shanghai, China
e-mail: Alice.wang2@astrazeneca.com

N. Yang
Evidence Generation and Decision Sciences-Asia Pacific Statistics, Sanofi (China) Investment Co. Ltd, Beijing, China
e-mail: na3.yang@Sanofi.com

L. Liang
Biostatistics and Research Decision Sciences, MSD R&D (China), Beijing, China
e-mail: li.wen.liang@merck.com

J. Wei et al. (eds.), *Estimands in Clinical Trials*, Springer Series in Pharmaceutical Statistics, https://doi.org/10.1007/978-3-032-02192-2_13

mand attributes, along with common intercurrent events in specific disease areas and estimand strategies, are discussed. These insights contribute significantly to trial design, data collection, and selection of analysis methods.

13.1 Introduction

In May 2021, the United States Food and Drug Administration (FDA) adopted the ICH E9(R1) guideline on estimands and sensitivity analyses in clinical trials (ICH, 2019). Consequently, sponsors are now recommended to apply the estimand framework and describe relevant estimands for their clinical trials. To facilitate the implementation of this guideline across a range of disease areas, the FDA subsequently published multiple disease-specific guidelines. These additional instructions offer further details on estimand considerations.

The objective of this chapter is to summarize the FDA's perspectives on the application of estimands and consideration for addressing intercurrent events in clinical trials. The following sections outline the implementation of the estimand framework across various therapeutic areas, as detailed within the corresponding FDA guidelines. Section 13.2 discusses estimand considerations for acute myeloid leukemia. Section 13.3 provides estimand considerations and statistical analysis plans for chronic rhinosinusitis with nasal polyps. Section 13.4 discusses estimands and suggested statistical analysis for the coronavirus disease. Section 13.5 provides an overview of estimand considerations for eosinophilic esophagitis. Concluding remarks are given in Sect. 13.6.

Owing to space limitations, this chapter does not cover all published FDA guidelines that provide definitions and/or examples of estimands. For example, the FDA's guidelines on graft-versus-host disease (FDA, 2023a) and Ulcerative Colitis (FDA, 2022a), which include the explicit discussion of estimands, are not covered in detail here. Readers interested in a comprehensive understanding of estimands across various therapeutic areas and the latest regulatory perspective are encouraged to download the relevant documents directly from the FDA's official website.

13.2 Acute Myeloid Leukemia

13.2.1 Introduction to Guideline Principles

In 2022, the FDA released a guideline on developing drugs and biological products to treat acute myeloid leukemia (AML) (FDA, 2022b). This guideline outlines the FDA's current perspective on various aspects of AML drug development, including general considerations, efficacy variables, trial design, and regulatory submission requirements. It covers the overall development program and clinical trial designs for drugs and biological products intended to support specific treatment phases, such as maintenance therapies or preparative regimens for transplantation.

Additionally, it addresses topics related to general drug development, including the selection of efficacy variables and consideration of exploratory and confirmatory trials within the context of AML. This section provides an overview of the relevant content related to the estimand framework, as outlined in this guideline.

13.2.2 Disease Background

AML is a cancer that originates in myeloid cells and is characterized by the uncontrolled proliferation and accumulation of abnormal myeloid cells in the bone marrow, leading to a decrease in healthy blood cells. AML is highly heterogeneous, with various subtypes classified based on morphological, clinical, and genetic features. AML can affect patients across all ages; the median age of diagnosis is 68 years.

Traditionally, intensive treatments like cytotoxic chemotherapy and following hematopoietic stem cell transplantation (HSCT) have been the standard treatment for AML, with the goal of achieving a cure. However, not all patients are suitable candidates for these intensive therapies, particularly those with mild pathological or age-related organ impairment. These patients are at a higher risk of treatment-related complications (e.g., life-threatening organ toxicity) and may instead be offered palliative treatments or might not be eligible for any active treatment.

Recent advancements have focused on developing targeted therapies that target specific genetic mutations or epigenetic abnormalities as alternatives to cytotoxic drugs. Although these newer treatments may not provide a cure, they can improve survival and offer meaningful benefits for patients with limited life expectancy. Additionally, temporary disease control and symptom palliation are considered crucial therapeutic goals in certain circumstances (refer to Section III in FDA, 2022b).

13.2.3 Considerations for Estimands

The scientific questions in clinical trials in AML vary depending on the disease stage and treatment phase. During the induction phase, the primary focus is on improving response rates, overcoming resistance to therapy, and achieving complete remission. In the consolidation stage, the critical clinical questions focus on preventing relapse and assessing the long-term outcomes of different regimens. The maintenance phase is to determine the optimal duration of therapy and its effect on long-term disease control. For continued treatment, the focus shifts to understanding resistance mechanisms, managing toxicity, and preventing disease recurrence following an initial response.

These scientific questions can be better addressed through the application of the estimand framework, which defines the precise treatment effect being measured in each trial. The guideline (FDA, 2022b) comprehensively provides the recommendation on estimand considerations, including population, variables, treatment, intercurrent events, and strategies, as well as population-level summary.

(a) Population
Patients with AML should be classified using the most recent diagnostic criteria and categorized based on the disease stage, such as newly diagnosed AML, late first relapse (e.g., first remission >6 months), and other relapsed or refractory AML (e.g., primary refractory, early first relapse, and any second or later relapse). Trials should be designed to independently support each indication, either through separate trials or separate cohorts within a single trial.

(b) Variable
The choice of the variables in AML clinical trials depends on the treatment's intended purpose. Table 13.1 provides more details on variable selection. Other commonly used efficacy variables include variables based on minimal residual disease, alternative biomarkers or measures of efficacy variables, and patient-focused outcomes.

(c) Treatment
AML treatments could be single treatments, combinations of treatments (e.g., add-ons to standard of care), or complex regimens involving a series of treatments. For example, the first-line treatment typically includes induction therapy, consolidation, and allogeneic HSCT.

(d) Intercurrent Events
For AML trials, it is common for patients to receive subsequent anti-AML treatments post-randomization, which include HSCT and/or anti-AML drugs (not to be confused with concomitant therapies). As use of subsequent treatments is consistent with the practice of medicine, the FDA recommends that the primary analysis of a time-to-event endpoint (e.g., OS, EFS) not censor for subsequent treatments. This approach implies that HSCT and/or subsequent anti-AML treatments are viewed as part of the as-needed AML treatment regi-

Table 13.1 Variables with different intended purposes of treatment

Category	Treatment's intended purpose	Variables
Traditional approvable clinical variables	Treatment of AML with curative intent	Overall survival (OS)
		Event-free survival (EFS)
		Relapse-free survival
	Treatment of AML without curative intent	Overall survival
		Event-free survival
	Treatment of AML with palliative intent	Complete remission
		Complete remission with partial hematologic recovery
		Transfusion independence

Note: OS is defined as the time from randomization to the date of death from any cause. EFS in AML is defined as the time from randomization to the date of induction treatment failure, relapse (for those with successful induction treatment), or death from any cause, whichever occurs first. Relapse-free survival is defined as the time from randomization to the date of relapse or the date of death from any cause, whichever occurs first. Transfusion independence is defined as the absence of red blood cell and platelet transfusions for a prespecified period during continued treatment. Detailed definitions of additional variables can be found in Section III.B of FDA, (2022b)

men taken after the initial study drug and that the treatment effect is the result of both the study drug and the subsequent anti-AML treatment. Therefore, a treatment policy strategy is recommended.

FDA (2022b) also discussed the reasons why the hypothetical strategy is not suggested; for example, the assumptions are difficult to justify, and the clinical relevance of such an estimand is still an open question if it cannot be realized in practice. More details can be found in Appendix 2 of the guideline.

(e) Population-Level Summary
The choice of the population-level summary depends on the type of variable being analyzed. For time-to-event variables, hazard ratios with 95% confidence intervals are typically presented. For binary variables, the summary includes the difference in response rate, ratio of response rate, or odds ratio, along with their 95% confidence intervals.

13.2.4 Statistical Analysis

For time-to-event variables, the FDA generally accepts the log-rank test as the primary analysis method, although alternative methods may be considered in appropriate cases.

For binary variables, primary analysis may employ Fisher's exact test or the Cochran-Mantel-Haenszel test (or an exact version) when stratification factors are used at randomization.

FDA (2022b) emphasizes the importance of adhering to a predetermined statistical analysis plan that includes sensitivity and supplementary analyses. These additional analyses may involve alternative definitions for variables and populations, different analysis methods, or varied approaches for addressing intercurrent events. For example, in cases of nonproportional hazards (e.g., plateauing effects), the FDA is open to considering alternative approaches such as weighted Cox regression or other weighted methods. Additionally, summarizing the treatment effect using restricted mean survival time or landmark survival analysis is also considered a viable option.

13.3 Chronic Rhinosinusitis with Nasal Polyps

13.3.1 Introduction to Guideline Principles

In 2023, the FDA released a guideline for developing drugs or biological products to treat chronic rhinosinusitis with nasal polyps (CRSwNP) (FDA, 2023b). This guideline outlines the FDA's current recommendations regarding trial populations, trial design, statistical analysis, efficacy, and safety considerations for CRSwNP drug development.

13.3.2 Disease Background

Chronic rhinosinusitis is characterized by inflammation of the nasal mucosa and paranasal sinuses and is classified into two subtypes: CRSwNP and chronic rhinosinusitis without nasal polyps (CRSsNP). Nasal polyps are inflammatory hyperplastic growths that protrude into the nasal passages, causing symptoms like nasal congestion, discharge, facial pain, and loss of smell.

For clinical trials of CRSwNP, randomized, double-blind, placebo-controlled, parallel-arm trial designs are generally recommended. Sponsors should incorporate the standard of care, which typically includes intranasal corticosteroids, antibiotics, and, when necessary, rescue systemic corticosteroids and surgery.

13.3.3 Considerations for Estimands

FDA (2023b) discusses the considerations for estimands with respect to population, variable, treatment, intercurrent events and strategies. Although a specific population-level summary is not explicitly outlined in the guideline, it can be inferred from the proposed analysis methods.

(a) Population
The target population of CRSwNP clinical trials should reflect the intended use of the drug. For drugs intended as an add-on to the standard of care, FDA (2023b) recommends including a population with more severe disease.

FDA (2023b) encourages diversity in the trial population, incorporating a wide range of demographic characteristics. Additionally, FDA (2023b) encourages early inclusion of pediatric patients (at least 12 years of age) in adult trials, when appropriate, based on safety data and potential benefits. Furthermore, FDA (2023b) recommends evaluating the feasibility of enrolling pregnant patients in clinical trials.

(b) Variable
The efficacy of CRSwNP treatment is typically assessed by measuring its treatment effect on nasal polyps and chronic rhinosinusitis. FDA (2023b) recommends using co-primary variables, the endoscopic nasal polyp score, and the nasal congestion score.

For these co-primary variables, either the change from baseline to a landmark time point or the absolute score at a landmark time point can be considered. Given the chronic nature of CRSwNP, FDA (2023b) recommends a trial duration of at least 24 weeks, preferably extending to 52 weeks. To account for day-to-day variability in patient-reported symptoms, FDA (2023b) suggests using an average score over several days or weeks to establish the score at baseline and at a landmark time point for each patient. This approach ensures a more accurate assessment of the drug efficacy over a sufficient time frame.

(c) Treatment
Treatment for CRSwNP may differ depending on the disease severity. Mild cases are often managed with intranasal corticosteroids and saline irrigation, whereas more severe cases may require systemic corticosteroids, monoclonal antibodies, or, in certain instances, surgery.

The primary treatment goals are to reduce symptoms, minimize the use of systemic corticosteroids, avoid surgery, and improve the overall quality of life for CRSwNP patients.

(d) Intercurrent Events
FDA (2023b) provides recommendations for addressing key intercurrent events in clinical trials, as outlined in Table 13.2.

(e) Population-Level Summary
The population-level summary is not explicitly outlined in the FDA guideline (FDA, 2023b).

Table 13.2 Intercurrent events and estimand strategies

Intercurrent events	Strategies	Comments
Treatment discontinuation	Treatment policy strategy	Treatment discontinuation reflects real-world treatment practices. FDA (2023b) recommends a treatment policy strategy without distinguishing the reason for discontinuation
Surgery	Composite variable strategy	FDA (2023b) recommends incorporating surgery into the endpoint and considering it as an unfavorable outcome. One reasonable approach is to assign the worst possible score for the co-primary endpoints (nasal polyp score and nasal congestion score)
Use of rescue systemic corticosteroids for CRSwNP in trials evaluating intranasal corticosteroids	Composite variable or treatment policy strategy	The choice between a composite variable or treatment policy strategy depends on the trial design or the relative impact of the intercurrent event on Interpretation of study results
Use of rescue systemic corticosteroids for CRSwNP in trials evaluating therapeutic biological products and comorbid conditions	Treatment policy strategy	A treatment policy strategy allows evaluation of the drug efficacy in the context of rescue systemic corticosteroid use
Switch from one study treatment to another treatment (e.g., a different intranasal corticosteroid spray or biologic therapy) for CRSwNP	Composite variable strategy	Treatment switching indicates an unfavorable outcome

13.3.4 *Statistical Analysis*

For the primary analysis, FDA (2023b) recommends adjusting for prespecified prognostic baseline covariates, such as the baseline value of the outcome measure, asthma or nonsteroidal anti-inflammatory drug-exacerbated respiratory disease status, and prior surgical history. A regression-based approach is recommended for comparing means between treatment arms.

To address missing data for key estimands, the protocol should clearly distinguish between treatment discontinuation and trial withdrawal. The protocol should also include plans for continued data collection following treatment discontinuation or the use of rescue therapies to ensure all relevant data are captured.

FDA (2023b) recommends prespecifying a sensitivity analysis plan to systematically assess the robustness of conclusions, considering potential deviations from the assumptions underlying the primary analysis.

For supplementary analysis, the FDA recommends exploring alternative estimands by using different strategies to address intercurrent events (e.g., using a treatment policy instead of a composite variable strategy). Additionally, it is recommended to explore different implementations of a given strategy (e.g., using a clinically justified alternative value instead of the worst possible score when applying a composite variable strategy) in supplementary analyses.

13.4 COVID-19

13.4.1 *Introduction to Guideline Principles*

In 2021, the FDA released the guideline for developing drugs and biological products for the treatment or prevention of the coronavirus disease (COVID-19) (FDA, 2021). This guideline excluded preventive vaccines and convalescent plasma from its scope. A final version of this guideline was released in 2023 (FDA, 2023c). This section primarily focuses on the estimand framework used in clinical trials for COVID-19 treatment, as detailed in the 2023 guideline (FDA, 2023c). Given that both the 2021 and 2023 versions discuss estimands, this section primarily presents the 2023 guideline.

13.4.2 *Disease Background*

COVID-19 is a highly infectious respiratory disease caused by the novel coronavirus, severe acute respiratory syndrome coronavirus 2 (SARS-CoV-2). Symptoms can range from mild, such as fever, cough, and shortness of breath, to severe, including respiratory failure, multiorgan failure, and even death.

The virus is primarily transmitted through respiratory droplets and close contact, although airborne transmission is also possible. Both symptomatic and asymptomatic patients can spread the virus.

While the prognosis is generally favorable for most, certain high-risk groups, such as the elderly, patients with chronic diseases (such as heart disease, lung disease, diabetes, or obesity), and immunocompromised patients, are more likely to experience severe or critical conditions or long-term complications.

13.4.3 Considerations for Estimands

The FDA (2023c) guideline primarily outlined estimand considerations in treatment trials, covering the suggestion on population, variable, treatment, intercurrent events and strategies, and statistical analysis. While variable selection for prevention trials is briefly outlined, this section will concentrate on interpreting estimands within the context of the treatment trials, aligning with the FDA (2023c) recommendations.

(a) Population

The target population for COVID-19 should clearly reflect the intended use of the drug and be categorized by disease severity, such as hospitalized or nonhospitalized patients at high or standard risk of progression to serious disease. FDA (2023c) recommended categorizing the population based on the baseline disease severity, with detailed examples provided in Appendix A of the guideline. The severity categories are as follows:

1. SARS-CoV-2 infection without symptoms: positive test for SARS-CoV-2 but no symptoms.
2. Mild COVID-19: Mild symptoms (e.g., fever, cough) without shortness of breath.
3. Moderate COVID-19: shortness of breath but saturation of oxygen (SpO_2) > 93% on room air.
4. Severe COVID-19: clinical signs indicating severe symptoms (e.g., $SpO_2 \leq 93\%$ on room air, high respiratory rate).
5. Critical COVID-19: Evidence of respiratory failure, Shock, and/or multi-organ dysfunction failure.

Nonhospitalized patients typically present with mild or moderate symptoms, while hospitalized patients often have severe or critical symptoms. FDA (2023c) also emphasizes the importance of enrolling a diverse population, including patients at high risk of complications, such as the elderly, those with chronic diseases (e.g., cardiovascular and respiratory diseases, diabetes, and chronic kidney disease), immunocompromised patients (e.g., organ transplant recipients or patients receiving cancer chemotherapy), and pregnant or postpartum women.

(b) Variable
Efficacy variables should be chosen to reflect the effect of the experimental drug compared to placebo or active control drugs. Currently, there is no universally recognized primary variable for COVID-19 treatment trials. Sponsors are encouraged to engage in close communication with regulatory agencies during development. The choice of efficacy variables depends on several factors such as the drug's mechanism of action, trial population, clinical setting, phase of drug development, and baseline disease severity. Table 13.3 provides examples of appropriate variables for different populations in the COVID-19 treatment trials.

(c) Treatment
The FDA (2023c) strongly recommends the use of superiority designs in randomized, placebo-controlled, double-blinded clinical trials for COVID-19 treatments.

Common treatment strategies include antiviral therapy, immunotherapy, and supportive care (e.g., oxygen supply, mechanical ventilation, and extracorporeal membrane oxygenation). The FDA (2023c) also includes the use of preventive vaccines as part of clinical management.

Moreover, it emphasizes collecting baseline and concomitant medication data, including COVID-19 standard of care, to support additional analysis of vaccination status and concomitant medication effects, which are further discussed in Sect. 13.4.4.

(d) Intercurrent Events
FDA (2023c) provides recommendations for addressing key intercurrent events in clinical trials. Table 13.4 summarizes these strategies.

(e) Population-Level Summary
The choice of the population-level summary depends on the type of variables being analyzed; FDA (2023c) does not provide a detailed discussion on it.

Table 13.3 Examples of appropriate variables based on trial population and disease severity

Trial Population	Nonhospitalized patients with mild and/or moderate COVID-19	Hospitalized patients with severe and/or critical COVID-19
Considerations	Focus on variables related to preventing hospitalization or severe/critical illness, or death, as well as alleviating symptoms	Focus on variables related to survival and respiratory function and other critical organ functions
Examples of variables	Proportion of hospitalization or death from any cause by appropriate time points (e.g., at least 28 days) Time to sustained clinical recovery is assessed at appropriate time points Virologic variables may be acceptable as the primary variable in the phase II clinical trials but are not recommended as primary variables for phase III trials	All-cause mortality by appropriate time points (e.g., 4–8 weeks; at least 28 days for hospitalized noncritically ill patients and 60 days for critically ill patients). Proportion of patients alive and free of respiratory failure or first occurrence of symptomatic thromboembolism at appropriate time points (e.g., at least 28 days for hospitalized noncritically ill patients and 60 days for critically ill patients)

Table 13.4 Intercurrent events and strategies

Intercurrent events	Strategies	Comments
Death	Composite variable strategy	Death is considered a very unfavorable outcome, not missing data
Hospitalization	Composite variable strategy	Hospitalization is a serious outcome for outpatient populations
Other intercurrent events	Treatment policy strategy	FDA prefers a treatment policy strategy but recommends consulting regulatory authorities for alternative strategies in advance

13.4.4 Statistical Analysis

The FDA (2023c) does not reiterate commonly used methods but instead provides more detailed and updated recommendations on covariate adjustment and analysis requirements for diverse populations with varying baseline characteristics.

To improve the precision of treatment effect estimation and inference, the guideline recommends adjusting for prespecified baseline prognostic covariates (such as age, baseline severity, comorbidities, baseline medications, and COVID-19 vaccination status) in the primary efficacy analysis. For binary endpoints, it gave the examples of methods to assess the unconditional treatment difference in proportion using covariate adjustment (Steingrimsson et al., 2017; Ye et al., 2023).

If a trial enrolls patients with diverse baseline severity levels, baseline medication use, and/or vaccination statuses, FDA (2023c) suggests conducting the subgroup and/or interaction analyses to evaluate potential treatment differences. It also indicates the necessity of including all randomized patients in the primary analysis, even if they have already completed vaccination or received other concomitant medication (including standard of care). Additionally, FDA (2023c) requires the descriptive analyses of concomitant medication use and changes in vaccination status throughout the trial.

Sensitivity analysis is critical for assessing the robustness of the clinical trial results. FDA (2023c) recommends that sponsors prepare the statistical analysis plan to include sensitivity and supplementary analysis methods. While it emphasizes the importance of sensitivity analysis, specific implementation recommendations are not provided in detail.

13.5 Eosinophilic Esophagitis

In 2020, the FDA published a guideline for developing drugs for the treatment of eosinophilic esophagitis (FDA, 2020). Eosinophilic esophagitis is a chronic immune or antigen-mediated esophageal disease characterized by symptoms of esophageal dysfunction and eosinophil-predominant inflammation, which can vary independently following treatment. The variability in symptoms between pediatric and adult patients adds complexity to clinical outcome assessments.

The FDA (2020) introduces estimands as a key concept but does not explicitly specify strategies for addressing intercurrent events. Instead, the guideline (FDA, 2020) advises sponsors to prespecify a primary estimand for each variable, provide justification, and describe strategies for addressing key intercurrent events, such as the initiation of systemic corticosteroid treatment, use of rescue medications, and changes in diet and eating behaviors.

Addressing these intercurrent events is critical, as they can significantly impact study results. Dietary restriction is an established and effective treatment for eosinophilic esophagitis. Since the disease's symptoms can alter dietary habits, it is essential for patients to maintain a stable diet both before and throughout the trial. Additionally, to minimize the impact of other treatments, patients should consistently maintain stable doses of proton pump inhibitors or locally acting corticosteroids for comorbid conditions, such as asthma and allergic rhinitis, throughout the trial.

13.6 Concluding Remarks

This chapter systematically reviews recent FDA guidelines concerning the recommendation of the estimand framework across various therapeutic areas, including acute myeloid leukemia, chronic rhinosinusitis with nasal polyps, COVID-19, and eosinophilic esophagitis. These guidelines outline the FDA's general recommendations for the strategies to address the intercurrent events for key efficacy variables.

While the FDA provides the general recommendation, it also allows flexibility, thereby encouraging sponsors to propose alternative strategies with solid justifications. Ensuring effective communication with the FDA and alignment on estimand selection early in the trial planning phase is crucial for the trial design, data collection, analysis approaches, and result interpretation of the clinical trials.

References

FDA. (2020). *Eosinophilic esophagitis: developing drugs for the treatment guidance for industry.* https://www.fda.gov/

FDA. (2021). *COVID-19: developing drugs and biological products for treatment or prevention.* https://www.fda.gov/

FDA. (2022a). *Ulcerative colitis: developing drugs for treatment.* https://www.fda.gov/

FDA. (2022b). *Acute myeloid leukemia: developing drugs and biological products for treatment.* https://www.fda.gov/

FDA. (2023a). *Graft-versus-Host diseases: developing drugs, biological products, and certain devices for prevention or treatment.* https://www.fda.gov/

FDA. (2023b). *Chronic rhinosinusitis with nasal polyps: developing drugs for treatment.* https://www.fda.gov/

FDA. (2023c). *COVID-19: developing drugs and biological products for treatment or prevention.* https://www.fda.gov/

ICH. (2019). *ICH E9 (R1) addendum on estimands and sensitivity analysis in clinical trials to the guideline on statistical principles for clinical trials*. Step 4 document. https://ich.org/

Steingrimsson, J., Hanley, D., & Rosenblum, M. (2017). Improving precision by adjusting for prognostic baseline variables in randomized trials with binary outcomes, without regression model assumptions. *Contemporary Clinical Trials, 54*, 18–24.

Ye, T., Bannick, M., Yi, Y., & Shao, J. (2023). Robust variance estimation for covariate-adjusted unconditional treatment effect in randomized clinical trials with binary outcomes. *Statistical Theory and Related Fields, 7*, 159–163.

Chapter 14
NMPA Guidelines and Their Relationship to the Estimand Framework

Yuhan Huang, Jie Chen, Jun Zhao, Xiaoni Liu, Mingli Heng, Yan Hou, Jun Wang, and Pingyan Chen

Abstract The China National Medical Products Administration (NMPA) adopted the ICH E9(R1) guideline on estimands and sensitivity analysis in clinical trials in early 2021. Considering the growing importance of well-defined estimands in clinical trials, this chapter discusses the NMPA's implementation of the estimand framework across various guideline documents, focusing primarily on drug development for Crohn's Disease (CD) and Uclcerative Colitis (UC), real-world studies (RWS), and pediatric extrapolation. We first discuss key principles embedded within the NMPA guidelines for drug development in CD and UC, emphasizing the treatment goal, rigorous trial designs, and considerations for estimands regarding population, variable, treatment, and intercurrent events. The chapter also illustrates the complexities of establishing estimands in RWS, highlighting considerations of diverse patient populations, treatment regimens, and intercurrent events related to behavior

Y. Huang (✉)
Statistics & Decision Sciences, J&J Innovative Medicine, R&D, Shanghai, China
e-mail: yhuang72@its.jnj.com

J. Chen
Department of Data Science, Taimei Intelligence Biopharma, Shanghai, China
e-mail: jie.chen8@taimei.com

J. Zhao · M. Heng · J. Wang
Statistics & Clinical Pharmacology, Center for Drug Evaluation, NMPA, Beijing, China
e-mail: zhaojun@cde.org.cn; hengml@cde.org.cn; wangj@cde.org.cn

X. Liu
Advanced Quantitative Sciences, Novartis Institutes for Biomedical Research Co., Shanghai, China
e-mail: xiaoni.liu@novartis.com

Y. Hou
Department of Biostatistics, Peking University, Beijing, China
e-mail: houyan@bjmu.edu.cn

P. Chen
Department of Biostatistics, Southern Medical University, Guangzhou, China
e-mail: chenpy99@126.com

J. Wei et al. (eds.), *Estimands in Clinical Trials*, Springer Series in Pharmaceutical Statistics, https://doi.org/10.1007/978-3-032-02192-2_14

and nonbehavioral factors. Drawing attention to recent suggestions for pediatric extrapolation, we emphasize the necessity of clear definitions of estimands aligning with trial objectives. In closure, the chapter ascertains the importance of proactive communication between sponsors and the NMPA to ensure adherence to these guidelines and successful implementation of estimands in China.

14.1 Introduction

In January 2021, the China National Medical Products Administration (NMPA) adopted the International Council for Harmonization (ICH) E9(R1) guideline on estimands and sensitivity analysis in clinical trials (ICH, 2019). This guideline was formally implemented in China as of January 2022. In response to this transition, pharmaceutical sponsors in China conducting confirmatory studies have begun integrating the estimand framework in clinical trial development. Underscoring its significance, the Center for Drug Evaluation (CDE) under the NMPA released a revised version of the guideline for data management and statistical analysis plans in clinical trials (NMPA, 2021) in December 2021. The purpose of this update was to streamline the alignment with the ICH E9(R1) framework from a practical perspective.

In this chapter, we explore several guidelines from the NMPA that relate to the estimand framework. The subsequent sections focus on specific disease areas and scenarios. In Sect. 14.2, we focus on the considerations of estimands in the clinical development of drugs to treat Crohn's Disease (CD) and Ulcerative Colitis (UC). In Sect. 14.3, we discuss the considerations for constructing estimands in real-world studies (RWS). Section 14.4 then focuses on pediatric extrapolation. Section 14.5 provides the concluding remarks of this chapter.

14.2 Crohn's Disease and Ulcerative Colitis

14.2.1 Introduction to Guideline Principles

In 2022, the NMPA released two guidelines on developing drugs for the treatment of inflammatory bowel disease, which includes two types: guideline on the development of drugs for the treatment of CD (NMPA, 2022a) and guideline on the development of drugs for the treatment of UC (NMPA, 2022b). These two guidelines mainly discuss the key considerations in the clinical development of drugs to treat CD and UC.

14.2.2 Disease Background and Trial Design

CD and UC are two types of inflammatory bowel disease that are characterized by chronic inflammation of the gastrointestinal tract, the cause of which remains unknown. CD can affect any part of the gastrointestinal tract discontinuously from the mouth to the anus. UC, on the other hand, primarily affects the rectum and can extend to all or part of the colon.

The treatment goal of CD and UC is to induce and maintain symptomatic and endoscopic remission, control complications, and improve quality of life. For both CD and UC, the NMPA guidelines recommend a randomized, double-blind, placebo-or active-controlled design. The choice of control arm is based on whether the drug is being developed as a first-or second-line treatment (refer to Sect. 14.2.3 for details). Stratified randomization can be considered, with stratification factors such as previous treatment.

To demonstrate induction and maintenance efficacy (induction and maintenance of remission), it is recommended to conduct induction and maintenance trials separately or conduct a single trial that evaluates both short-term induction and long-term maintenance efficacy. This can be achieved by a treat-through or a randomized withdrawal design. The treat-through design is to continue the trial for long-term maintenance of efficacy following the short-term induction while maintaining blinding and randomization. The randomized withdrawal design is to re-randomize patients who have achieved response or remission at the end of short-term induction. These patients are then assigned to either the experimental or control arm in a maintenance trial. The duration of the induction trial is usually 6–12 weeks, and the total trial duration should be at least 12 months (including the induction phase).

14.2.3 Considerations for Estimands

This section summarizes the considerations for estimands in the NMPA guidelines for clinical trials of developing drugs to treat CD/UC in terms of population, variable, treatment, and intercurrent events. It is recommended that the primary estimand should estimate treatment effects based on the achievement (induction of remission/short-term treatment) or maintenance (maintenance of remission/long-term treatment) of symptomatic and endoscopic remission.

(a) Population
Active CD/UC refers to patients who exhibit evidence of active disease based on clinical signs and symptoms, along with endoscopic findings made within 3 months (for CD only) or 1 month (for UC only) before enrollment. For UC, histological findings within 1 month before enrollment are also considered. If the target population with moderate to severe CD/UC includes both patients who have failed conventional therapy and those who have had biologic failures,

it is recommended to prespecify the proportion of these different population groups.

(b) Variable

In clinical trials for both CD and UC, it is recommended by the NMPA to use primary endpoints evaluating the drug's effect on signs and symptoms (symptomatic remission) and underlying mucosal inflammation (endoscopic remission). Specifically, for CD clinical trials, the NMPA recommends using co-primary endpoints to assess both the proportion of responders achieving symptomatic remission and the proportion of responders achieving endoscopic remission. For UC clinical trials, the NMPA suggests two types of endpoints. The first is co-primary endpoints for both symptomatic remission and endoscopic remission, similar to CD clinical trials; the second is a single primary endpoint, clinical remission, which evaluates the proportion of responders achieving both symptomatic remission and endoscopic remission.

Table 14.1 summarizes the considerations for primary endpoints and the instruments used for evaluation of primary endpoints in CD and UC clinical trials.

(c) Treatment

When determining the control arm for first-line indications in the treatment of active CD/UC, it is necessary to provide a direct comparison with the current generally accepted standard first-line treatment. For second-line indications (after failure or intolerance to primary therapy), a placebo or active comparator can be considered.

For considerations on background therapy, when patients receive treatment for CD/UC at enrollment, they are generally allowed to continue using these treatments during the trial as background therapy and maintain stable doses (except for glucocorticoids). Patients entering an early treatment phase while

Table 14.1 Considerations for primary endpoints in CD and UC clinical trials

CD	UC
The NMPA recommends co-primary endpoints for both symptomatic remission and endoscopic remission (endoscopic response may be acceptable)	The NMPA recommends co-primary endpoints for both symptomatic remission and endoscopic remission, or a single primary endpoint of clinical remission (achieving both symptomatic and endoscopic remission)
A different time point for the assessment of symptomatic remission and endoscopic remission in the co-primary endpoints can be acceptable	
Symptomatic remission: Evaluated by PRO2, or SF and AP, or CDAI	Symptomatic remission: Evaluated by RB and SF
Endoscopic remission: Evaluated by SES-CD or CDEIS	Endoscopic remission: Evaluated by UCEIS or Mayo subscore

Note: *SF* Stool Frequency, *AP* Abdominal Pain, *RB* Rectal Bleeding, *PRO2* For CD, this is a patient-reported outcome measure focusing on SF and AP, *SES-CD* Simple Endoscopic Score for CD, *CDAI* Crohn Disease Activity Index, *CDEIS* CD Endoscopic Index of Severity, *UCEIS* UC Endoscopic Index of severity

Table 14.2 Intercurrent events and estimand strategies

Intercurrent events	Strategies	Comments
Treatment discontinuation (due to lack of tolerability, lack of efficacy, or disease progression)	If the therapeutic intent is to induce remission in the short term: Treatment policy strategy	
	If the therapeutic intent is maintaining remission in the long term: Composite variable strategy	CD/UC is a chronic disease requiring long-term treatment, and discontinuation from treatment is considered as being unsuccessfully treated
Use of rescue medication	Composite variable strategy	The use of rescue medication, and in particular the initiation of corticosteroid treatment, should be considered as a failure of the assigned drug
Failing to taper steroids according to the protocol-planned fixed schedule	Composite variable strategy	A failure to taper steroids according to the protocol-planned fixed schedule can be considered as a special case of rescue medication
Use of prohibited medication	Not available	Intercurrent event mentioned but not discussed in the guidelines
Change in background therapy	Not available	Intercurrent event mentioned but not discussed in the guidelines

on steroids should remain on a fixed dose and then have their steroids tapered according to a fixed schedule.

(d) Intercurrent Events
Table 14.2 summarizes the intercurrent events that need to be considered and the estimand strategies mentioned in the guidelines.

(e) Population-Level Summary
This is not discussed in the guideline.

14.2.4 Statistical Analysis

According to the NMPA guidelines, statistical analysis (including the handling of missing data) should be aligned with the prespecified estimand and fully justified in the trial protocol.

It is important to make every effort to collect the necessary data to align with the prespecified estimand. For the primary estimand, if using a composite variable strategy to consider the occurrence of a specific intercurrent event as treatment failure, data for the clinical outcome variable after the intercurrent event is not needed for analysis. However, these data might still be required for estimands addressing other scientific questions of interest. It is also important to distinguish between intercurrent events and missing data, as suggested in both guidelines.

14.2.5 Summary and Discussion

Both guidelines intend to address the NMPA position on clinical development of new drugs in the treatment of CD/UC; they provide general recommendations on trial design, population, variable, treatment, and intercurrent events we need to consider in the clinical trials, which are fully aligned with the estimand framework.

Given the variety of trial designs that can be considered and the evolving understanding of instruments for evaluating primary endpoints in CD/UC clinical trials, early interaction between sponsors and regulators would be beneficial in achieving alignment on trial objectives, clinical questions of interest, and corresponding estimands.

14.3 Real-World Studies

14.3.1 Introduction to Guideline Principles

Although the ICH E9 (R1) guideline is primarily formulated for randomized clinical trials, its principles can also be applied to studies aiming at generating real-world evidence. In early 2023, the NMPA released the guideline on the design and protocol development of real-world studies (NMPA, 2023b).

This guideline discusses the complexity of constructing estimands in real-world studies (RWS). In particular, it describes how the estimand attributes can be precisely defined in RWS by considering the heterogeneity of the population, the distinction of endpoint selection, the flexibility of treatment regimes, the diversity of intercurrent events, and the sophistication of analytical methods (including primary and sensitivity analyses).

14.3.2 Considerations for Estimands

This guideline discusses the considerations of estimands in RWS regarding population, variable, treatment, and intercurrent events.

(a) Population
A precise definition of the target patient population in RWS may not be as straightforward as one would think. This is primarily due to, for example, a complex pattern of phenotypes (e.g., disease spectrum, use of concomitant medications, demographics, location, healthcare system) and genotypes (e.g., gene expression, existence/lack of a receptor) of the target population.

(b) Variable
The choice of endpoint(s) depends not only on the research question but also on the available data sources. Two broad categories of commonly used endpoints in clinical research can be considered: surrogate and clinical endpoints. While both types of endpoints can be used in clinical trials, the latter is usually preferred, as they are more likely to be captured in RWS. Furthermore, a single specific clinical endpoint (e.g., hospitalization, death) is always preferred over a composite clinical endpoint (e.g., a composite of death or myocardial infarction or stroke) because not all individual components might be captured in RWS.

(c) Treatment
The treatment regimen in the real world could be quite complicated, for example, concomitant medications, dosage adjustment, and dynamic treatments including treatment switching back and forth over time, due to, for example, comorbidities, product-induced treatment changes, and personal preferences. The availability of many therapeutically similar products and the complexity of treatment regimens may create many comparison groups in RWS. Therefore, it is important to clearly articulate the treatment regimens of primary interest when defining the estimands in the protocol.

(d) Intercurrent Events
The ICH E9(R1) guideline states that intercurrent events should be considered explicitly in the description of a clinical question. To account for intercurrent events in RWS, it is important to consider not only events related to safety, intolerability, lack of efficacy, and terminal events (e.g., death), but also events related to behavioral factors and nonbehavioral factors. For example, the behavior factors may include patient preference, inconvenience of use for the current product, and physician–patient relationship. Additionally, nonbehavioral factors may include a change of health insurance program that contradicts the use of the current therapy and an improvement of health conditions.

(e) Population-Level Summary
This is not discussed in the guideline.

14.3.3 *Summary and Discussion*

The construction of estimands for an RWS may differ from that for a randomized clinical trial. It is important to understand the stakeholders' questions and the utility of the corresponding policy before applying relevant frameworks to construct appropriate estimands. This may be an iterative process requiring a revisit of the original research question and redefining the estimand's attributes to ensure identifiability of the causal estimand using the available data.

14.4 Pediatric Extrapolation

In 2023, the NMPA released its guideline on quantitative approaches for pediatric extrapolation from adults (NMPA, 2023a), which provides recommendations for pediatric extrapolation to support pediatric drug development from a quantitative perspective.

For each different stage of clinical development, clinical trials are designed to answer different scientific questions of interest. The more precisely the scientific question is articulated, the more definitively the primary estimand can be determined. In cases where pediatric trials are a part of the extrapolation plan, adherence to principles detailed in the ICH E9(R1) guideline is important. This ensures that the estimands are aligned with the trial objectives and guarantees that trial design (including sample size determination), data collection, and analysis reflect the primary estimand to answer the scientific questions of interest.

In terms of the uncertainty of extrapolation and borrowed information, a sound scientific understanding and justification are essential. They should be reflected in the justification and definitions of the primary estimand.

It is important to note that estimands in pediatric trials and reference groups will inevitably differ (as the 'population' attribute will always differ). In fact, every attribute of the estimands in pediatric trials and reference groups might differ. However, this does not undermine the concept of extrapolation. Indeed, trying to align estimands in the pediatric and reference populations is not necessarily the best way of justifying extrapolation and may not even be scientifically desirable.

When considering estimands in the pediatric extrapolation plan, the first step is to determine at a high level what pediatric trials are needed to mitigate the knowledge gaps identified in the extrapolation concept. Estimand thinking process can be particularly useful at this stage, as it helps to translate the research question—aimed at filling a knowledge gap—into a precisely defined quantity of interest. Subsequently, the design and analysis of the pediatric trial are aligned with the specified estimand.

If we consider augmenting the pediatric trial with external data (e.g., leveraging controls from adult trials to supplement the control arm in a randomized clinical trial), having a well-defined estimand can inform our decisions about what external data to leverage and how heavily it should be weighted.

14.5 Concluding Remarks

In summary, the implementation of the ICH E9(R1) guideline, viewed from a regulatory perspective, denotes a remarkable progression in clinical trial conduct. With its focus on clear definitions of estimands, appropriate strategies for addressing intercurrent events, and emphasis on sensitivity analyses, the guideline enhances the transparency, reliability, and interpretability of trial results. This progress can optimize and strengthen the decision-making processes in drug development and regulatory review, ultimately expediting the provision of safe and efficacious treatments to patients.

This chapter highlights the essential aspects of estimands based on specific disease areas and scenarios as outlined in the guidelines issued by the NMPA. For disease areas such as CD and UC, the NMPA offers general recommendations on trial design and considerations for defining key attributes of estimands. In scenarios involving RWS and pediatric extrapolation, sponsors should give additional attention and consideration.

It is important for sponsors to engage in proactive communication and seek alignment with the NMPA during the early planning stages of the trials. This will facilitate the successful implementation of estimands in accordance with the NMPA guidelines, ultimately leading to the generation of robust and meaningful clinical evidence.

References

ICH (2019) ICH E9 (R1) addendum on estimands and sensitivity analysis in clinical trials to the guideline on statistical principles for clinical trials. Step 4 document. https://ich.org/

NMPA. (2021). *Guideline for data management and statistical analysis plans in clinical trials*. https://www.cde.org.cn/

NMPA. (2022a). *Guideline on the development of drugs for the treatment of Crohn's Disease*. https://www.cde.org.cn/

NMPA. (2022b). *Guideline on the development of drugs for the treatment of Ulcerative Colitis*. https://www.cde.org.cn/

NMPA. (2023a). *Guideline on quantitative approaches for pediatric extrapolation from adult trials*. https://www.cde.org.cn/

NMPA. (2023b). *Guideline on the design and protocol development of real-world studies*. https://www.cde.org.cn/

Part IV
Statistical Analysis Under the Estimand Framework

This part of the book provides an overview of statistical analysis methods under the estimand framework, with a focus on various types of endpoints and strategies for addressing intercurrent events. It begins with a discussion of continuous endpoints, including considerations for implementation and missing data handling in alignment with the estimand of interest. This is followed by a discussion of binary and recurrent event endpoints, highlighting the unique analytical challenges each presents in the context of the estimand framework. Next, strategies for addressing intercurrent events and handling of missing data are discussed for time-to-event endpoints, along with other key elements such as variable definitions, population-level summaries, and sensitivity analyses. A dedicated chapter introduces readers to handling the complexities of treatment noncompliance and posttreatment complications using principal stratification. The final chapter focuses on covariate adjustment, illustrating how the estimand framework supports the appropriate use of covariates to improve the precision and interpretability of treatment effect estimates.

Chapter 15
Statistical Analysis Under the Estimand Framework: Continuous Endpoints

Chen Lu, Vladimir Dragalin, Elena Polverejan, Björn Bornkamp, Marcel Wolbers, , Longshen Xie, and Na Yang

Abstract For a given estimand, an appropriate analysis method or estimator should be employed to provide an estimate that allows for a reliable interpretation. This chapter serves as a practical guide to the application of the estimand framework in analyzing continuous endpoints in clinical trials. It focuses on addressing issues arising from intercurrent events, which are the post-randomization events that may be related to treatment and outcome. We provide a detailed discussion of the treatment policy, hypothetical, and composite variable strategies for addressing intercurrent events under the estimand framework, their aligned estimators, and sensitivity

C. Lu (✉)
Global Biostatistical Science, Amgen Inc., Thousand Oaks, CA, USA
e-mail: chelu@amgen.com

V. Dragalin
Quantitative Sciences and Clinical Pharmacology, Johnson & Johnson, Spring House, PA, USA
e-mail: vdragali@its.jnj.com

E. Polverejan
Quantitative Sciences and Clinical Pharmacology, Johnson & Johnson, Titusville, NJ, USA
e-mail: EPolvere@its.jnj.com

B. Bornkamp
Advanced Quantitative Sciences, Novartis Pharma AG, Basel, Switzerland
e-mail: bjoern.bornkamp@novartis.com

M. Wolbers
Methods, Collaboration, and Outreach; Pharma Development Science and Analytics, Roche, Basel, Switzerland
e-mail: marcel.wolbers@roche.com

L. Xie
Department of Biometrics and Data Management, Shenyang Sunshine Pharmaceutical Co., Ltd., Shanghai, China
e-mail: xielongshen@3sbio.com

N. Yang
Evidence Generation and Decision Sciences, Sanofi, Beijing, China
e-mail: Na3.yang@sanofi.com

J. Wei et al. (eds.), *Estimands in Clinical Trials*, Springer Series in Pharmaceutical Statistics, https://doi.org/10.1007/978-3-032-02192-2_15

analysis methods. A case study on asymptomatic Alzheimer's disease serves to illustrate the steps of the estimand thinking process. Meanwhile, it demonstrates how different questions of interest can lead to different strategies being specified in the estimand definition for the intercurrent events of treatment discontinuation and initiation of treatment with cholinesterase inhibitors.

15.1 Introduction to Continuous Endpoints

Continuous variables, which are a type of quantitative variable obtained through measurement or quantification, may take on any value within a certain range. For example:

- Drug concentration measurements, such as maximum serum concentration observed and area under the serum concentration used in pharmacokinetic studies.
- Lipid measurements, such as low-density lipoprotein cholesterol (LDL-C), in cardiovascular studies.
- Respiratory measurements, such as change in forced expiratory volume in the first second (FEV1) trough value from baseline at week 24 in chronic obstructive pulmonary disease or asthma studies.
- Patient-reported outcomes measurements, such as change in the total symptom score of the Kansas City Cardiomyopathy Questionnaire (KCCQ-TSS) from baseline at week 16 in heart failure with preserved or mildly reduced ejection fraction (HFpEF, HFmrEF) studies.

Common descriptive statistics for continuous variables include the arithmetic mean, geometric mean, standard deviation, median, maximum, and minimum values, etc. Continuous variables are usually assumed to follow a normal or log-normal distribution. For single measurement endpoints, the most common statistical model in trials is to take the target measurement as the dependent variable, with treatment, baseline, and all stratification factors acting as covariates. The ordinary least squares linear regression method (also known as analysis of covariance (ANCOVA)) is often applied for analysis. For repeated measures endpoints, the most common statistical method employed is the mixed-effects model repeated measures (MMRM) approach (Mallinckrodt et al., 2008), where the target measurement is the dependent variable, whereas treatment, baseline, all stratification factors, visit, visit by treatment interaction, and occasionally, visit by baseline or other interactions are included as covariates in the model. The form of the covariance structure for the repeated outcome measures also needs to be prespecified, together with what alternative types are planned to be used in case of non-convergence.

When there is missing data, the ANCOVA model assumes missing outcome data are missing completely at random (MCAR), meaning that the probability of missingness is unrelated to the observed and unobserved outcome data but could depend on baseline covariates in the model. On the other hand, the MMRM model assumes missing outcome data are missing at random (MAR), meaning that the probability of missingness is related only to the observed outcome and baseline covariate data but not the unobserved data. This indicates that the missingness can be predicted or explained by the observed variables in the model.

Regarding covariate selection in analysis, the EMA (2015) guideline on adjustment for baseline covariates in clinical trials states that if there is "a strong or moderate association between a baseline covariate(s) and the primary outcome measure, adjustment for such baseline covariate(s) generally improves the efficiency of the analysis and avoids conditional bias from chance covariate imbalance." To ensure the analysis is consistent with the design, stratification factors should normally be included as covariates as well. FDA (2023a) and NMPA (2020) also have relevant guidelines. For more details about covariate adjustment, please see Chapt. 20.

The remainder of this Chapter is structured as follows. In Sect. 15.2, we discuss different strategies for addressing intercurrent events under the estimand framework and the aligned analysis methods. In Sect. 15.3, we consider a long-term prevention trial in patients who are asymptomatic and at risk of developing Alzheimer's dementia. This illustrates the definition of different estimands, which correspond to different clinical questions of interest, and how to define estimators that are aligned with these estimands.

15.2 Addressing Intercurrent Events and Missing Data

In this section, we discuss different strategies for addressing intercurrent events under the estimand framework and the aligned analysis methods. We focus on analysis for treatment policy, hypothetical, and composite variable strategies. Subsequently, the while on treatment and principal stratum strategies, as well as sensitivity analyses, are briefly discussed. For more details on the principal stratum strategy, please refer to Chap. 19.

15.2.1 Treatment Policy Strategy

For the treatment policy strategy, the ICH E9(R1) guideline states that "... the occurrence of the intercurrent event is considered irrelevant in defining the treatment effect of interest...." and that "... in relation to whether or not a patient continues treatment, and whether or not a patient experiences changes in other treatments (e.g., background or concomitant treatments), the intercurrent event is considered to be part of the treatments being compared ..." (ICH, 2019).

Using a treatment policy strategy for intercurrent events means that all observed values of the relevant variables at the final time point will be used, regardless of whether the intercurrent event occurs. The scientific question of interest often effectively incorporates the intercurrent event into the treatment definition, so it investigates a treatment policy rather than the pure effect of the investigational treatment alone. Since data after the occurrence of intercurrent events will be used, it is important to collect all data until the primary endpoint has been observed, regardless of the occurrence of intercurrent events. If all data is available (i.e., an ideal but unlikely situation), the analysis can be performed using the models mentioned earlier, such as ANCOVA or MMRM, as appropriate.

However, usually, not all data may have been collected as planned, resulting in a missing data problem. Under this situation, a common approach is to impute the missing observations. Besides model-based approaches that impute the missing data implicitly (e.g., MMRM), various methods exist to explicitly impute missing data within a multiple imputation framework. All imputation methods rely on untestable assumptions. It is necessary to consider reasonable assumptions under the treatment policy strategy, including clinically plausible assumptions and sufficient statistical modeling assumptions. Once a set of assumptions has been selected for the primary analysis of a particular estimand, we can then vary them in the sensitivity analysis so that the robustness of statistical inference based on different modeling assumptions can be assessed.

Suppose there is a need to impute missing data after study withdrawal when the intercurrent event of treatment discontinuation is addressed with the treatment policy strategy. One commonly used imputation method is based on retrieved dropout (RDO) data. It assumes that patients with missing data after discontinuation of treatment would behave similarly to those who remain in the trial and continue to be followed up after discontinuation of treatment, namely, RDO patients. This is a plausible assumption for treatment policy, since it models the outcome of patients with missing data after discontinuation of treatment based on observed data after discontinuation of treatment, as well as measurement history and model covariates. There are multiple publications on this topic that can be referred to for more details. Polverejan and Dragalin (2020) and Noci et al. (2023) explored the operating characteristics of multiple imputation methods using RDO data and compared them with other methods, such as reference-based multiple imputation. Wang et al. (2023) also explored the operating characteristics of several methods aligned with the treatment policy strategy and expressed their preference for the use of an RDO approach. Drury et al. (2023) explored the operating characteristics of several RDO-based sequential multiple imputation methods, where missing data at each timepoint is imputed using previous outcomes based on the status of on/off treatment or the pattern of treatment discontinuation history. Bell et al. (2025) introduced likelihood-based versions of RDO-based methods and compared them to existing approaches in an extensive simulation study. In general, the bias of the RDO-based methods was observed to be small in simulation studies described in the referenced papers. However, one limitation of an RDO-based method is that it requires sufficient RDO data to be available to reliably fit the RDO model. If there is not enough RDO data available, using this method may result in increased variance in the estimates relative to all other methods, leading to a reduction in power (Roger et al., 2019; Polverejan & Dragalin, 2020; Wang et al., 2023, and Bell et al., 2025). There is no clear cutoff for "having sufficient RDO data"; however, increased variance impairing power was observed for scenarios with 50% or less available data after treatment discontinuation (Polverejan & Dragalin, 2020; Bell et al., 2025). Similarly, Guizzaro et al. (2021) showed that in an MAR setting, estimation methods increase their performance when a variable representing compliance is used in the model. For an example of using treatment policy strategy to address intercurrent events with an estimator using the RDO approach, please see Sect. 15.3.3.

When we believe that the outcome measures of patients with missing data after discontinuation of treatment could be modeled based on the control/reference group, we can use reference-based imputation methods, such as copy reference (CR), jump-to-reference (J2R), and copy increment in reference (CIR). Under CR, a patient's whole distribution, both pre- and posttreatment discontinuation, is assumed to be the same as the reference (typically, but not necessarily, control) group. Under J2R, the patient ceases randomized treatment, and the patient's mean response distribution is now that of a "reference" group of patients (typically, but not necessarily, control patients). If the reference group is chosen as the control, patients on active treatment will lose the effect of their period on treatment. Under this method, if a patient's observed outcomes are better/worse than those of patients in the patient's own treatment arm, the mean for imputations for that patient at the imputed visit will tend to be better/worse than those observed for the control group at that visit. Similar descriptions were included in the Estimand 1 example of Polverejan et al. (2023). Under CIR, after the patient discontinues treatment, the patient's mean increments copy those from the reference group (typically, but not necessarily, control patients). If the reference is chosen to be the control arm, the patient's mean profile following deviation tracks that of the mean profile in the control arm, but starting from the benefit already obtained. This method could be considered in disease-modifying settings. For detailed descriptions of these methods, please refer to Carpenter et al. (2013), O'Kelly and Ratitch (2014), and Cro et al. (2019, 2020). Comprehensive figures are given in Sect. 7.3.5 of O'Kelly and Ratitch (2014).

White et al. (2020) suggested a causal modeling framework for reference-based imputation, and Wolbers et al. (2022) proposed a deterministic implementation of reference-based imputation. A recent ongoing discussion in the literature on reference-based imputation methods focuses on which variance estimator to use; see Bartlett (2023), Liu et al. (2022), and the recent letter by Cro et al. (2024) with a rejoinder by Wolbers et al. (2024). Depending on the assumptions considered, other methods for missing data imputation can be utilized. These include the return-to-baseline or last observation-like multiple imputation as discussed in Qu and Dai (2022) and in Sect. 7.4.4. of O'Kelly and Ratitch (2014). Furthermore, delta-based methods can be considered, as highlighted in Cro et al. (2019), where a worsening effect is applied on imputed values derived from other methods. This is specifically common in delta-based multiple imputation sensitivity analysis used as a tipping point method, as noted in Ratitch et al. (2013) and García-Hernandez et al. (2023).

Numerous software tools exist for implementing the treatment policy strategy. For instances with minimal missing data where the MMRM is appropriate, SAS PROC MIXED or the R package `mmrm` can be applied, as described in Sabanes

Bove et al. (2022). For SAS code and examples of implementing RDO methods, please refer to the "Stepwise imputation for marginal model based on previous residuals" and "Template code treatment policy using SAS PROC MI and the MISTEP macro" developed by the Drug Information Association (DIA) Scientific Working Group on Estimands and Missing Data. (https://www.lshtm.ac.uk/research/centres-projects-groups/missing-data#dia-missing-data). The DIA missing data website also includes several SAS macros for reference-based imputation methods. In R, the `rbmi` package (Gower-Page & Noci 2022, Gower-Page et al., 2022) implements imputation approaches under basic and enriched MAR assumptions, alongside reference-based imputation and delta-based imputation for sensitivity analyses. This package supports Bayesian, maximum likelihood-based, and deterministic imputation methods with the addition of detailed help files and vignettes. For users of Stata, the new command "mimix" supports reference-based sensitivity analyses as highlighted in Cro et al. (2016).

15.2.2 Hypothetical Strategy

According to the ICH E9(R1) guideline, under a hypothetical strategy, "a scenario is envisaged in which the intercurrent event would not occur," and the outcome value is that which "the variable would have taken in the hypothetical scenario defined" (ICH, 2019).

The guideline emphasizes that from clinical and/or regulatory perspectives, some hypothetical scenarios are of more interest than others. For instance, hypothetical scenarios corresponding to different treatment conditions from those that can be carried out in a trial are considered of greater regulatory importance. An example presented in the guideline is a hypothetical scenario where additional medication is unavailable, even though, ethically, it must be provided. Conversely, scenarios that assume a change in patient behavior, such as hypothetically not experiencing an adverse event and treatment discontinuation after having done so, are considered of less regulatory relevance. Therefore, a clear justification of the relevance of each proposed hypothetical scenario is necessary.

The following considerations on estimation under this strategy have been expanded from those presented in Table 1 of Polverejan et al. (2023). In the estimation process aligned with the hypothetical strategy, data collected after the intercurrent event is typically deemed irrelevant for estimation and consequently excluded from analysis. Model-based approaches (such as MMRM or other likelihood-based models if the MAR assumption is appropriate) or imputation methods (like multiple imputation) can be considered. Several multiple imputation methods mentioned under the treatment policy strategy could be applied under the hypothetical strategy, such as MAR or reference-based multiple imputation, if appropriate for the hypothetical scenario under consideration.

Different hypothetical scenarios could lead to different assumptions, which in turn could affect the aligned estimators. Refer to Sect. 15.3.2 for an example of using a hypothetical strategy to address the intercurrent event "initiation of treatment with cholinesterase inhibitors." This hypothetical scenario assumes the intercurrent event would not have occurred because treatments with cholinesterase inhibitors were not available. Consequently, values of outcomes collected post this intercurrent event are not utilized for estimation, and a "similar to placebo" assumption is employed. The proposed main estimator uses a reference-based multiple imputation method. If an estimand applies a hypothetical scenario in which patients would continue treatment as assigned (e.g., rather than starting alternative treatments for the same target population), a MAR assumption could be considered, and a corresponding estimator under this assumption could be MMRM or MAR multiple imputation.

Regardless of the assumptions linked to the described hypothetical scenario, sensitivity analyses are important to assess the robustness of inferences when the assumptions deviate from the proposed main estimators, as described in the forthcoming subsection on sensitivity analysis.

Different types of approaches have been proposed to define estimators for hypothetical estimands, with varying levels of causal formalization. These include Bayesian approaches and methods that apply adjustments to post-intercurrent event data to model the patient trajectory under the envisaged hypothetical scenario (Olarte Parra et al., 2023; Olarte Parra et al., 2025; Lasch et al., 2023; Michiels et al., 2021). In particular, Olarte Parra et al. (2023) contrast traditional likelihood-based longitudinal models with more formal causal inference-based estimation models. They show that using outcome data after the occurrence of intercurrent events being addressed by the hypothetical strategy could lead to more precise estimates but requires stronger modeling assumptions. Lasch et al. (2023) evaluated several estimators under a hypothetical strategy dealing with the intercurrent event of initiation of symptomatic treatment in the context of disease-modifying treatment for Alzheimer's disease. Their study revealed that the MMRM estimator, which discarded the post-intercurrent event data, exhibited reduced power and biased estimates under the alternative hypothesis. Liu et al. (2022) proposed a Bayesian approach to address hypothetical estimands in longitudinal clinical trials with normally distributed outcomes.

15.2.3 Composite Variable Strategy

The ICH E9(R1) guideline notes that composite variable strategies affect the variable attribute of the estimand: "... An intercurrent event that is considered in itself to be informative about the patient's outcome and is therefore incorporated into the definition of the variable ..." (ICH, 2019). The original outcome variable is combined with the information that the intercurrent event occurred (and possibly when it occurred). The new composite variable, hence, no longer measures the original variable of interest but reflects a combination of two (or more) outcomes.

The new composite variable can be seen as a utility function, trading off efficacy and intercurrent events. Permutt (2016) highlights this interpretation in the context of HbA1c measurements and the intercurrent event of death. The definition of such a utility function requires the judgment of "equivalent" events, meaning the occurrence of the intercurrent event needs to be equated to a particular value on the scale of the original variable. For binary and time-to-event outcomes, this tends to be relatively straightforward. In a binary endpoint, treatment discontinuation might be reflected as a "non-response" on the original binary variable of interest. For time-to-event outcomes, the intercurrent event of death may be reflected as an event. An example of this is the assessment of time to hospitalization in cardiovascular research. For continuous endpoints, due to the finer scale of measurement, the definition of "equivalent" events is more difficult and potentially more arbitrary. This has led to the development of a variety of approaches. In what follows, some examples of composite strategies are presented; see also Keene (2019) for further approaches.

Despite well-known caveats in terms of information loss (see Cox, 1957; Senn & Julious, 2009; Fedorov et al., 2009), dichotomization is a commonly used approach. Here, a new binary variable U is defined based on the underlying continuous variable Y with

$$U = \begin{cases} 1 & \text{if } Y \geq c \; AND \; no \; intercurrent \; event \\ 0 & \text{if } Y < c \; OR \; intercurrent \; event \end{cases}$$

If no well-established cut off c exists, the specification of the cut off from a clinical but also statistical perspective can be a challenge.

Another common strategy is the assignment of specific values for the occurrence of intercurrent events.

$$U = \begin{cases} Y & \text{if } no \; intercurrent \; event \\ \tau & \text{if } intercurrent \; event \end{cases}$$

An example of this would be the nasal polyp score, where patients who undergo surgery would receive the worst possible score on the scale (Keene, 2019; FDA, 2023b). Usage of the worst value on a scale appears to be a commonly used approach. Note that the distance of τ to the bulk of the observations Y implicitly drives the trade-off/utility of intercurrent events versus the magnitude of the original variable, so selection of τ should be carefully considered in each situation.

Darken et al. (2020) discuss strategies for selection of τ by time point (in a longitudinal setting) based on sufficiently unfavorable population quantiles observed in the control arm in a single or multiple imputation strategy. Note, however, that under a multiple imputation strategy, the variable attribute of the estimand may be difficult to describe, as τ may differ across imputations.

In addition to the variable, the composite variable strategy can also impact the summary measure. While use of the difference in means is common for continuous endpoints, the utilized worst value τ may have a potentially undesired large impact on this summary measure if there is a non-negligible number of intercurrent events. An alternative summary measure is the median, which is less sensitive to the tail observations (Holzhauer et al., 2015).

A further alternative is the Mann–Whitney probability. Denoting by $U(1)_i$, $U(0)_j$ the potential outcomes of the utility U above (defined in terms of τ) for different patients i and j, the Mann–Whitney probability is defined as

$$P\left(U(1)_i > U(0)_j\right) + \frac{1}{2} P\left(U(1)_i = U(0)_j\right)$$

Here, P is the probability distribution over all pairs of patients i, j from the investigational arm and the control arm. A value of 0.5 for the Mann–Whitney probability corresponds to no treatment effect, whereas 1 is the largest possible treatment effect. Note that this summary measure does not require a concrete definition of τ if it is desired to reflect a "worst" value. Statistical testing can be performed with the Wilcoxon-Mann–Whitney test (Mann & Whitney, 1947) or the Brunner-Munzel test (Brunner & Munzel, 2000). A disadvantage of this summary measure is that the scale of the original variable is lost, and defining a clinically meaningful effect size on the scale of the Mann–Whitney probability can be challenging. Furthermore, the Mann–Whitney probability is a relative measure, without a corresponding summary measure available per treatment arm, making comparisons beyond the trial of interest challenging. Closely related summary measures are the win odds, which is the odds of the Mann–Whitney probability (Gasparyan et al., 2021; Brunner et al., 2021), and the win ratio (Pocock et al., 2012), which is defined as $WR = P(U(1)_i > U(0)_j)/P(U(1)_i < U(0)_j)$. Note that traditionally the win ratio uses time-to-event and recurrent event outcomes, but it could also be used to combine a continuous variable with intercurrent events.

The final summary measure we present is the trimmed mean per treatment arm (Permutt & Li, 2017; Ocampo & Bather, 2023). The idea is to compare the mean of the continuous variable among the fraction of (1-p) "best" patients in both treatment arms, where patients with intercurrent events are ranked as worst (again without a need to explicitly specify τ). In the adaptive version of the trimmed mean, p is selected equal to the proportion of patients with intercurrent events for the treatment arm with the highest proportion of intercurrent events. The arm with fewer intercurrent events is thus implicitly favored, as the best values are selected from a larger pool of intercurrent event-free observations compared to the other arm, where all observations that are without intercurrent events are used. A graphical visualization, which is aligned with the trimmed means summary, is to plot the proportion of "responders" against the cutoff, as proposed in Farrar et al. (2006). This plot is closely related to the empirical distribution function, but here patients with intercurrent events get an unspecified worst value assigned so that the distribution functions do not converge toward 1 but toward 1-p in each treatment arm. The area between the two distribution functions is proportional to the difference in trimmed means (Permutt & Li, 2017).

Under the composite variable strategy, the number of missing observations is usually smaller than under alternative strategies: the intercurrent events become part of the variable definition, so that common intercurrent events such as permanent treatment discontinuation do not cause missing data. Strategies for handling missing data when the outcome variable is a binary composite variable are discussed in Pham et al. (2021).

15.2.4 While on Treatment Strategy

The while on treatment strategy, when applied to intercurrent events, focuses on the treatment effect before the event occurs. As such, any outcomes after the intercurrent event are not considered of interest and are excluded from statistical analysis. In the estimand definition, this strategy is reflected in the "variable" attribute. Since only pre-intercurrent event measurements are of interest, the "variable" cannot relate to a fixed time point, as treatment duration varies between patients. For example, consider the original variable as a change from baseline at week 16. Under the while on treatment strategy for death (i.e., while alive strategy), the variable definition changes to the change from baseline at week 16 or the time of death, whichever occurs first. As described in Polverejan et al. (2023), other examples of suitable variables could include the area under the curve (refer to Estimand 7a example in the paper and Estimand 3 in Sect. 15.3 in this chapter), the average or a slope derived from pre-intercurrent event measurements, or the last measurement before or at the time of the event. This variable has to be meaningful in the clinical context. Notably, this strategy reduces the amount of missing data, as the variable is mainly established on observed data (Little & Kang, 2015).

15.2.5 Principal Stratum Strategy

The principal stratum strategy may be used to address the relevant intercurrent events when the population of interest is defined by these intercurrent events. It is critical to distinguish between the principal stratum and subgroups. The former stratifies the population based on the occurrence, or likelihood thereof, of the intercurrent event. In contrast, subgroups typically divide the population based on events that have occurred before the start of treatment—generally baseline characteristics. A case study featuring an example of this strategy is available in Sect. 15.3. For a more detailed analysis of the principal stratum strategy, please refer to Chap. 19.

15.2.6 *Sensitivity and Supplementary Analyses*

After identifying the estimand, a key consideration when selecting the appropriate analysis methods and estimators is evaluating the underlying assumptions. These assumptions should be clearly stated and documented. Appropriate sensitivity analysis should be identified to explore the robustness of inferences when assumptions deviate from the primary analysis. Sensitivity analysis should be structured, indicating which assumptions have been changed and what alternative assumptions have been used. Sometimes multiple sensitivity analyses are needed, but it is often preferable to alter only one aspect at a time to establish how each assumption impacts the results. For example, when using the hypothetical strategy to address treatment discontinuation, ANCOVA (following an adequate imputation of the measurements after treatment discontinuation, assuming missing outcomes are MAR) can be utilized as the main estimator. Sensitivity analysis can then be conducted to explore the potential impact of violating the MAR assumption by modifying the imputation model from MAR, for example, using a tipping point analysis.

The ICH E9(R1) distinguishes sensitivity analyses from supplementary analyses. Sensitivity analyses address the same questions under different assumptions, and to qualify, it must be possible to change inference from the primary analysis (Morris et al., 2014). Supplementary analyses, on the other hand, address different but related questions. Therefore, supplementary analyses can include different estimands that involve the primary outcome (e.g., using different strategies for intercurrent events) or an estimand based on another outcome. For example, it may be helpful to supplement the analysis of a continuous endpoint with an analysis that compares the percentage of patients with clinically relevant improvements on that continuous endpoint, such as a responder rate analysis.

15.3 Case Study

15.3.1 *Background*

Alzheimer's disease is categorized into several stages, starting from the asymptomatic or preclinical stage without clinical manifestations, to prodromal or mild cognitive impairment, followed by mild, moderate, and severe stages. For more details, see Sect. 9.5 in Chap. 9. The estimand framework for an asymptomatic Alzheimer's disease study was first explored in Polverejan and Dragalin (2020), and we expand the case study in this section.

Health authorities have approved medications that fall into two categories: drugs that change disease progression in people living with early Alzheimer's disease and drugs that may temporarily mitigate some symptoms of Alzheimer's dementia. An example of the latter medications is cholinesterase inhibitors, which do not stop the damage Alzheimer's causes to brain cells but may help lessen or stabilize symptoms for a limited time by affecting certain chemicals involved in carrying messages among and between the brain's nerve cells. Initiation of cholinesterase inhibitors could signal the transition of a patient from asymptomatic to symptomatic disease.

In clinical trials of long-term treatment for patients with asymptomatic Alzheimer's disease, the initiation of treatment with cholinesterase inhibitors could be allowed, if medically indicated, leading to potential therapeutic benefit due to the symptomatic effects of these medications. Consequently, initiation of treatment with cholinesterase inhibitors should be considered as an intercurrent event that should be addressed in the definition of estimands. Treatment discontinuation is also considered an intercurrent event. A different type of intercurrent event is the treatment switching to another Alzheimer's disease-modifying treatment. To avoid complex estimand definitions, this intercurrent event will not be included in the estimand discussion below. For more detailed descriptions of the Health Authorities' guidelines for Alzheimer's disease, see Sect. 12.3 in Chap. 12.

The format of the estimand definitions and some of the estimand and estimator descriptions are based on Polverejan et al. (2023). This format follows the steps of the estimand thinking process described in Chap. 4.

Four estimand examples are discussed in this section. Their differing questions of interest lead to different corresponding strategies being specified in the estimand definition for the intercurrent events of treatment discontinuation and initiation of treatment with cholinesterase inhibitors: Estimand 1 (Treatment policy, Hypothetical), Estimand 2 (Treatment policy), Estimand 3 (While on treatment, Treatment policy), Estimand 4 (Principal stratum). No applicable question of interest in this case was linked to a composite variable strategy.

15.3.2 Estimand 1 (Treatment Policy, Hypothetical)

Estimand 1 addresses the treatment discontinuation intercurrent event with the treatment policy strategy and the initiation of treatment with cholinesterase inhibitors with the hypothetical strategy, as shown in Table 15.1 below.

We now discuss an alternative hypothetical strategy to deal with the intercurrent event "initiation of treatment with cholinesterase inhibitors" (indicating the transition from asymptomatic to symptomatic phases in an adult with this intercurrent event). As the target population includes asymptomatic adults at risk for developing Alzheimer's dementia, a different kind of estimand could capture a treatment effect while the adults maintain their asymptomatic status. The hypothetical strategy can be formulated "as if patients would remain asymptomatic." This is different from the hypothetical scenario of "cholinesterase inhibitor events would not occur." Cholinesterase inhibitor events may occur, but one might not be interested in the patient's outcome after that because the patient has transitioned into a new stage of clinical disease for which the treatment is not developed. The situation is more similar to the "while on treatment" strategy, but it is "while asymptomatic" to emphasize the population, not the treatment. The estimand variable could be defined as the

Table 15.1 Estimand 1

<table>
<tr><td>Context</td><td>Disease-modifying treatment in Alzheimer’s dementia</td></tr>
<tr><td>Stakeholder</td><td>Health authority agency</td></tr>
<tr><td>Decision to be made</td><td>Determine if the study contributes substantial evidence of long-term efficacy for Drug X</td></tr>
<tr><td>Objective</td><td>To assess the superiority of Drug X versus placebo on long-term cognitive impairment</td></tr>
<tr><td>Intercurrent events</td><td>Treatment discontinuation
Initiation of treatment with cholinesterase inhibitors</td></tr>
<tr><td>Question of interest</td><td>For asymptomatic adults at risk for developing Alzheimer’s dementia, what would be the expected effect of assigning Drug X on cognitive impairment at month 54 if no treatments with cholinesterase inhibitors were available?</td></tr>
<tr><td>Estimand definition</td><td>Population: Asymptomatic adults at risk for developing Alzheimer’s dementia
Variable: Change from baseline to month 54 in the Alzheimer’s Disease Cooperative Study-Preclinical Alzheimer Cognitive Composite (ADCS-PACC) score
Treatment: Drug X vs. placebo, at the selected dose and frequency of administration, regardless of treatment discontinuation and as if treatments with cholinesterase inhibitors were not available
Intercurrent Events:
<table>
<tr><td>Intercurrent events</td><td>Strategies</td><td>Description</td></tr>
<tr><td>Treatment discontinuation</td><td>Treatment policy strategy, as reflected in the treatment definition</td><td>Strategy targeting the effect of treatment assignment, regardless of the occurrence of this intercurrent event</td></tr>
<tr><td>Initiation of treatment with cholinesterase inhibitors</td><td>Hypothetical strategy, as reflected in the treatment definition</td><td>A scenario is considered in which the event would not have occurred because treatments with cholinesterase inhibitors were not available</td></tr>
</table>
Population-Level Summary: Difference in mean change from baseline between treatment conditions</td></tr>
</table>

(continued)

Table 15.1 (continued)

Context	Disease-modifying treatment in Alzheimer's dementia
Utility of this question of interest and corresponding estimand to stakeholder	Answering this question requires an estimate of the expected effect of treatment under trial conditions as close as possible to real-world use. The evaluation of the assignment to either Drug X or a placebo is of practical importance, as treatment discontinuation occurs not only in trials but also in clinical practice and a treatment effect in an ideal condition, where there is perfect compliance, would be unrealistic due to the long treatment period. On the other hand, under this estimand, the effect of cholinesterase inhibitors that might be used following assignment to either Drug X or placebo is not of interest in this population of asymptomatic adults
Trial design	Parallel, double-blind, placebo-controlled, and randomized trial design
Key implementation elements needed to address this estimand	Efficacy outcome data after treatment discontinuation are directly relevant to this estimand, and efforts should be made to collect them. Efficacy data after cholinesterase inhibitors are not relevant to this estimand, but study protocols should plan to collect the information because the data may be relevant to a different or supplementary estimand. The date of occurrence of each intercurrent event should be clearly documented in the electronic case report form (eCRF)
Estimand and estimator aligned analysis set	Values of the outcome measure collected from baseline to month 54 in all randomized patients, including the values collected after treatment discontinuation
Data not used	Values of the outcome measure collected after the intercurrent event of cholinesterase inhibitors, addressed by a hypothetical strategy
Missing data	After study withdrawal or missing due to missed visits or missed data collections not related to study withdrawal
Assumptions for data not used and missing	For intermittent missing: MAR assumption, implying that measurements are assumed similar to those from the other patients from the same treatment arm, who do not have intermittent missing measurements For data not used and monotone missing data: Conditional on observed baseline attributes and on observed post-baseline outcomes, outcomes are assumed similar to those in the placebo arm Note: the "similar to placebo" assumption is considered an option under the hypothetical scenario of cholinesterase inhibitors not being available and for missing data due to study withdrawal
Main estimator	• Impute intermittent missing based on Markov Chain Monte Carlo, assuming MAR • Impute data not used and monotone missing data based on the CR method • Analysis based on MMRM or ANCOVA models • Combine results based on Rubin's rules Under the CR method, a patient's whole distribution, both pre- and posttreatment discontinuation, is assumed to be the same as the placebo arm. Patients in the control group are imputed under the MAR assumption Note: Multiple imputation based on RDO could be considered as an alternative estimator (Guizzaro et al., 2021; see also the template code and macros available on the DIA Scientific Working Group on Estimands and Missing Data website)

(continued)

Table 15.1 (continued)

Context	Disease-modifying treatment in Alzheimer's dementia
Sensitivity estimator(s), including what assumptions change from the main estimator	Sensitivity estimator: Same steps as in the main estimator, except that in the second step a J2R method is used instead Change in the assumptions for missing data: Under J2R, patient's mean response distribution after treatment discontinuation is assumed to be the same as the control group
Analysis used for decision-making, mentioning if it is different or same as the main estimator	Decision for establishing superiority for Drug X versus placebo is made based on the p-value from the contrast test for month 54 visit, using main estimator as above

slope based on the change from baseline in ADCS-PACC. Outcome values collected after the intercurrent event of cholinesterase inhibitors would not be used in the estimation. See Estimand 3 for an example of how an estimator can be selected when the estimand variable is a slope.

Another estimand could be based on the time to initiation of cholinesterase inhibitors, given that initiation of cholinesterase inhibitors signals the transition from asymptomatic disease, which one hopes to prevent with the treatment.

15.3.3 Estimand 2 (Treatment Policy)

The following examples highlight only the components that are different from Estimand 1 example. For this estimand, the question of interest is changed to "For asymptomatic adults at risk for developing Alzheimer's dementia, what would be the expected effect of assigning Drug X on cognitive impairment at month 54?"

Under this estimand, the treatment of interest is Drug X or placebo, at the selected dose and frequency of administration, regardless of treatment discontinuation and initiation of treatment with cholinesterase inhibitors.

Both treatment discontinuation and initiation of treatment with cholinesterase inhibitors intercurrent events are addressed with the same treatment policy strategy targeting the effect of treatment assignment, regardless of the occurrence of these intercurrent events. Treatment with cholinesterase inhibitors can be considered as part of the treatment regimen, used for symptomatic relief if the initially asymptomatic adults start having symptoms. One could argue that treatment policy for cholinesterase inhibitors is closer to the "real world treatment effect," in which the new drug is added to the current "standard of care." All other attributes of the estimand definition remain the same as in Estimand 1.

The key estimation elements for this estimand differ from those in Estimand 1. In this case, efficacy data after treatment discontinuation and after cholinesterase inhibitors are directly relevant to this estimand, and efforts should be made to collect them. The date of occurrence of each intercurrent event should be clearly documented in the eCRF. The analysis set should include values of the outcome measure collected from baseline to month 54 in all randomized patients, including the values collected after treatment discontinuation and cholinesterase inhibitors. Missing data occurs after study withdrawal or due to missed visits or missed data collections.

For intermittent missing data, **a** MAR assumption is used, implying that measurements are assumed similar to those from the other patients from the same treatment arm who do not have intermittent missing measurements.

For data not used and monotone missing data, **a** MAR assumption is used, conditional on baseline value, post-baseline observed measurements, and treatment.

Four types of patterns are defined as follows:

1. Patients who complete study treatment without using cholinesterase inhibitors
2. Patients who discontinue treatment without using cholinesterase inhibitors
3. Patients who complete study treatment and use cholinesterase inhibitors
4. Patients who discontinue treatment and use cholinesterase inhibitors

The main estimator is the same as for Estimand 1, except that the monotone missing data are imputed based on the MAR multiple imputation method performed within each of the patterns. Patients from the different patterns could be considered different from each other. However, not having enough patients in a pattern could lead to an increase in the estimated variability and potential non-convergence. In this case, patterns could be merged, or alternative methods could be used (such as reference-based methods).

15.3.4 Estimand 3 (While on Treatment, Treatment Policy)

For this estimand, the question of interest is changed to "For asymptomatic adults at risk for developing Alzheimer's dementia, what would be the expected effect of assigning Drug X on the rate of cognitive decline, while treatment is taken and regardless of initiation of treatment with cholinesterase inhibitors?"

Capturing a treatment effect while treatment is being administered could be of interest in long-term trials. Moreover, if the treatment is disease-modifying, post-treatment patient trajectories could be influenced by the attained effect while on treatment.

Under this estimand, the treatment of interest is Drug X or placebo, at the selected dose and frequency of administration, regardless of initiation of treatment with cholinesterase inhibitors. The variable is defined as the slope of change in the ADCS-PACC score from baseline up to month 54 or treatment discontinuation, whichever occurs first. Population-level summary is the difference in means of the slopes between treatment conditions.

The treatment discontinuation intercurrent event is addressed by the while on treatment strategy, as reflected in the variable definition. The cholinesterase inhibitors' intercurrent events are addressed by the treatment policy strategy, as reflected in the treatment definition. All other attributes of the estimand definition remain the same as for Estimand 1.

The key implementation elements needed to address this estimand are different from those in Estimands 1 and 2. For example, only efficacy data while the study treatment is taken (so before any treatment discontinuation) are relevant to this estimand. Efficacy data after cholinesterase inhibitors are directly relevant to this estimand, and efforts should be made to collect them. The date of occurrence of each intercurrent event should be clearly documented in the eCRF. The analysis set should include values of the outcome measure collected while on treatment (from baseline to either month 54 or treatment discontinuation, whichever is earlier) in all randomized patients, including the values collected after cholinesterase inhibitors.

The MAR-based main estimator is based on a mixed-effect model for the change from baseline in the ADCS-PACC score while on treatment, treating time as a continuous variable. The model will include fixed effects of time, treatment, and time-by-treatment interaction, as well as random effects for both time and intercept. Additionally, fixed effects of several prespecified baseline covariates will be included. The difference in mean slopes between treatment conditions is estimated using restricted maximum likelihood (REML) for this model. This is a more efficient approach (Pinheiro & Bates, 2000) than fitting individual regression lines for each patient and then applying a weighted average estimate of the difference between mean slopes.

Options for sensitivity estimators include using a different set of baseline covariates or using a non-proportional treatment effect over time.

15.3.5 Estimand 4 (Principal Stratum)

Estimating the treatment effect in the stratum of patients who would take Drug X for a certain duration could be of interest to a prescriber or a patient, and it may also be of interest to a health authority agency and/or payers.

The decision of a prescriber, for example, is to determine if the study provides sufficient evidence of efficacy to prescribe Drug X to patients in the target population by understanding the treatment effect in patients who would adhere to Drug X for a certain duration.

The trial objective is to assess the superiority of Drug X vs placebo on long-term cognitive impairment in patients who would adhere to Drug X for a certain duration.

The question of interest is "For asymptomatic adults at risk for developing Alzheimer's dementia, who would take Drug X as prescribed and would not initiate cholinesterase inhibitors for 18 months, what would be the expected effect of Drug X on cognitive impairment at month 54?"

The principal stratum estimand is defined as following:

(a) Population: Stratum of asymptomatic adults at risk for developing Alzheimer's dementia, who would complete treatment with Drug X and not start treatment with cholinesterase inhibitors for 18 months.

(b) Variable: Change from baseline to month 54 in the ADCS-PACC score.
(c) Treatment: Drug X vs placebo, at the selected dose and frequency of administration.
(d) Intercurrent events of treatment discontinuation and cholinesterase inhibitors, if assigned to Drug X, are both addressed with the principal stratum strategy, as reflected in the population definition.
(e) Population-Level Summary: Difference in means change from baseline between treatment conditions.

The key implementation element needed to address this estimand is a comprehensive collection of baseline variables potentially predicting intercurrent events. The date of occurrence of each intercurrent event should be clearly documented in the eCRF. The analysis set should include values of the outcome measure collected from baseline to month 54 for patients with no intercurrent events within the first 18 months and from baseline to intercurrent event for patients with intercurrent events within the first 18 months. Values of the outcome measure after any of the intercurrent events in either treatment arm will not be used in the analysis.

Missing data is due to study withdrawal or missing due to missed visits or missed data collections not related to study withdrawal. For patients on placebo, the probability that they would not experience intercurrent events if they had been assigned Drug X instead is assumed to be estimable based on the predetermined baseline variables. The estimation is done using the multiple imputation model from the first two steps of the main estimator described below.

The main estimator is defined by the following steps (for implementation, see Estimating Principal Strata, site of the Drug Information Association Scientific Working Group on Estimands and Missing Data):

- Define a multiple imputation model for the presence/absence of intercurrent events based on the observed intercurrent events (response) and the predetermined baseline characteristics from Drug X group (explanatory variables).
- For each patient in the placebo arm, multiply impute M times the presence/absence of intercurrent events had the patient been assigned to Drug X instead, using the patient's observed baseline characteristics.
- In each of the M imputed datasets, select the patients in the principal stratum of patients not experiencing intercurrent events under Drug X. They include the patients from the Drug X group who did not experience intercurrent events and the patients from the placebo arm who were imputed not to have any intercurrent events had they been assigned to Drug X instead.
- Estimate treatment difference in each of the M principal strata (apply MMRM) and combine results using Rubin's rules.

Standard model testing measures will be used to assess the bias and variance of the multiple imputation model for intercurrent event presence/absence based on the treatment arm. The average number of patients modeled as present in the principal stratum will be presented by the treatment arm. Summary statistics for the model explanatory variables of patients from the principal stratum will also be presented by treatment arm.

Several sensitivity estimators can be used. One could, for example, define multiple imputation models using a different set of baseline characteristics (e.g., a subset of the initial set) or use alternative analysis methods other than MMRM. In addition, Wang and Hu (2022) proposed sensitivity analysis based on a joint model that multiply imputes the principal stratum membership and the outcome variable while allowing different levels of violation of the principal ignorability assumption. DiazOrdaz and Carpenter (2019) proposed a substantive model compatible with the multiple imputation method to impute the latent compliance class and missing data in the model.

15.4 Concluding Remarks

This chapter focused on appropriate statistical models and analysis techniques to implement the intercurrent event strategies introduced in the ICH E9(R1) guideline for continuous outcome data. We provided an overview of each of the intercurrent event strategies from a more methodological perspective. We then conceptually illustrated the application of the estimand framework, including intercurrent event strategies and analysis methods, using a case study in asymptomatic Alzheimer's disease.

When working with estimands, employing continuous variables presents both advantages and challenges in terms of estimation and sensitivity analysis, in comparison to binary and time-to-event variables. Continuous variables offer a more comprehensive and detailed understanding of the data due to their ability to provide a wider range of values, ultimately enabling a more nuanced analysis compared to binary or time-to-event variables. Moreover, continuous variables tend to be more sensitive to even slight variations in the treatment effect, allowing for the detection of smaller effects or changes. Additionally, the flexibility inherent in the use of continuous variables facilitates the application of diverse statistical models and techniques, thereby capturing complex relationships and interactions.

However, while continuous variables provide benefits such as more information, higher statistical power, and modeling flexibility, they also introduce challenges and increased complexity. For example, the composite variable strategy is more challenging to implement for continuous variables. The definition of a sufficiently unfavorable outcome on a continuous scale (reflecting the occurrence of an intercurrent event) can be perceived as more arbitrary compared to situations where the outcome is already on a categorical or binary scale (such as occurrence or nonoccurrence of an event). Furthermore, assumptions about the underlying distribution, measurement precision, and sensitivity to outliers are some of the potential complications associated with continuous variables. Researchers must carefully account for these factors when conducting estimation and sensitivity analysis within the framework of estimands. As highlighted in this chapter, there are many ongoing active research areas on methods for a continuous endpoint, such as performing reliable estimation under the treatment policy strategy when missing data occurs, advantages of using post-intercurrent event outcome data for estimation under the hypothetical strategy, reliable methods for sensitivity analysis under the principal stratum or while on treatment strategies, or addressing the challenges of applying a composite variable strategy.

References

Bartlett, J. W. (2023). Reference-based multiple imputation—What is the right variance and how to estimate it. *Statistics in Biopharmaceutical Research, 15*(1), 178–186.

Bell, J., Drury, T., Mütze, T., Pipper, C. B., Guizzaro, L., Mitroiu, M., & Wright, D. (2025). Estimation methods for estimands using the treatment policy strategy; a simulation study based on the PIONEER 1 trial. *Pharmaceutical Statistics, 24*(2), e2472.

Brunner, E., & Munzel, U. (2000). The nonparametric Behrens-fisher problem: Asymptotic theory and a small-sample approximation. *Biometrical Journal, 42*, 17–25.

Brunner, E., Vandemeulebroecke, M., & Mütze, T. (2021). Win odds: An adaptation of the win ratio to include ties. *Statistics in Medicine, 40*, 3367–3384.

Carpenter, J. R., Roger, J. H., & Kenward, M. G. (2013). Analysis of longitudinal trials with protocol deviation: A framework for relevant, accessible assumptions, and inference via multiple imputation. *Journal of Biopharmaceutical Statistics, 23*(6), 1352–1371.

Cox, D. R. (1957). Note on grouping. *Journal of the American Statistical Association, 52*, 543–547.

Cro, S., Morris, T. P., Kenward, M. G., & Carpenter, J. R. (2016). Reference-based sensitivity analysis via multiple imputation for longitudinal trials with protocol deviation. *The Stata Journal, 16*(2), 443–463.

Cro, S., Carpenter, J. R., & Kenward, M. G. (2019). Information-anchored sensitivity analysis: Theory and application. *Journal of the Royal Statistical Society Series A: Statistics in Society, 182*(2), 623–645.

Cro, S., Morris, T. P., Kenward, M. G., & Carpenter, J. R. (2020). Sensitivity analysis for clinical trials with missing continuous outcome data using controlled multiple imputation: A practical guide. *Statistics in Medicine, 39*(21), 2815–2842.

Cro, S., Morris, T. P., Roger, J. H., & Carpenter, J. R. (2024). Comments on 'standard and reference-based conditional mean imputation': Regulators and trial statisticians be aware! *Pharmaceutical Statistics, 23*, 598.

Darken, P., Nyberg, J., Ballal, S., & Wright, D. (2020). The attributable estimand: A new approach to account for intercurrent events. *Pharmaceutical Statistics, 19*, 626–635.

DiazOrdaz, K., & Carpenter, J. (2019). Local average treatment effects estimation via substantive model compatible multiple imputation. *Biometrical Journal, 61*(6), 1526–1540.

Drury, T., Abellan, J. J., Best, N., & White, I. R. (2023). *Estimation of treatment policy estimands for continuous outcomes using off treatment sequential multiple imputation*. arXiv preprint arXiv:2308.10857.

Drug Information Association Scientific Working Group on Estimands and Missing Data (https://www.lshtm.ac.uk/research/centres-projects-groups/missing-data#dia-missing-data): J Roger MISTEP macro (see Stepwise imputation for marginal model based on previous residuals); Template code treatment policy using SAS PROC MI and the MISTEP macro.

EMA. (2015). *Guideline on adjustment for baseline covariates in clinical trials*. Committee for Medicinal Products for Human Use, European Medicines Agency (EMA). https://www.ema.europa.eu/

Farrar, J. T., Dworkin, R. H., & Max, M. B. (2006). Use of the cumulative proportion of responders analysis graph to present pain data over a range of cut-off points: Making clinical trial data more understandable. *Journal of Pain and Symptom Management, 31*, 369–377.
FDA. (2023a). *Adjusting for covariates in randomized clinical trials for drugs and biological products*. Guidance for industry. https://www.fda.gov/
FDA (2023b) Chronic rhinosinusitis with nasal polyps: Developing drugs for treatment. Guidance for industry FDA
Fedorov, V., Mannino, F., & Zhang, R. (2009). Consequences of dichotomization. *Pharmaceutical Statistics, 8*, 50–61.
García-Hernandez, A., Pérez, T., Pardo, M. D. C., & Rizopoulos, D. (2023). A flexible analytical framework for reference-based imputation, Delta adjustment and tipping-point stress-testing. *Statistics in Biopharmaceutical Research, 15*, 1–13.
Gasparyan, S. B., Folkvaljon, F., Bengtsson, O., Buenconsejo, J., & Koch, G. G. (2021). Adjusted win ratio with stratification: Calculation methods and interpretation. *Statistical Methods in Medical Research, 30*, 580–611.
Gower-Page C, Noci A (2022). *_rbmi: Reference Based Multiple Imputation*. R package version 1.2.3, (CRAN - Package rbmi (r-project.org)).
Gower-Page, C., Noci, A., & Wolbers, M. (2022). Rbmi: A R package for standard and reference-based multiple imputation methods. *Journal of Open Source Software, 7*(74), 4251.
Guizzaro, L., Pétavy, F., Ristl, R., & Gallo, C. (2021). The use of a variable representing compliance improves accuracy of estimation of the effect of treatment allocation regardless of discontinuation in trials with incomplete follow-up. *Statistics in Biopharmaceutical Research, 13*(1), 119–127.
Holzhauer, B., Akacha, M., & Bermann, G. (2015). Choice of estimand and analysis methods in diabetes trials with rescue medication. *Pharmaceutical Statistics, 14*, 433–447.
ICH. (2019). *ICH E9(R1) addendum on estimands and sensitivity analysis in clinical trials to the guideline on statistical principles for clinical trials*. Step 4 document. www.ich.org
Keene, O. N. (2019). Strategies for composite estimands in confirmatory clinical trials: Examples from trials in nasal polyps and steroid reduction. *Pharmaceutical Statistics, 18*(1), 78–84.
Lasch, F., Guizzaro, L., Petavy, F., & Gallo, C. (2023). A simulation study on the estimation of the effect in the hypothetical scenario of no use of symptomatic treatment in trials for disease-modifying agents for Alzheimer's disease. *Statistics in Biopharmaceutical Research, 15*(2), 386–399.
Little, R., & Kang, S. (2015). Intention-to-treat analysis with treatment discontinuation and missing data in clinical trials. *Statistics in Medicine, 34*(16), 2381–2390.
Liu, G. F., Liu, J., Chen, F., Gutman, R., & Lu, K. (2022). Bayesian approaches for handling hypothetical estimands in longitudinal clinical trials with gaussian outcomes. *Statistics in Biopharmaceutical Research, 14*(4), 626–635.
Mallinckrodt, C. H., Lane, P. W., Schnell, D., Peng, Y., & Mancuso, J. P. (2008). Recommendations for the primary analysis of continuous endpoints in longitudinal clinical trials. *Drug Information Journal, 42*(4), 303–319.
Mann, H. B., & Whitney, D. R. (1947). On a test of whether one of two random variables is stochastically larger than the other. *Annals of Mathematical Statistics, 18*, 50–60.
Michiels, H., Sotto, C., Vandebosch, A., & Vansteelandt, S. (2021). A novel estimand to adjust for rescue treatment in randomized clinical trials. *Statistics in Medicine, 40*(9), 2257–2271.
Morris, T. P., Kahan, B. C., & White, I. R. (2014). Choosing sensitivity analyses for randomised trials: Principles. *BMC Medical Research Methodology, 14*, 1–5.
NMPA. (2020). *Guidelines on covariate adjustment in clinical trials*. https://www.cde.org.cn
Noci, A., Wolbers, M., Abt, M., Baayen, C., Burger, H. U., Jin, M., & Robieson, W. Z. (2023). A comparison of estimand and estimation strategies for clinical trials in early parkinson's disease. *Statistics in Biopharmaceutical Research, 15*(3), 491–501.
Ocampo, A., & Bather, J. R. (2023). Single-world intervention graphs for defining, identifying, and communicating estimands in clinical trials. *Statistics in Medicine, 42*, 3892–3902.

O'Kelly, M., & Ratitch, B. (2014). *Clinical trials with missing data: A guide for practitioners*. Wiley.

Olarte Parra, C., Daniel, R. M., & Bartlett, J. W. (2023). Hypothetical estimands in clinical trials: A unification of causal inference and missing data methods. *Statistics in Biopharmaceutical Research, 15*(2), 421–432.

Olarte Parra, C., Daniel, R. M., Wright, D., & Bartlett, J. W. (2025). Estimating hypothetical estimands with causal inference and missing data estimators in a diabetes trial case study. *Biometrics, 81*(1)

Permutt, T. (2016). A taxonomy of estimands for regulatory clinical trials with discontinuations. *Statistics in Medicine, 35*(17), 2865–2875.

Permutt, T., & Li, F. (2017). Trimmed means for symptom trials with dropouts. *Pharmaceutical Statistics, 16*(1), 20–28.

Pham, T. M., White, I. R., Kahan, B. C., Morris, T. P., Stanworth, S. J., & Forbes, G. (2021). A comparison of methods for analyzing a binary composite endpoint with partially observed components in randomized controlled trials. *Statistics in Medicine, 40*, 6634–6650.

Pinheiro, J., & Bates, D. (2000). *Mixed-effects models in S and S-PLUS*. Springer.

Pocock, S. J., Ariti, C. A., Collier, T. J., & Wang, D. (2012). The win ratio: A new approach to the analysis of composite endpoints in clinical trials based on clinical priorities. *European Heart Journal, 33*(2), 176–182.

Polverejan, E., & Dragalin, V. (2020). Aligning treatment policy estimands and estimators—A simulation study in Alzheimer's disease. *Statistics in Biopharmaceutical Research, 12*(2), 142–154.

Polverejan, E., O'Kelly, M., Hefting, N., Norton, J. D., Lim, P., & Walton, M. K. (2023). Defining clinical trial Estimands: A practical guide for study teams with examples based on a psychiatric disorder. *Therapeutic Innovation & Regulatory Science, 57*, 1–29.

Qu, Y., & Dai, B. (2022). Return-to-baseline multiple imputation for missing values in clinical trials. *Pharmaceutical Statistics, 21*(3), 641–653.

Ratitch, B., O'Kelly, M., & Tosiello, R. (2013). Missing data in clinical trials: From clinical assumptions to statistical analysis using pattern mixture models. *Pharmaceutical Statistics, 12*(6), 337–347.

Roger, J. H., Bratton, D. J., Mayer, B., Abellan, J. J., & Keene, O. N. (2019). Treatment policy estimands for recurrent event data using data collected after cessation of randomised treatment. *Pharmaceutical Statistics, 18*(1), 85–95.

Sabanes Bove, D., Dedic, J., Kelkhoff, D., Kunzmann, K., Lang, B., Li, L., Wang, Y. (2022). *mmrm: Mixed Models for Repeated Measures*. R package version 0.2.2, <https://CRAN.R-project.org/package=mmrm>

Senn, S., & Julious, S. (2009). Measurement in clinical trials: A neglected issue for statisticians? *Statistics in Medicine, 28*(26), 3189–3209.

Wang, S., & Hu, H. (2022). Impute the missing data using retrieved dropouts. *BMC Medical Research Methodology, 22*(1), 82.

Wang, Y., Tu, W., Kim, Y., Sinks, S., He, J., Cambon, A., & Clark, J. (2023). Statistical methods for handling missing data to align with treatment policy strategy. *Pharmaceutical Statistics, 22*, 650.

White, I., Joseph, R., & Best, N. (2020). A causal modelling framework for reference-based imputation and tipping point analysis in clinical trials with quantitative outcome. *Journal of Biopharmaceutical Statistics, 30*(2), 334–350.

Wolbers, M., Noci, A., Delmar, P., Gower-Page, C., Yiu, S., & Bartlett, J. W. (2022). Standard and reference-based conditional mean imputation. *Pharmaceutical Statistics, 21*(6), 1246–1257.

Wolbers, M., Noci, A., Delmar, P., Yiu, S., & Bartlett, J. W. (2024). Rejoinder to the letter: 'Standard and reference-based conditional mean imputation': Regulators and trial statisticians be aware! *Pharmaceutical Statistics, 25*, 604–610.

Chapter 16
Statistical Analysis Under the Estimand Framework: Binary Endpoints

Longshen Xie, Yongming Qu, and Hongying Li

Abstract In this chapter, we explore statistical analysis of binary endpoints under the estimand framework. While the consideration for addressing intercurrent events and the principle for missing data imputation for binary endpoints are similar to the continuous variables, the statistical methods and the summary statistics for binary endpoints need further discussion. We briefly introduce the common statistical methods for binary endpoints and review three commonly used summary measures: risk difference, relative risk, and odds ratio. We delve into the similarities and differences among these summary measures from the logic-respecting perspective and provide recommendations. Additionally, we illustrate the tipping point analysis, which is commonly used for binary endpoints in the sensitivity analysis. Finally, we present and compare the original analysis method and the analysis method under the estimand framework from a real case study.

16.1 Introduction to Binary Endpoints

A variable is a discrete variable if it can only take on a finite or countably infinite set of outcomes. A discrete variable that only has two possible outcomes, such as "response" (success) or "no response" (failure), is known as a binary variable. In clinical studies, binary variables are frequently used as primary endpoints.

L. Xie (✉)
Department of Biometrics and Data Management, Shenyang Sunshine Pharmaceutical Co., Ltd., Shanghai, China
e-mail: xielongshen@3sbio.com

Y. Qu
Department of Global Statistical Sciences, Eli Lilly and Company, Indianapolis, IN, USA
e-mail: qu_yongming@lilly.com

H. Li
China Statistical Sciences, Eli Lilly and Company, Shanghai, China
e-mail: li_hong_ying@lilly.com

J. Wei et al. (eds.), *Estimands in Clinical Trials*, Springer Series in Pharmaceutical Statistics, https://doi.org/10.1007/978-3-032-02192-2_16

Researchers can generate binary outcomes in two ways: (1) those derived from one or more continuous outcomes and (2) those collected directly as the original outcomes. Common population-level summaries for binary endpoints include odds ratio, risk difference, and relative risk. The chi-squared test (Pearson, 1900) and Fisher's exact test (Fisher, 1922) are commonly used statistical tests for binary data. Additionally, the Cochran-Mantel-Haenszel (CMH) method (Mantel & Haenszel, 1959) can be used when there are stratification factors, and logistic regression (Hosmer Jr et al., 2013) can be used to adjust for baseline covariates. The generalized linear mixed model (GLMM) (Stroup, 2012) can be considered in repeated measures studies. In this chapter, we delve into the considerations of analyzing and handling binary endpoints under the estimand framework, with a particular focus on strategies for addressing intercurrent events and population-level summary. Additionally, we introduce a case study that uses the American College of Rheumatology 50% (ACR50) response criteria (Felson et al., 1995) as the primary endpoint to illustrate how to define estimands and select analysis methods for a binary endpoint.

The remainder of this chapter is structured as follows. In Sect. 16.2, we discuss different strategies for addressing intercurrent events under the estimand framework and the aligned analysis methods. In Sect. 16.3, we discuss key considerations of population-level summaries for binary endpoints. In Sect. 16.4, we illustrate sensitivity analysis, especially the tipping point analysis method for binary endpoints. In Sect. 16.5, we present and compare the original analysis method and the analysis method under the estimand framework from a real case study. We conclude with a discussion in Sect. 16.6.

16.2 Addressing Intercurrent Events and Missing Data

For binary endpoints, the principles for choosing a strategy for an intercurrent event remain the same as for continuous endpoints in Chap. 15. The composite variable strategy has advantages under binary endpoints, as it naturally defines the patients with intercurrent events as nonresponders. It is thus frequently used in practice. For the principal stratum strategy, we refer to Chap. 19. Typically, in a clinical trial, several strategies may be used to address different types of intercurrent events in one estimand (Darken et al., 2020; Qu & Lipkovich, 2021; Qu et al., 2021). For example, the treatment policy strategy may be used for treatment discontinuations due to adverse events or lack of efficacy, and a hypothetical strategy may be used for treatment discontinuations due to reasons not related to study efficacy and safety.

To facilitate understanding of the subsequent sections, we now introduce several commonly used imputation methods and models for binary endpoints. As mentioned earlier, binary outcomes can be generated from one or more continuous outcomes or collected directly as the original outcomes. The first type is common, with examples including ACR50, weight loss $\geq$ 10%, HbA1c reaching the treatment target of 7.0%, and others. In cases where we have this type of binary outcome, it is recommended to impute the underlying continuous outcomes first and then define the binary outcome based on the imputed data. Ma et al. (2022) showed that imputing the underlying continuous outcome is better than directly imputing the binary outcome or estimating the parameter directly via a GLMM, particularly when the continuous outcome is normally distributed. When the binary outcome is directly collected as the source data, such as death or not, the missing values can be imputed based on the fully conditional specification (e.g., "`mice`" R package) (Van Buuren, 2007; Van Buuren & Groothuis-Oudshoorn, 2011). Furthermore, regardless of directly imputing the binary outcome or imputing the underlying continuous outcome, the missing data imputation should be consistent with the potential outcome defined in the estimands (Lipkovich et al., 2020). For example, if the treatment policy strategy to address intercurrent events is used in defining estimands, using retrieved dropouts (RDO) data (EMA, 2010) may be an appropriate approach to impute the missing data; more details of imputation by RDO data can be found in Chap. 15.

16.2.1 Treatment Policy Strategy

For the treatment policy strategy, the primary focus is to assess the treatment effect while the intercurrent event is considered to be part of the treatments being compared. Therefore, researchers will include data after the occurrence of intercurrent events in the analysis and collect it as much as possible. However, missing data is often unavoidable. Some methods for handling missing data in the treatment policy strategy for continuous endpoints in Chap. 15, such as imputation based on RDO data or based on reference arm data (Carpenter et al., 2013), are also applicable to binary endpoints.

16.2.2 Hypothetical Strategy

When the clinical question of interest is the treatment effect in the absence of intercurrent events, the hypothetical strategy is appropriate. Similar to continuous endpoints, data after the occurrence of intercurrent events are not used. Instead, imputation methods will be adopted to predict the data under specific hypothetical scenarios. For example, if the hypothetical scenario is when the intercurrent events do not occur, patients would behave similarly to those without intercurrent events. We can then employ a multiple imputation approach based on regression models (Little & Rubin, 2019) that assume the missing data are missing at random (MAR).

16.2.3 Composite Variable Strategy

As mentioned in the composite variable strategy section of the ICH E9(R1) guideline (2019), "an intercurrent event is considered in itself to be informative about the patient's outcome and is therefore incorporated into the definition of the variable." Therefore, under the composite variable strategy, the intercurrent events are reflected in the variable definition, and the application is straightforward, where patients experiencing intercurrent events are directly labeled as nonresponders.

Since the intercurrent events become part of the variable, it avoids the imputation of missing data. For multi-category ordinal endpoints, the composite variable strategy can also be considered. For example, if researchers categorize the efficacy outcomes of the multi-category ordinal endpoint as relief, maintenance, and no improvement, then patients who withdraw from the trial due to intercurrent events, such as toxicity, can be classified as having a no improvement outcome. Notably, summarizing the occurrence of intercurrent events in each treatment arm is particularly useful for the composite variable strategy to facilitate the interpretation of the analysis results.

16.2.4 While on Treatment Strategy

If the focus is on the treatment effect prior to the occurrence of intercurrent events, we can use the while on treatment strategy. Although this strategy no longer uses data after the occurrence of intercurrent events, like the hypothetical strategy, it differs by not assuming the absence of the intercurrent events. Instead, it exclusively relies on data obtained prior to the occurrence of intercurrent events. Similar to the composite variable strategy, the while-on-treatment strategy can also influence the definition of the variable.

Since the response to treatment before the occurrence of intercurrent events is of interest, the while on treatment strategy typically does not generate a missing data issue. Like continuous endpoints, when a binary endpoint is repeatedly measured, not only the observed values at the prespecified fixed time point but also all values up to the time of intercurrent events may be considered relevant for the clinical question. Moreover, it requires specific attention when the times and/or frequencies of the occurrences of intercurrent events are different between treatment arms. Hence, providing a summary of the time and frequency of the occurrence of intercurrent events in each treatment arm is crucial for the while on treatment strategy.

16.3 Population-Level Summary

One key difference between binary and continuous endpoints lies in the population-level summary. A continuous endpoint generally uses the mean difference as the population-level summary of treatment effect, while for a binary endpoint, summary measures such as risk difference, relative risk, or odds ratio are used. Let random variables Y^t and Y^c be the outcomes that would have been observed under the investigational and control arms. The causal risk difference in the population corresponds to the average causal effect across individuals on the difference scale, which indicates that $E(Y^t) - E(Y^c) = E(Y^t - Y^c)$. In contrast, the causal risk ratio, including relative risk and odds ratio, is not the average of the individual causal effects on the ratio scale. This means that they are a measure of causal effect in the population but do not represent the average of individual causal effects, such as $E(Y^t)/E(Y^c) \neq E(Y^t/Y^c)$ (Hernán & Robins, 2020). Each summary measure has its own applicability. For example, the risk difference is useful in benefit-risk assessments compared to other summary measures like odds ratio (Nie, 2021) and sometimes preferred by regulatory agencies. The relative risk is a typical summary measure for a log-linear model, while the odds ratio is more commonly used in a logistic regression model. The robust estimation of relative risk and risk difference can be found in the Food and Drug Administration (FDA) (2023) and Ye et al. (2023). In terms of interpretation, the risk difference and relative risk tend to be more intuitive than the odds ratio; the latter can be difficult to interpret for clinicians and even for statisticians.

Covariate adjustment with nonlinear models is often used in the analysis of a binary endpoint. Although this is an acceptable method, the FDA covariate adjustment guideline (FDA, 2023) pointed out that additional issues should be considered before using nonlinear models. Under the estimand framework, it is important to define whether the treatment effect to be estimated is marginal or conditional. In the context of binary endpoints, a marginal treatment effect involves comparing response probabilities obtained by averaging over the entire covariate space. On the other hand, one can interpret a conditional treatment effect as the treatment parameter in a generalized linear regression with specific covariate values (Xi & Bretz, 2021a). Both marginal and conditional treatment effects allow for a causal interpretation in accordance with the ICH E9(R1) guideline, and the choice between them should be guided by the clinical meaningfulness of the resulting treatment effects (Xi & Bretz, 2021a).

Researchers can employ the CMH method to analyze clinical trial data with binary endpoints when aiming to estimate a conditional odds ratio that is assumed to remain consistent across subgroups defined by a covariate with discrete levels. The generalized linear model (GLM) (Dobson & Barnett, 2018) extends the CMH method by allowing adjustment for continuous covariates.

According to the FDA covariate adjustment guideline (FDA, 2023), there are two important considerations when applying a GLM. Firstly, the FDA recommends that sponsors account for covariates that are expected to have a significant association with the outcome of interest. The selection of covariates can be based on scientific literature or previous project experience. However, as we never know the exact true regression model (i.e., which covariates are to be included), the conditional treatment effect generally requires stronger assumptions, as the corresponding estimands may be different when conditioning on different covariates. In contrast, the marginal treatment effect is robust to the estimation methods and the covariates to be adjusted. Even when the covariates are misspecified in the regression model, the marginal treatment effect can still be consistently estimated (Ye et al., 2023). Notably, for the odds ratio, although the magnitude of the treatment effect is generally larger for the conditional treatment effect compared to the marginal treatment, the statistical powers for the conditional and marginal treatment effects are asymptotically equivalent (Rosenblum & Steingrimsson, 2016). Secondly, unlike the linear model, certain conditional and marginal summary measures are different in the GLM. For instance, the odds ratio lacks logic-respecting or collapsibility, as illustrated in the FDA covariate adjustment guideline (FDA, 2023).

The concept of logic-respecting was introduced by Lin et al. (2019) and Liu et al. (2022). A summary measure is logic-respecting if $\theta_{\{c^-,c^+\}} \in \left[\theta_{c^-}, \theta_{c^+}\right]$, where θ_{c^-}, θ_{c^+}, and $\theta_{\{c^-,c^+\}}$ denote the true (unknown) treatment effect in subgroups c^-, c^+, and all-comers, respectively. A summary measure comparing two treatment arms for a binary endpoint is collapsible on a covariate with weights $w_c \geq 0$ and $\sum_c w_c = 1$ if $\theta_{\{c^-,c^+\}} = \theta_{c^-} w_{c^-} + \theta_{c^+} w_{c^+}$. Collapsibility has been extensively studied by many researchers (Greenland et al., 1999; Agresti, 2002; Huitfeldt et al., 2019; Lin et al., 2019). Logic-respecting and collapsibility are population-level definitions and are not tied to specific models. They do not affect whether the statistic is a causal quantity or not; however, they do impact the interpretation of subgroup results (Xi & Bretz, 2021b). Table 16.1 (Liu et al., 2023) lists the logic-respecting summary measures for different types of endpoints. The risk difference and relative risk are both logic-respecting and collapsible, whereas the odds ratio is not. Consequently, we

Table 16.1 Logic-respecting summary measures for all endpoint types (Liu et al., 2023)

Endpoint type	Summary measures	Logic-respecting?
Continuous	Difference of means	Yes
Binary	Risk difference	Yes
	Relative risk	Yes
	Odds ratio	No
Time-to-event	Hazard ratio	No
	Difference of medians	No
	Ratio of medians	Yes[a]
	Difference of RMSTs	Yes
	Ratio of RMSTs	Yes
	Difference of milestone probabilities	Yes
	Ratio of milestone probabilities	Yes

[a] When there are proportional hazards within each subgroup under the Weibull model

Table 16.2 An example of responders and nonresponders' probabilities given treatment in different subpopulations and the all-comers population

	Subpopulation c^+		Subpopulation c^-		Population	
	R	NR	R	NR	R	NR
E	0.8/100	0.2/100	0.4/100	0.6/100	0.6/200	0.4/200
P	0.6/100	0.4/100	0.2/100	0.8/100	0.4/200	0.6/200

may observe a counterintuitive scenario in which an odds ratio for a population is not bounded by the odds ratio in each subgroup. For example, in Table 16.2, $RR_{c^-} = \frac{12}{6}$, $RR_{c^+} = \frac{8}{6}$, $RR = \frac{9}{6}$, and $RR \in \left[RR_{c^-}, RR_{c^+}\right]$. However, $OR_{c^-} = \frac{32}{12}$, $OR_{c^+} = \frac{32}{12}$, and $OR = \frac{27}{12}$. OR is not within the range of $\left[OR_{c^-}, OR_{c^+}\right]$. These properties suggest the risk difference and relative risk may be more attractive in interpretation and can be more robustly estimated. More detailed discussions on this topic can be found in Chap. 20.

E and P denote investigational and placebo arms, respectively. R and NR represent responders and nonresponders. X/Y denotes response probability/number of patients.

16.4 Sensitivity Analysis

Researchers should plan sensitivity analysis to explore the robustness of inferences from the main estimator when assumptions deviate from the primary analysis. Tipping point analysis (Liublinska & Rubin, 2014) is a widely used sensitivity analysis method for binary endpoints under the missing not at random (MNAR) assumption. This method introduces a sensitivity parameter or multiple sensitivity parameters and identifies at what values of the sensitivity parameters the treatment effect is not statistically significant anymore. This helps to evaluate the robustness of the treatment effect estimated under the primary analysis method.

For binary endpoints, tipping point analysis can be performed by systematically enumerating the response rate of missing outcomes in a stepwise manner. An example is used to illustrate this method below (Fig. 16.1). Suppose there are ten and seven missing efficacy outcomes in the control arm and the investigational arm, respectively.

The first step of tipping point analysis involves generating a matrix of all possible imputation combinations for the missing data, resulting in a matrix of dimensions 11*8 in this example. Each element $P_{i,j}$ in the matrix represents the p-value obtained from a statistical test on the binary endpoint after imputation, where $i = \{1,..,11\}$ and $j = \{1,..,8\}$. For example, $P_{2,6}$ represents the p-value calculated using the imputation scenario where the control arm has one response and the investigational arm has five responses. By the same token, we can calculate all 88 possible combinations of p-values and generate Fig. 16.1.

By observing the proportion of statistically significant p-values, we can assess the confidence in the trial's success. A higher proportion indicates greater confidence. In practice, we can also perform calculations in a fixed order of steps without computing all 88 p-value combinations (Yan et al., 2009). For instance, we can begin by calculating $P_{1,1}$ in the first row and the first column. If $P_{1,1}$ is statistically significant, we continue to calculate $P_{2,1}$, $P_{3,1}$, and so on, until we encounter the first p-value without statistical significance. Subsequently, we proceed to the first row and the second column, calculating $P_{1,2}$, $P_{2,2}$, $P_{3,2}$, without calculating the remaining p-values in the first column. This approach is based on the observation that, following the first p-value that does not exhibit statistical significance, subsequent p-values obtained by incrementally increasing the number of imputed responses in the control arm typically do not demonstrate statistical significance as well.

Note that for certain methods, such as the chi-squared test or Fisher's exact test, the p-values may not exhibit a monotonic trend. That is, p-values may change from significant to nonsignificant and later become significant again. However, this does

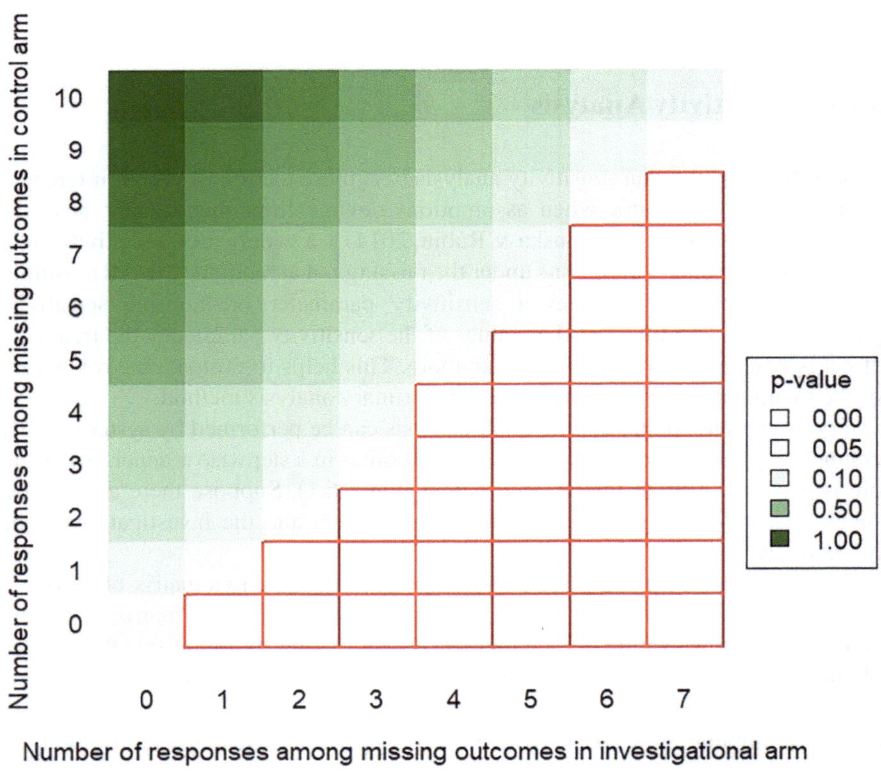

Fig. 16.1 Heat map of p-values for binary endpoint tipping point using simulated data

not affect our use of the tipping point method, as the change from nonsignificant to significant is typically caused by the imputation of missing outcomes in the control group as responses. For the one-sided test methods, such as the Fisher randomization test (Rubin, 1980), this monotonic trend can be clearly observed, as shown in Fig. 16.1. Hence, for each column in the matrix, it is sufficient to calculate the first nonsignificant p-value, which serves as the tipping point for that column. As a result, this analysis is referred to as tipping point analysis.

Nevertheless, as the assumed response rate pertains to the population level without individual-level imputation, the aforementioned approach is unable to adjust for covariates, except in some extreme cases. For example, in the worst-best case analysis (Jakobsen et al., 2017), missing outcomes are assumed to be nonresponders in the investigational group and responders in the control group. Feedback from regulatory agencies regarding this approach suggests that it fails to account for imputation uncertainty (Sui et al., 2023). Therefore, the multiple imputation approach is recommended for conducting tipping point analysis for binary endpoints. To this end, we can use a direct Bernoulli sampling approach for performing tipping point analysis proposed by Sui et al. (2023).

16.5 Case Study

In this section, we demonstrate the statistical analysis of binary endpoints within the estimand framework using a real clinical case study named PREMIER (ClinicalTrials.gov identifier NCT00195663). The interpretation of this case study is based on a regulatory agency's publicly disclosed review document (FDA-Approved Drugs, BLA 125057/SUPPL-46) and involves the consideration of several elements. We begin with a description of the clinical background and trial design, then move on to an introduction to the original analysis and the regulatory agency review. Although this trial was conducted before the publication of the ICH E9(R1) guideline, we can discern the initial semblance of the estimand framework from the review report. At last, we reframe the analysis under the estimand framework.

16.5.1 Background

The case study is a phase III, parallel, multicenter, randomized controlled clinical trial designed to evaluate the efficacy and safety of adalimumab and methotrexate (MTX) combination therapy compared to MTX monotherapy in patients with recent onset (disease duration less than 3 years) rheumatoid arthritis not previously treated with MTX. Additionally, the trial includes an adalimumab arm to assess efficacy against the adalimumab + MTX arm, resulting in a total of three treatment arms. The trial consists of two periods: a 2-year double-blind treatment period followed by an 8-year open-label extension period, with a total planned duration of 10 years.

As rheumatoid arthritis is usually incurable, clinical treatment aims to alleviate joint inflammation and inhibit disease progression. This trial has two primary endpoints. One is the number of patients meeting ACR50 response criteria at week 52. This is a binary endpoint to measure clinical symptom improvement, including the alleviation of joint inflammation and the inhibition of disease progression. The other is the change from baseline in the modified Total Sharp Score (mTSS) at week 52, which is a continuous endpoint and assesses radiological improvement. The primary comparison is between the combination therapy treatment and the MTX monotherapy treatment. Since this chapter is about binary endpoints, we will focus on the primary endpoint ACR50 in the following content. For an alternative estimand discussion in rheumatoid arthritis, we refer to Sect. 8.3.

16.5.2 Original Analysis and Regulatory Agency Review

Before defining the primary estimand, we first review the statistical analysis conducted by the sponsor and the FDA's review comments on the results. The primary analysis was based on an intention-to-treat analysis set. Patients who withdrew early prior to week 52 or missed the week 52 results were imputed as nonresponders. The chi-squared test was used to test the treatment difference between the combination treatment and the MTX monotherapy treatment. Sensitivity analyses were performed using both the last observation carried forward (LOCF) imputation method and no imputation. The observed ACR50 responses at week 52 demonstrated statistical significance for adalimumab + MTX vs MTX and adalimumab + MTX vs adalimumab.

However, the trial experienced a high dropout rate. Out of the 799 initially recruited patients, 189 (23.7%) withdrew from the trial before week 52. The primary reasons for dropout were attributed to lack of efficacy or adverse events. Furthermore, the dropout rates varied among the three treatment arms, with the lowest rate observed in the adalimumab + MTX arm (17.9% (48/268)), followed by the MTX arm (23.7% (61/257)), and the highest rate observed in the adalimumab arm (29.2% (80/274)).

Accordingly, the FDA reviewers used the partial imputation method to evaluate the impact of the unbalanced dropout rates as a sensitivity analysis for the primary endpoints. They imputed the missing data so that the sample distribution of the follow-up time in the three arms became comparable (Wei & Shih, 2001). The partial imputation method is appropriate for dependent dropout (Glidden & Wei, 1999) or informative censoring (Wu & Carroll, 1988), whose dropout process depends on the response variable. After imputation, the completion rates at week 52 were comparable among the three arms: 81.7% (210/257) in the MTX arm, 82.1% (225/274) in the adalimumab arm, and 82.0% (220/268) in the adalimumab + MTX arm. The results based on the partial imputation method provided by the FDA reviewers were consistent with those from the sponsor (Table 16.3). Ultimately, the FDA regarded the sponsor's analysis results as robust, as indicated

Table 16.3 The FDA reviewers' analyses for ACR50

ACR50 responses at week 52	MTX (1)	Adalimumab (2)	Adalimumab + MTX (3)	*P*-values (2) vs (3)	(1) vs (3)
Partial imputation responses/n (%)	118/210 (56.2)	113/225 (50.2)	165/220 (75.0)	<0.0001	<0.0001

in the FDA-Approved Drugs document (FDA-Approved Drugs, BLA 125057/SUPPL-46). This case demonstrates the FDA's consideration of the impact of missing data on efficacy assessment.

16.5.3 Analysis Under the Estimand Framework

One of the primary objectives of the ICH E9(R1) guideline is to foster consensus between the reviewers and sponsors regarding clinical questions of interest during the trial design stage. While the ICH E9(R1) guideline had not yet been released at the time of the case study review, similar thoughts have already been reflected in FDA review reports. With a comprehensive understanding of the entire review background, we now define intercurrent events and their corresponding strategies under the estimand framework. Following the recommended estimand thinking process outlined in Chap. 3, we need to engage in discussions and decision-making regarding strategies to address intercurrent events in collaboration with physicians and other functional roles. We have assessed the feasibility of implementing remedial treatment in clinical practice and its potential impact on efficacy; it is reasonable to treat remedial treatment as one of the intercurrent events. Table 16.4 outlines the specific details and considerations related to intercurrent events and estimand strategies.

For the primary estimand, the primary clinical question of interest is: in patients with recent onset (disease duration less than 3 years) rheumatoid arthritis not previously treated with MTX, where patients who died or early terminated treatment due to lack of efficacy (without using remedial treatment) or adverse events are considered as nonresponders, what is the treatment difference between the Adalimumab + MTX and the MTX monotherapy assessed by ACR50 after 52 weeks of treatment, without the effect of remedial therapy?

Then we define attributes for the primary estimand.

(a) Population: Patients with recent onset (disease duration less than 3 years) rheumatoid arthritis not previously treated with MTX.
(b) Variable: Number of patients meeting ACR50 response criteria at week 52 without death or early termination of treatment due to lack of efficacy or adverse events.
(c) Treatment: MTX $\leq$20 mg/week or Adalimumab 40 mg + MTX $\leq$20 mg/week, without using remedial therapy. Dose adjustment due to adverse events is permitted.

Table 16.4 Proposed estimand strategies

Intercurrent events	Strategies	Comments
Remedial treatment is used due to lack of efficacy	Hypothetical	Not interested in the effect after remedial treatment
Death or early termination of treatment due to lack of efficacy (without using remedial treatment) or adverse events	Composite variable	Treatment failure, assuming that continuing the previous treatment will not provide any clinical benefits
Early termination of treatment due to other reasons (without using remedial treatment)	Treatment policy	The imperfect compliance issue reflecting clinical practice
Dose adjustment due to adverse events	Treatment policy	The imperfect compliance issue reflecting clinical practice

(d) Intercurrent Events and Strategies: See Table 16.4.
(e) Population-Level Summary: Difference in the proportion of ACR50 responses at week 52 between the Adalimumab + MTX and the MTX monotherapy.

Clinical rationales and statistical considerations for choosing this estimand are listed as follows: (1) The effect of remedial treatment is not of interest, so we chose the hypothetical strategy. (2) Death or early termination of treatment due to lack of efficacy or adverse events is regarded as treatment failure, thus using the composite variable strategy. (3) Early termination of treatment due to other reasons and dose adjustment due to adverse events are considered imperfect compliance issues in clinical practice; therefore, we used the treatment policy strategy.

For the statistical analysis, we need to define the primary analysis, sensitivity analysis, and supplementary analysis if necessary. The primary analysis methods involve the chi-squared test for hypothesis testing and the GLMM for estimation. The model includes treatment group, visit, and treatment-by-visit interaction. For patients with missing data after early termination of treatment due to other reasons or dose adjustment due to adverse events, RDO-based multiple imputation is used. If there are not enough RDOs, multiple imputation based on reference arm data (jump to reference) will be adopted. For missing data after remedial treatment or other intermittent missing, we use multiple imputation based on regression models with the MAR assumption, which indicates that efficacy is assumed to be similar to that of non-missing patients in the same treatment group. The choice of analysis methods is guided by the following considerations: the primary analysis method chooses multiple imputation instead of partial imputation because multiple imputation is commonly used in such cases and its assumptions are well understood, facilitating subsequent sensitivity analyses. We conduct two sensitivity analyses: tipping point analysis (Sui et al., 2023) and nonresponder imputation (considering all those missing as nonresponders).

For the supplementary analysis, if using remedial treatment due to lack of efficacy is regarded as clinical practice and the effect should be included in the estimation, we can select the treatment policy strategy for this intercurrent event. Or we can apply different strategies based on whether remedial treatment was administered within 1 week before week 52 or outside of this time window. In the former scenario, the composite variable strategy is appropriate, considering these cases as indicating no improvement. In the latter scenario, we can use the hypothetical strategy.

16.6 Concluding Remarks

As one of the most commonly used endpoints in clinical trials, binary endpoints share many similarities with continuous endpoints in the context of the estimand framework. Therefore, in this chapter, we focus on highlighting the differences between them, such as the logic-respecting and collapsibility of summary measures. Additionally, we provide a detailed introduction to the application of the tipping point method to binary endpoints. Finally, this chapter presents a complete statistical analysis process of a real rheumatoid arthritis clinical trial within the estimand framework. This case study also demonstrates the differences and limitations in statistical analysis when estimands are not considered. We aim for this chapter to serve as a reference and assistance for readers in future analyses of binary endpoints within the estimand framework.

References

Agresti, A. (2002). Categorical data analysis. In *Wiley series in probability and statistics* (Vol. 721). Wiley.

Carpenter, J. R., Roger, J. H., & Kenward, M. G. (2013). Analysis of longitudinal trials with protocol deviation: A framework for relevant, accessible assumptions, and inference via multiple imputation. *Journal of Biopharmaceutical Statistics, 23*(6), 1352–1371.

Darken, P., Nyberg, J., Ballal, S., & Wright, D. (2020). The attributable estimand: A new approach to account for intercurrent events. *Pharmaceutical Statistics, 19*(5), 626–635.

Dobson, A. J., & Barnett, A. G. (2018). *An introduction to generalized linear models*. CRC Press.

EMA. (2010). *Guideline on missing data in confirmatory clinical trials*. https://www.ema.europa.eu/

FDA. (2023). *Guidance for industry adjusting for covariates in randomized clinical trials for drugs and biological products*. https://www.fda.gov/

Felson, D. T., Anderson, J. J., Boers, M., Bombardier, C., Furst, D., Goldsmith, C., & Kieszak, S. (1995). American College of Rheumatology preliminary definition of improvement in rheumatoid arthritis. *Arthritis & Rheumatism: Official Journal of the American College of Rheumatology, 38*(6), 727–735.

Fisher, R. A. (1922). On the interpretation of χ 2 from contingency tables, and the calculation of P. *Journal of the Royal Statistical Society, 85*(1), 87–94.

Glidden, D. V., & Wei, L. J. (1999). Rank estimation of treatment differences based on repeated measurements subject to dependent censoring. *Journal of the American Statistical Association, 94*, 888–895.

Greenland, S., Pearl, J., & Robins, J. M. (1999). Confounding and collapsibility in causal inference. *Statistical Science, 14*(1), 29–46.

Hernán, M. A., & Robins, J. (2020). *Causal inference: What if*. Chapman & Hall/CRC.

Hosmer, D. W., Jr., Lemeshow, S., & Sturdivant, R. X. (2013). *Applied logistic regression* (Vol. 398). John Wiley & Sons.
Huitfeldt, A., Stensrud, M. J., & Suzuki, E. (2019). On the collapsibility of measures of effect in the counterfactual causal framework. *Emerging Themes in Epidemiology, 16*, 1–5.
ICH. (2019). *ICH E9 (R1) addendum on estimands and sensitivity analysis in clinical trials to the guideline on statistical principles for clinical trials*. Step 4 document. https://ich.org/
Jakobsen, J. C., Gluud, C., Wetterslev, J., & Winkel, P. (2017). When and how should multiple imputation be used for handling missing data in randomised clinical trials–a practical guide with flowcharts. *BMC Medical Research Methodology, 17*(1), 1–10.
Lin, H. M., Xu, H., Ding, Y., & Hsu, J. C. (2019). Correct and logical inference on efficacy in subgroups and their mixture for binary outcomes. *Biometrical Journal, 61*(1), 8–26.
Lipkovich, I., Ratitch, B., & Mallinckrodt, C. H. (2020). Causal inference and estimands in clinical trials. *Statistics in Biopharmaceutical Research, 12*(1), 54–67.
Little, R. J., & Rubin, D. B. (2019). *Statistical analysis with missing data* (Vol. 793). John Wiley & Sons.
Liu, Y., Wang, B., Yang, M., Hui, J., Xu, H., Kil, S., & Hsu, J. C. (2022). Correct and logical causal inference for binary and time-to-event outcomes in randomized controlled trials. *Biometrical Journal, 64*(2), 198–224.
Liu, Y., Yang, M., Kil, S., Li, J., Mondal, S., Shentu, Y., & Yung, G. (2023). From logic-respecting efficacy estimands to logic-ensuring analysis principle for time-to-event endpoint in randomized clinical trials with subgroups. *Statistics in Biopharmaceutical Research, 15*, 1–14.
Liublinska, V., & Rubin, D. B. (2014). Sensitivity analysis for a partially missing binary outcome in a two-arm randomized clinical trial. *Statistics in Medicine, 33*(24), 4170–4185.
Ma, C., Shen, X., Qu, Y., & Du, Y. (2022). Analysis of an incomplete binary outcome dichotomized from an underlying continuous variable in clinical trials. *Pharmaceutical Statistics, 21*(5), 907–918.
Mantel, N., & Haenszel, W. (1959). Statistical aspects of the analysis of data from retrospective studies of disease. *Journal of the National Cancer Institute, 22*(4), 719–748.
Nie, L. (2021). Discussant: Logical causal inference for binary and time-to-event Estimands. In *ASA biopharmaceutical section regulatory-industry statistics workshop*. https://www.amstat.org/meetings/asa-biopharmaceutical-section-regulatory-industry-statistics-workshop
Pearson, K. (1900). On the criterion that a given system of deviations from the probable in the case of a correlated system of variables is such that it can be reasonably supposed to have arisen from random sampling. *Philosophical Magazine, Series 5, 50*(302), 157–175.
Qu, Y., & Lipkovich, I. (2021). Implementation of ICH E9 (R1): A few points learned during the COVID-19 pandemic. *Therapeutic Innovation & Regulatory Science, 55*(5), 984–988.
Qu, Y., Shurzinske, L., & Sethuraman, S. (2021). Defining estimands using a mix of strategies to handle intercurrent events in clinical trials. *Pharmaceutical Statistics, 20*(2), 314–323.
Rosenblum, M., & Steingrimsson, J. A. (2016). *Matching the efficiency gains of the logistic regression estimator while avoiding its interpretability problems, in randomized trials.*
Rubin, D. B. (1980). Randomization analysis of experimental data: The Fisher randomization test comment. *Journal of the American Statistical Association, 75*(371), 591–593.
Stroup, W. W. (2012). *Generalized linear mixed models: Modern concepts, methods and applications*. CRC Press.
Sui, Y., Bu, X., Li, Y., & Wang, X. (2023). *Application of tipping point analysis in clinical trials using the multiple imputation procedure in SAS*. https://www.pharmasug.org/
Van Buuren, S. (2007). Multiple imputation of discrete and continuous data by fully conditional specification. *Statistical Methods in Medical Research, 16*(3), 219–242.
Van Buuren, S., & Groothuis-Oudshoorn, K. (2011). Mice: Multivariate imputation by chained equations in R. *Journal of Statistical Software, 45*, 1–67.
Wei, L., & Shih, W. J. (2001). Partial imputation approach to analysis of repeated measurements with dependent drop-outs. *Statistics in Medicine, 20*(8), 1197–1214.

Wu, M. C., & Carroll, R. J. (1988). Estimation and comparison of changes in the presence of informative right censoring by modeling the censoring process. *Biometrics, 44*, 175–188.
Xi, D., & Bretz, F. (2021a). Discussion on 'correct and logical causal inference for binary and time-to-event outcomes in randomized controlled trials'. *Biometrical Journal. Biometrische Zeitschrift, 64*(2), 243–245.
Xi, D., & Bretz, F. (2021b). Conditional vs. marginal estimands: From collapsibility to logic respect. In *ASA Biopharmaceutical Section regulatory-industry statistics workshop*. https://www.amstat.org/meetings/asa-biopharmaceutical-section-regulatory-industry-statistics-workshop
Yan, X., Lee, S., & Li, N. (2009). Missing data handling methods in medical device clinical trials. *Journal of Biopharmaceutical Statistics, 19*(6), 1085–1098.
Ye, T., Bannick, M., Yi, Y., & Shao, J. (2023). Robust variance estimation for covariate-adjusted unconditional treatment effect in randomized clinical trials with binary outcomes. *Statistical Theory and Related Fields, 7*(2), 159–163.

Chapter 17
Statistical Analysis Under the Estimand Framework: Recurrent Events

Tobias Mütze and Tianmeng Lyu

Abstract This chapter discusses the statistical analysis of recurrent events within the estimand framework. Recurrent events are those that can occur repeatedly for a single patient, such as heart failure hospitalizations, relapses in multiple sclerosis, or exacerbations in chronic obstructive pulmonary disease (COPD) or asthma. Focusing on a two-arm clinical trial scenario where discontinuation of the randomized treatment for any reason is the only intercurrent event, this chapter illustrates how to define the corresponding estimand attributes when addressing the intercurrent event using one of the five strategies outlined in the ICH E9(R1) guideline. For each estimand, appropriate estimation methods are presented. The methods are illustrated with a case study using synthetic data from a clinical trial in asthma. The chapter concludes with a review of the literature on estimands for recurrent events in the presence of death and remarks on software solutions for the presented estimation approaches.

17.1 Introduction

An event is called recurrent when it can occur repeatedly for a single patient. For many diseases, the disease burden in clinical trials is measured through recurrent events, for example, heart failure hospitalizations in chronic heart failure (Solomon et al., 2019), relapses in multiple sclerosis (Hauser et al., 2020), exacerbations in chronic obstructive pulmonary disease (COPD) or asthma (Keene et al., 2007;

T. Mütze (✉)
Advanced Methodology and Data Science, Novartis Pharma AG, Basel, Switzerland
e-mail: tobias.muetze@novartis.com

T. Lyu
Advanced Methodology and Data Science, Novartis Pharmaceuticals Corporation, East Hanover, NJ, USA
e-mail: tianmeng.lyu@novartis.com

J. Wei et al. (eds.), *Estimands in Clinical Trials*, Springer Series in Pharmaceutical Statistics, https://doi.org/10.1007/978-3-032-02192-2_17

Keene et al., 2008), headaches after transcatheter atrial septal defect closures (Rodés-Cabau et al., 2015), or flares in acute gouty arthritis (Schlesinger et al., 2011).

Chapter 12 of this book discusses guidelines from the European Medicines Agency (EMA) that have embraced the estimand framework. We refer to Sect. 12.5 for an overview of guidelines for chronic diseases with recurrent event endpoints that include estimand-related guidance.

The underlying premise of this chapter is that recurrent events are appropriate for defining the clinical question of interest and for measuring disease burden. In practice, the discussion is often about whether the time to the occurrence of the first event or the recurrence of the event is more appropriate. Such discussions are disease-specific, as outlined by Anker and McMurray (2012) in the context of trials in patients with heart failure. For estimands for time-to-event outcomes, we refer to Chap. 18 of this book.

When defining an estimand for a recurrent event, it is key to consider the definition of an event and how this relates to the disease that is studied. This usually includes determining if and how event severity, event duration, and proximity of event occurrences are handled. For example, in patients with asthma, exacerbations are categorized into mild, moderate, or severe (National Heart, Lung, and Blood Institute, 2007), but for the assessment of a treatment's efficacy, only moderate to severe exacerbations might be relevant (Brightling et al., 2021). In some settings, when two recurrent events occur in proximity, they might be combined into a single occurrence. Finally, events are often based on granular criteria and adjudicated by an independent committee. The exact definition of an event needs to be specified in the clinical trial protocol (Carson et al., 2023).

When defining an estimand for a clinical trial where the primary endpoint is based on a recurrent event, only the definition of the variable and the summary measure are specific to recurrent events. Defining the other attributes and their general considerations is discussed in Chap. 2. In the following, we will illustrate in a simplified setting of a two-arm clinical trial without any intercurrent events, focusing on the discussion of general types of variable definitions and summary measure definitions for recurrent events. The variable attribute describes what is measured for a single trial patient. The following two variable definitions are potentially of interest:

- Number of recurrent events between randomization and time T^*;
- Timing of the recurrent events occurrences between randomization and time T^*.

The main difference between these definitions of the variable is whether only the number of events up to T^* or also their timing is of interest. The second definition includes additional information about the timing of the events, which may be needed to calculate certain choices of summary statistics. If the definition of the summary measure does not depend on the timing of the individual recurrent events, then there is no need to include the timing of the recurrent events in the variable.

The time frame T^* is determined based on clinical considerations and describes the period for which the trial compares the two treatment conditions. As part of the estimand definition, the time frame is identical for each patient. Differences in the follow-up between trial patients are handled as part of the analysis.

To describe common summary measures for recurrent event data, we first introduce some notations. Let $N_i(t)$ denote the number of events between randomization and time t for a patient in trial arm $i = 1, 2$ and let $\mu_i(t) = E[N_i(t)]$ be the mean function, that is, the expected number of events up to a given time t. The rate $\rho_i(t) = d\mu_i(t)/dt$ is the first derivative of the mean function with respect to time. Summary measures can be defined to be univariate (i.e., a single number), to be multivariate, or to be a function. The common univariate summary measures for recurrent event data are:

- Expected number of recurrent events up to time T^*: $\mu_i(T^*)$ for $i = 1, 2$ indexing the trial arm.
- Expected number of recurrent events per time unit, $\mu_i(T^*)/T^*$, up to time T^* for $i = 1, 2$ indexing the trial arm.

For each of these summary measures, the between-arm comparison may be based on the difference or the ratio. Which summary measure to use depends on the clinical question of interest and how the treatment effect is planned to be quantified. From the definition of the summary measures, it is clear that these two summary measures can easily be transformed into each other and that they result in identical between-arm ratios. Summary measures based on the expected number of events up to time T^* take all prior events into account and are, as such, reflecting the complete patient journey up to time T^*.

Alternatively, there might be settings in which interest is not in the expected number of events or the rate at a single time point, but rather in any time point $t \in [0, T^*]$. In these settings, the summary measures could also be defined to be a function, for example, the mean function $\mu_i(t)$ for $t \in [0, T^*]$. Especially when interest is in the rate, it is common that interest is not in the rate at a particular timepoint, but in the rate function $\rho_i(t)$, $i = 1, 2$, in the time interval $[0, T^*]$. Regardless of whether the summary measure is univariate or a function, it needs to include a time frame to be precise and unambiguous.

An alternative summary measure is the intensity function (Cook & Lawless, 2007). While the intensity function can be used to fully describe the data-generating process and, thus, is in some sense the most informative summary measure, intensity functions is generally difficult to interpret for the purpose of comparing treatments since it is defined conditional on the event history and, therefore, are not recommended to be used to define estimands in clinical trials.

It is important that the summary measure and consequently the estimand be defined to be free of statistical assumptions; that is, assumptions such as the proportionality of rates or means should be part of the analysis and not be part of the estimand definition. Statistical assumptions as part of the estimand raise concerns about the existence of the defined treatment effect, as the assumption might not be true.

The remainder of this section is structured as follows: In Sect. 17.2, we introduce recurrent event models that are commonly used to analyze clinical trials. In Sect. 17.3, we discuss estimands and estimand-aligned analysis for recurrent events for the setting where treatment discontinuation is the only intercurrent event. In Sect.

17.4, we illustrate different estimands and their estimation through synthetic data from a clinical trial with recurrent events. In Sect. 17.5, we discuss the setting where death is an intercurrent event. We conclude with a discussion in Sect. 17.6.

17.2 Common Recurrent Event Models

The estimand thinking process (ICH, 2021), see also Chap. 3, emphasizes the importance of separating the clinical question of interest as specified through the estimand from the statistical analysis method. The estimand is defined first, and then the statistical analysis is selected accordingly and in alignment with the estimand. In particular, comparisons of statistical analysis methods (Gregson et al., 2023) that target different estimands are generally not sensible, as they correspond to comparing apples with oranges.

In the following, we will recapitulate the negative binomial model and the Andersen–Gill model with robust variance estimation (i.e., the Lin Wei Yang Ying (LWYY) model) as two of the most common analysis models for recurrent event data in clinical trials. For an in-depth discussion of recurrent event models, we refer to Cook and Lawless (2007). We discuss when and how these models can be used to estimate estimands commonly of interest in clinical trials with recurrent events in Sect. 17.3.

17.2.1 *Negative Binomial Model*

For illustration purposes, we introduce the standard negative binomial model with a time-homogeneous rate first and then discuss various extensions. The standard negative binomial model is a Poisson-Gamma mixture model: for each patient, it is assumed that the number of recurrent events up to time t follows a Poisson distribution conditional on the patient-specific rate. In detail, let $N_{ij}(t)$ be the number of events up to time t for patient j in arm i and let the patient-specific event rate λ_{ij} follow a Gamma distribution with shape $\alpha = 1/\phi$ and rate $\beta = 1/(\phi\mu_i)$ parameterized such that the expected value and the variance are μ_i and $\phi\mu_i^2$, respectively. Let the number of events $N_{ij}(t)$ follow a conditional Poisson distribution, that is $N_{ij}(t) \mid \lambda_{ij} \sim Pois(t\lambda_{ij})$. Then the marginal distribution of $N_{ij}(t)$ is a negative binomial distribution with mean $t\mu_i$ and variance $t\mu_i(1 + \phi t\mu_i)$. The probability function of a negative binomial distribution is given by

$$P\left(N_{ij}(t)=n\right)=\frac{\Gamma\left(n+\frac{1}{\phi}\right)}{\Gamma\left(\frac{1}{\phi}\right)n!}\left(\frac{1}{1+\phi t\mu_i}\right)^{\frac{1}{\phi}}\left(\frac{\phi t\mu_i}{1+\phi t\mu_i}\right)^n.$$

The negative binomial distribution can be extended to a negative binomial regression model, which allows modeling the effect of a covariate vector $\boldsymbol{X}$ on the mean through an exponential link function, that is $\mu_i = \exp(\boldsymbol{X}'\boldsymbol{\beta}_i)$. For a more detailed discussion of the negative binomial regression model, we refer to Lawless (1987a). The negative binomial model introduced above assumes that the rate is constant over time, which might be an assumption that is violated in some clinical settings. An extension to time-dependent rates (i.e., a Poisson-Gamma mixture model with a time-dependent baseline function) was introduced by Lawless (1987b).

17.2.2 Andersen–Gill Model with Robust Variance Estimation (LWYY Model)

Andersen and Gill (1982) proposed an extension of the Cox proportional hazard model for counting processes, that is, for modeling recurrent events. The Andersen–Gill model makes two key assumptions: (1) any influence of past events on future events is mitigated through time-dependent covariates; in other words, the intensity function at time t depends on the process history only through the covariates at time t; (2) the covariates influence the intensity function through an exponential link function with an unspecified baseline intensity function. The estimation of the unknown parameters in an Andersen–Gill model follows the same partial likelihood approach as the estimation of the unknown parameters in a Cox proportional hazard model.

Lin et al. (2000) proposed a proportional rate model, the so-called LWYY model, that removes the first assumption from the Andersen–Gill model. This proportional rate model allows dependencies of future events on past events other than those captured by time-varying covariates. The score function for estimating the unknown parameters is the same as in the Andersen–Gill model and, as such, both models result in the same point estimates. However, for statistical inference, in the LWYY model, the standard errors are estimated with a robust sandwich variance estimator rather than a maximum-likelihood estimator.

17.3 Estimands and Estimand-Aligned Analysis for Recurrent Events

In this section, we discuss how to align the analysis with the estimand for recurrent event data. For illustration purposes, we focus on the simplified setting of a two-arm clinical trial where only a single nonterminal intercurrent event is expected. We consider discontinuation of the randomized treatment for any reason; in short, treatment discontinuation is the intercurrent event of interest. The case of a terminal intercurrent event is discussed in Sect. 17.5. The primary trial objective is to show superiority of the experimental treatment versus the control treatment in a chronic disease. In the following, we discuss different clinical questions of interest and the corresponding estimands based on the five strategies outlined in ICH (2019). It is worth noting that these are examples of potential questions of interest and that this section does not constitute an exhaustive list.

17.3.1 Treatment Policy Strategy

The treatment policy strategy is applied to an intercurrent event when the interest is in comparing treatment strategies that include the effect of the intercurrent event. For example, the clinical question of interest may be "What is the effect of the experimental treatment regardless of discontinuation compared to the control treatment regardless of discontinuation on the expected number of events of interest up to time T* in patients with 'disease'?" Here, "regardless of" implies that the observed outcome variable is of interest whether or not treatment discontinuation occurs. The corresponding estimand attributes are:

- Population: Patients with the disease of interest.
- Treatment conditions: Experimental treatment regardless of discontinuation, control treatment regardless of discontinuation.
- Variable: $N(T^*)$, with $N(t)$ the number of the event of interest between randomization and time t.
- Population-level summary: Expected number of events $E[N(T^*)]$; the between-arm comparison is performed based on the ratio of the expected number of events between arms.

When an intercurrent event is addressed through the treatment policy strategy, the events that occur after the intercurrent event contain information relevant to the treatment effect of interest and should be included in the estimation. Inference for the treatment policy estimand is straightforward if there is no missing data, for example, with methods of moments estimators, a negative binomial model, or an LWYY model. However, in practice, clinical trials almost never have complete data. In particular, missing data is more likely for patients who discontinue their randomized treatment since these patients tend not to remain on the trial, and as a consequence, the characteristics of patients having complete data and those having missing data are generally different. Therefore, as outlined in previous chapters (e.g., Sect. 2.5.2.1 for general considerations, Sect. 15.2.1 for continuous endpoints, Sect. 16.2.1 for binary endpoints, and Sect. 18.2.1 for time-to-event data), under these circumstances the estimation of treatment policy estimands is challenging, because the missing data must be imputed implicitly or explicitly under assumptions that are not verifiable. Missing data in the recurrent event setting is special in the sense that part of the variable $N(T^*)$ is observed (i.e., number of events until the time when missingness starts is known). Analysis models such as the negative binomial model or the LWYY model address nonintermittent missing data implicitly under a missing at random assumption when only the observed data is analyzed. However, this assumes that, conditional on baseline covariates, the patients' behavior after discontinuing the trial is similar to the behavior of those patients who remain on the trial. Especially when patients receive an active treatment, this assumption is implausible, because the patients with missing data and the patients without missing data generally have different characteristics, since the patients without missing data are predominantly on their randomized treatment. Therefore, unless the amount of missing data is so small that the missing data approach does not affect the analysis results relevantly, the missing data after treatment discontinuation must be addressed explicitly, for example, through multiple imputation (Rubin, 1987), inverse probability censoring weighting (Seaman & White, 2013), or modeling of the loss to follow-up process (Lawless & Cook, 2019). In current practice, missing data is commonly addressed through multiple imputation. Depending on the analysis model, the number of recurrent events or the event times must be imputed. This requires assumptions on how the patients who have missing data would have behaved had they not discontinued the trial. It is common to express such assumptions based on a reference arm, for example, the control arm, see Sect. 15.2.1 of this book and Carpenter et al. (2013), which results in the well-known reference-based imputation approaches such as jump-to-reference, copy reference, and copy increment references. For recurrent event data, these reference-based imputation approaches have been studied by Keene et al. (2014), Akacha and Ogundimu (2016), Diao et al. (2022), and Gao et al. (2017). For the imputation model, Keene et al. (2014) assumed a negative binomial model, Diao et al. (2022) used a semiparametric proportional intensity Gamma-frailty model, Gao et al. (2017) used a piecewise constant proportional rate Gamma-frailty model, and Akacha and Ogundimu (2016) used a parametric proportional Gamma-frailty model. The ideas of reference-based approaches can easily be extended to retrieved dropout imputation (Roger et al., 2019). An important aspect to consider when performing a reference-based imputation is how to estimate the variance (Bartlett, 2023). The mentioned imputation models focus on imputing the number of recurrent events but do not impute the event times, which would be necessary if the LWYY model were used for the analysis.

In terms of software implementation, Keene et al. (2014) outline how their method could be implemented in SAS, and their method is implemented in the R package `dejaVu` (Burkoff et al., 2021). A *C* implementation of the method discussed in Diao et al. (2022) is provided by the authors. An SAS implementation of the methods described by Roger et al. (2019) is provided by the authors online (https://www.lshtm.ac.uk/research/centres-projects-groups/missing-data#dia-missing-data). To the best of our knowledge, no implementation of an approach that imputes the event times, which is needed if the analysis is performed with an LWYY model, is publicly available.

17.3.2 Hypothetical Strategy

Under the hypothetical strategy, the clinical question of interest is about the treatment effect if an intercurrent event would not happen by time T^*, where T^* is the prespecified time frame as discussed in Sect. 17.1. As an example, the clinical question of interest may be "What is the effect of the experimental treatment compared to the control treatment if patients would not discontinue treatment by time T^* on the expected number of events of interest up to time T^* in patients with 'disease'?" The definition of the variable and summary measure stays the same as the estimand with the treatment policy strategy, while the treatment attribute is the experimental treatment and control treatment. ICH (2019) discussed what hypothetical scenarios might be of more clinical and regulatory interest compared to others. For example, the hypothetical setting, which can potentially be carried out by trial design, may be of more interest. On the other hand, the clinical relevance of hypothetical settings that may not be expected in practice, for example, the setting where patients would not discontinue treatment when they had adverse events, may be questionable. In practice, whether a hypothetical setting is of clinical interest should be discussed on a case-by-case basis and aligned within the trial team and with health authorities. For further discussions of the hypothetical strategy, we refer to Chap. 2 and Sect. 15.2.2.

Since the interest is in a treatment effect in the hypothetical setting where the intercurrent event would not happen, data collected after the occurrence of the intercurrent event (e.g., treatment discontinuation) are in current practice typically excluded from the analysis, even though statistical methods that target a hypothetical estimand and use post-intercurrent event data exist (Lasch & Guizzaro, 2022). Therefore, outcomes under the hypothetical setting can be considered as missing and need to be imputed, either explicitly or implicitly, and then used in the analysis to target the hypothetical estimand of interest. The explicit imputation methods (e.g., Keene et al., 2014; Akacha & Ogundimu, 2016; Diao et al., 2022; Gao et al., 2017) referenced in Sect. 17.3.1 can be used to model the hypothetical trajectory of patients. The negative binomial model and the LWYY model, where data after the occurrence of an intercurrent event are simply excluded, target the hypothetical estimand if the resulting missing data can be assumed to be missing at random conditional on the baseline covariates adjusted in the models. However, this assumption may not be true in practice because it is likely that the occurrence of intercurrent events depends on time-varying covariates that also impact the recurrent events (we call them time-varying confounders). Olarte Parra et al. (2023) discussed estimation methods targeting hypothetical estimands that properly adjust for time-varying confounders in continuous data. The methods discussed in the paper (e.g., g-computation, inverse probability weighting, etc.) may be applied to analysis models for recurrent events, but this has not yet been discussed in the existing literature. Missing data imputation approaches may be considered as well, under practical assumptions where both baseline and time-dependent confounders are considered. Note that with the imputation approach, only the number of recurrent events needs to be imputed if the standard negative binomial model is used, while the event times need to be imputed as well if the LWYY model is used in the final analysis. It is worth noting that Olarte Parra et al. (2023) also discussed the estimation approaches where data after the occurrence of intercurrent events are exploited to estimate hypothetical estimands. No matter which estimation method is used, the assumptions for the unobserved outcomes under a hypothetical setting with the chosen analysis method need to be clearly communicated. For a more general discussion on this topic, we refer to the paper from Olarte Parra et al. (2023).

17.3.3 Composite Strategy

The idea of a composite strategy is to include the intercurrent event in the definition of the variable, because the occurrence of the intercurrent event is informative about the patients' outcome (ICH, 2019). The FDA guideline on multiple endpoints in clinical trials (FDA, 2022) provides regulatory considerations for defining composite endpoints. In particular, it is stated that the effect of experimental treatment on the composite endpoint can only be interpreted as characterizing the overall effect of the experimental treatment if all components have similar clinical importance, and that the experimental treatment's benefit might be questioned if the experimental treatment has opposite effects on the different components of the composite endpoint. For a more in-depth discussion of the regulatory considerations of composite variables, we refer to the FDA (2022).

There are various ways to incorporate treatment discontinuation in the variable definition. For example, a hierarchical composite from the number of recurrent events, $N_i(t)$, and the time between randomization and treatment discontinuation can be specified, and the summary measure could be defined as a win ratio, win odds, or win probability (Pocock et al., 2012; Brunner et al., 2021). In the latter approach, the summary measure is generally difficult to interpret and not on the scale of the number of expected events or the rate scale. For a more thorough discussion on the interpretation of such summary measures, we refer to Sect. 15.2.3. An alternative approach is to consider the occurrence of treatment discontinuation as an additional event. In practice, this is unlikely to be of relevance as the clinical importance of treatment discontinuation generally differs from the recurrent event of interest. The interpretation is additionally complicated by the fact that the composite is not a recurrent event in the traditional sense since not all parts of the composite are recurrent in nature. However, since there might be clinical settings in which counting the occurrence of an intercurrent event as an event is meaningful, we discuss this in the following.

As an example, we define the estimand attributes as follows for the clinical question, "What is the effect of the experimental treatment compared to the control treatment on the expected number of composite events of event of interest and treatment discontinuation, which is counted as an additional event, at time T^* in patients with 'disease'?"

The population are patients with the particular disease of interest, and the treatment attributes are experimental treatment and control treatment. The variable and the summary measure are defined as follows:

- Variable: $N(T^*)+\mathbb{I}(T^*)$, with $N(t)$ as the number of the event of interest between randomization and time t of a patient, and $\mathbb{I}(t)$ as a step function that is 1 once the patient has discontinued treatment and 0 otherwise.
- Summary measure: Expected number of events $E\left[N(T^*)+\mathbb{I}(T^*)\right]$; the between-arm comparison is performed based on the ratio of the expected number of events between arms.

The analysis can, for example, be conducted with the negative binomial model or an LWYY model. A key issue in the analysis will be the handling of missing data, which has to be imputed either explicitly or implicitly. The missing data handling considerations are similar but not identical to those for the estimation of the treatment policy estimand. What makes it more complicated is that treatment discontinuation is counted as an additional event. In detail, let us, for example, assume that a patient takes the randomized treatment until $T^*/2$ and then discontinues the trial. Generally, if a patient discontinues the trial, it is expected that they simultaneously discontinue the treatment, which would mean that $\mathbb{I}\left[(t)\right]=1, t \geq T^*/2$, that is, the indicator for treatment discontinuation is not missing. Therefore, using independent censoring for the patients at the time that they leave the trial when analyzing the composite is not sensible, as only the recurrent event part of the composite is missing. Instead, the missing part of the composite must be imputed, for example, through an imputation model that jointly models the recurrent event part of the composite and the treatment discontinuation process. Joint models for recurrent event data and time-to-event data have been studied extensively in the literature; see, for example (Huang & Wang, 2004). Considerations about the off-treatment behavior of patients are the same as for the handling of missing data in the treatment policy setting.

17.3.4 While on Treatment Strategy

Under the while on treatment strategy, the clinical question of interest focuses on the treatment effect before the intercurrent event (e.g., treatment discontinuation) happens. For simplicity and for illustration purposes, in the following discussions, we will use the first of the two variable definitions discussed in Sect. 17.1, and, as before, we focus on the intercurrent event of treatment discontinuation.

Because the variable of interest is the number of events up to the minimum of time to discontinuation and the fixed follow-up time, under the while on treatment strategy, we inevitably simultaneously study the effect of treatment on the event of interest and on treatment discontinuation. If the experimental and control treatments have different effects on the occurrence of the treatment discontinuation, then care needs to be taken in the interpretation of the while on treatment estimand. For example, if patients in the investigational arm tend to discontinue treatment earlier than those in the control arm, then as time goes on, patients remaining in the investigational arm are those who tend to stay with the treatment longer (e.g., potentially healthier) compared to the patients who remained in the control arm. If we further assume that there is a positive correlation between time to treatment discontinuation and time to recurrent event, then those who tend to discontinue later (e.g., healthier) may have fewer events, leading to a positive impact on the treatment effect on recurrent events. This gives an example where a negative effect on time to intercurrent event (i.e., earlier treatment discontinuation in the previous example) may lead to a positive effect on the final summary measure, and thus we need to be cautious with the interpretation of the while on treatment estimand in such cases.

There are various approaches for mitigating the described concern. For example, a composite while on treatment strategy, whereby one event is added to the count for patients with the intercurrent event before T^*, could be considered. For a more detailed discussion of the composite while on treatment strategy, we refer to Schmidli et al. (2023) and Wei et al. (2023). Alternatively, the summary measure could be defined through the number of events prior to treatment discontinuation per time unit on treatment. This summary measure accounts for both the treatment effect on the event of interest and the treatment effect on the time to treatment discontinuation. An additional estimand for time to treatment discontinuation will provide a more complete picture and help with the interpretation.

As an example, we define the estimand attributes as follows for the clinical question "What is the effect of the experimental treatment compared to the control treatment on the expected number of the event of interest per the expected time on treatment up to time T^*, in patients with 'disease'?" The population are patients with the particular disease of interest, and the treatment attributes are experimental treatment and control treatment. The variable and the summary measure are defined as follows:

- Variable: $(N(\min(T^*, T^{ICE})), T^{ICE})$, that is, a tuple of the number of the event of interest before treatment discontinuation (T^{ICE}) or a fixed follow-up time T^*, whichever comes first, the time of treatment distribution T^{ICE}.
- Summary Measure: Expected number of events divided by the expected time at risk, that is, $E[N(\min(T^*, T^{ICE}))]/E[\min(T^*, T^{ICE})]$; the between-arm comparison is performed based on the ratio of this between arms.

For the estimation methods, Wei et al. (2023) discussed and compared different estimation methods under the setting of a joint frailty model for recurrent events and a terminal event. They showed that the negative binomial model does not target the while alive (i.e., while on treatment strategy when the intercurrent event is death) estimand, while the LWYY model only has a small bias for the while alive estimand under certain conditions. Mao (2023) proposed nonparametric inference for general while on treatment estimands in recurrent events.

17.3.5 Principal Stratum Strategy

The motivation for using the principal stratum strategy is to evaluate the treatment effect within a subgroup of patients defined based on the potential occurrence of an intercurrent event, for example, the occurrence of treatment discontinuation. For example, the clinical question of interest addressed by a principal stratum strategy could be: "What is the effect of experimental treatment versus control treatment on the expected number of recurrent events at time T^* in patients with *disease* who would not discontinue treatment under both arms?"

The principal stratum is defined based on potential outcomes instead of observed outcomes to ensure that the treatment effect is evaluated between the two arms with the same population. Because we can never observe both potential outcomes, the principal stratum effect is not identifiable, and further assumptions are needed in order to estimate a principal stratum estimand. The simple contrast to compare treatment effect within the subgroup of patients who did not discontinue treatment in the two arms is not a causal effect and thus not targeting the principal stratum estimand, because the occurrence of discontinuation may be impacted by the treatment. We refer to Chap. 19 for a more detailed discussion on the principal stratum and the estimation methods. Lyu et al. (2023) proposed a Bayesian modeling approach to estimate a principal stratum estimand in recurrent events with death as an intercurrent event. A similar idea may be extended and applied to principal stratum estimands defined based on other intercurrent events. The choice of assumptions and modeling approaches to estimate a principal stratum estimand depends on the specific question of interest and the clinical setting.

17.4 Case Study

In this section, we illustrate the estimation of estimands that address intercurrent events with a treatment policy and hypothetical strategy, respectively, using a synthetic data example simulated based on a Phase III trial in asthma.

In this synthetic trial example, 612 patients were randomized to Drug X and 609 patients were randomized to the control arm. All patients were expected to be followed for 26 weeks, but patients were allowed to discontinue treatment and/or drop out of the trial anytime during the trial. The endpoint of interest is the total number of asthma exacerbations (including all severity categories) up to Week 26. For illustration purposes, we focus on the intercurrent event of treatment discontinuation and present the estimand definition and the corresponding estimation methods for treatment policy and hypothetical strategies.

In this synthetic data set, four baseline covariates are available, including region, history of asthma exacerbations, forced expiratory volume in 1 second (FEV1) prior to inhalation, and FEV1 post inhalation.

One particularity of this synthetic trial data and the underlying trial is that the data collection finished prior to planned Week 26 for a portion of the patients due to administrative reasons ("administrative censoring"). Also, no data is available for the period after patients discontinued their randomized treatment. In other words, all observed data is on-treatment data. A patient can either discontinue their randomized treatment or be censored for administrative reasons. Table 17.1 shows, per trial arm, the number of patients randomized, with the intercurrent event, and with administrative censoring.

Table 17.2 shows the mean number of exacerbations and the mean number of days on the randomized treatment.

17.4.1 Treatment Policy Strategy

If we use a treatment policy strategy to address treatment discontinuation, the estimand can be defined as follows.

(a) Population: Symptomatic patients with a diagnosis of asthma.
(b) Variable: Total number of asthma exacerbations between baseline and Week 26.
(c) Treatment: Drug X and control, regardless of treatment discontinuation.
(d) Intercurrent event: Treatment discontinuation. Treatment discontinuation is addressed by treatment policy strategy, which is reflected in the definition of the "Treatment" attribute. It implies that data collected after treatment discontinuation should be included in the analysis. The estimand will be estimated with a negative binomial regression model with the randomized treatment as the only covariate.
(e) Population-Level Summary: Expected total number of asthma exacerbations between baseline and Week 26; the between-arm comparison is performed based on the ratio of the expected number of events between arms.

Treatment discontinuation is addressed by treatment policy strategy, which is reflected in the definition of the "Treatment" attribute. It implies that data collected after treatment discontinuation should be included in the analysis. The estimand

Table 17.1 Key patient counts for the trial arms

Arm	Number of randomized patients	Number of patients with the intercurrent event	Number of patients with administrative censoring
Control	609	42	45
Drug X	612	42	46

Table 17.2 Summary statistics for the total number of exacerbations and the time on randomized treatment

Arm	Mean number of exacerbations	Mean number of days on the randomized treatment
Control	0.384	169
Drug X	0.294	171

will be estimated with a negative binomial regression model with the randomized treatment as the only covariate.

Since in this data set patients dropped out of the trial at the same time as treatment discontinuation and since the data collection was stopped before some patients reached their Week 26 visit, we have a missing data problem. In the following, we illustrate a reference-based imputation approach and present the corresponding analysis results.

As the imputation model, we chose to fit a Bayesian Poisson-lognormal mixture model with a log-link function to all observed counts, that is, to the on-treatment data. This model includes a normally distributed patient-specific random effect. Using a normally distributed random effect instead of a Gamma-distributed random effect is generally computationally advantageous. The fixed effects are the randomized treatment, four baseline covariates as described before, and the interaction between the randomized treatment and any of the baseline covariates. The time on treatment (or time to trial discontinuation for those who have not had their Week 26 visit due to administrative reasons) is included in the model as an offset. All fixed-effect regression parameters have improper flat priors over the real line. The normally distributed random effect has a half student-t prior with three degrees of freedom and a scale parameter of 2.5. The model is fitted with the R package `brms` (Bürkner, 2018).

The missing values for the patients in the control arm are imputed under a missing at random assumption using the above imputation model. Through the patient-specific random effect, the imputed number of exacerbations is correlated with the observed number of exacerbations for a specific patient.

For patients in the Drug X arm who discontinue their treatment, the missing exacerbations are imputed using a jump-to-reference approach. This imputation is performed by changing the arm assignment from "Drug X" to "Control" when predicting the missing data using the above imputation model. Through the patient-specific random effect, the imputed and observed data for a single patient are correlated.

For patients in the Drug X arm who have missing data but did not discontinue their treatment, the missing exacerbations are imputed under a missing at random assumption using the above imputation model, that is, the same assumption as for missing data in the control arm. Through multiple imputation, we create 1000 complete data sets. Each data set is analyzed through a negative binomial regression model with the randomized treatment as the only covariate. The results are pooled using Rubin's rule.

The analysis approach yields a between-arm ratio of the expected number of total exacerbations at Week 26 of 0.766 (95%-CI: [0.575, 1.02]).

17.4.2 Hypothetical Strategy

If we use a hypothetical strategy to address treatment discontinuation, the corresponding estimand definition is as follows:

(a) Population: Symptomatic patients with a diagnosis of asthma.
(b) Variable: Number of asthma exacerbations up to Week 26.
(c) Treatment: Drug X and control, taken as indicated without the option to discontinue.
(d) Intercurrent event: Treatment discontinuation.
(e) Population-Level Summary: Expected total number of asthma exacerbations between baseline and Week 26; the between-arm comparison is performed based on the ratio of the expected number of events between arms.

To the best of our knowledge, the estimation of hypothetical estimands under the recurrent events setting has not been studied in the literature. Therefore, in this example, we present three ad hoc approaches. The first approach is fitting a standard negative binomial regression model with the randomized treatment as the only covariate to the observed data. This approach assumes that both missing data after treatment discontinuation and missing data due to administrative censoring are missing at random conditional on the randomized treatment. This is a strong assumption that is unlikely to be true, as treatment discontinuation generally depends on patient characteristics. The second approach is based on multiple imputation using the same imputation model as introduced for the estimation of a treatment policy estimand in Sect. 17.4.1. However, instead of using a jump-to-reference approach in the Drug X arm, the same missing at random assumption as in the control arm is employed. Lastly, a simple inverse probability weighting (IPW) analysis is conducted. The weight is the product of the censoring weight and treatment weight. The censoring weight is based on a logistic regression for the binary outcome of whether patients have missing data due to administrative censoring. The treatment weight is based on a logistic regression for the binary outcome of whether patients have discontinued their randomized treatment. In both logistic regressions, the effects are the randomized treatment, four baseline covariates, and the interaction between the randomized treatment and any of the baseline covariates. All effects are fixed effects. The final analysis is a weighted negative binomial regression run on all patients who neither discontinue their randomized treatment nor experience administrative censoring. An IPW analysis yields an asymptotically unbiased estimate if the model for the administrative censoring and the discontinuation of the randomized treatment are correctly specified, that is, all confounders are adjusted for. This is implemented using the glm.nb() function in the R package `MASS`. Robust standard errors, obtained from the sandwich() function in the R package `sandwich`, are used to calculate the confidence intervals. Table 17.3 shows the results from the three different analysis approaches.

Table 17.3 Results of the three estimation methods for the hypothetical estimand

Estimation approach	Ratio (95% CI)
Negative binomial model	0.740 [0.562, 0.973]
Negative binomial model after multiple imputation under MAR	0.749 [0.565, 0.992]
IPW	0.780 [0.577, 1.050]

The difference between the estimation approaches is the following. The negative binomial model implicitly predicts the hypothetical trajectories and the missing data that is due to administrative censoring using the missing at random assumption conditional on the randomized treatment. The analysis based on multiple imputation explicitly predicts the hypothetical trajectories and the missing data under the missing at random assumption conditional on the randomized treatment and the four baseline covariates. On the other hand, the IPW analysis creates a pseudo population in which the occurrence of treatment discontinuation and missing data due to administrative censoring, respectively, does not occur and is independent of the randomized treatment and the four baseline covariates. This is achieved by modeling the treatment discontinuation and missing data due to administrative censoring processes, respectively.

17.5 Death as an Intercurrent Event

So far, our focus has been on a setting with a nonterminal intercurrent event, that is, a setting where trial patients can still experience the recurrent event of interest after the occurrence of the intercurrent event. However, not all intercurrent events are nonterminal. Terminal intercurrent events prevent the occurrence of future (recurrent) events. The main example of a terminal intercurrent event is death. Clinical trials in chronic heart failure are one example where death plays an important role. The considerations about the relevant clinical question of interest are particularly challenging in settings with death as the intercurrent event, as treatment benefit has multidimensional aspects: for example, a low number of recurrent events does not necessarily indicate that a treatment is beneficial for patients if the low number of recurrent events is due to an early death. In particular, not all intercurrent event strategies outlined in ICH (2019) are applicable; that is, a treatment policy strategy for the intercurrent event of death does not make sense since death cannot be part of a treatment strategy. In the context of clinical trials in chronic heart failure, defining a relevant clinical question of interest has been discussed as part of an EMA qualification procedure (EMA, 2023), which resulted in a Qualification Opinion (EMA, 2020). The Qualification Opinion does not recommend any specific estimand but states that "the main therapeutic goals in the treatment of chronic heart failure are to reduce cardiovascular mortality and to prevent deterioration of the clinical status and heart failure events; these goals should represent the primary aim of new agents developed for the treatment of chronic heart failure." After the Qualification Opinion was issued, the applicant published three manuscripts (Schmidli et al., 2023; Wei et al., 2023; Fritsch et al., 2023). Schmidli et al. (2023) defined causal estimands for recurrent event endpoints in the presence of death and also outlined which estimands are implied by common statistical analysis methods, including, but not limited to, the LWYY model (Lin et al. 2000), the PWP model (Prentice et al., 1981), and the WLW model (Wei et al., 1989). Janvin et al. (2023a, 2023b) and Hung and Wang (2023) wrote letters to the editor providing their perspectives. Janvin et al. (2023a, 2023b) argue for the importance of subject matter expertise when choosing the estimand and discuss the role of identifying assumptions when selecting a method for estimating a causal estimand. Hung and Wang (2023) highlight that challenges of defining a treatment effect in the presence of death also arise in the time-to-event setting. In the applicant's second manuscript, Fritsch et al. (2023) compare the efficacy of analysis methods for recurrent event endpoints and time-to-event endpoints in the presence of death, respectively. Finally, Wei et al. (2023) define a while alive estimand and a composite while alive estimand and compare their properties. Since then, the topic of estimands for recurrent events in the presence of death has received additional attention, with Mao (2023) proposing nonparametric inference for the while alive estimand and Janvin et al. (2023a, 2023b) providing an in-depth discussion of causal estimands and their identifiability assumptions.

17.6 Concluding Remarks

In this chapter, we discussed estimands for two-arm clinical trials with a recurrent event endpoint. In Sect. 17.3, based on the five strategies for addressing intercurrent events described in ICH (2019), we discussed different clinical questions and the corresponding estimands that might be of interest in the setting with a nonterminal intercurrent event. In Sect. 17.4, we illustrate methods for estimating an estimand that addresses treatment discontinuation with a treatment policy and a hypothetical strategy, respectively. In Sect. 17.5, we reviewed the existing literature for estimands with a recurrent event endpoint and death as the intercurrent event.

Compared to continuous and binary data, the endpoint-specific literature on estimands and estimand-aligned estimation specifically for recurrent event data is limited. Future research in this area should focus on better understanding how estimand-aligned estimation approaches and ideas that are commonly employed for other endpoints can be used for recurrent event data. In particular, more practical experience is needed, and we encourage publication of case studies that discuss clinical trials with recurrent data in light of the estimand framework.

We also encourage the community to develop and maintain software for the estimand-aligned estimation methods. While some software tools exist, for example, the R package `dejaVu` (Burkoff et al., 2021), there is a general lack of well-established, documented, and easily accessible software tools for the analysis of recurrent events.

References

Akacha, M., & Ogundimu, E. O. (2016). Sensitivity analyses for partially observed recurrent event data. *Pharmaceutical Statistics, 15*(1), 4–14.

Andersen, P. K., & Gill, R. D. (1982). Cox's regression model for counting processes: A large sample study. *The Annals of Statistics, 10*, 1100–1120.

Anker, S. D., & McMurray, J. J. (2012). Time to move on from 'time-to-first': Should all events be included in the analysis of clinical trials? *European Heart Journal, 33*(22), 2764–2765.

Bartlett, J. W. (2023). Reference-based multiple imputation—What is the right variance and how to estimate it. *Statistics in Biopharmaceutical Research, 15*(1), 178–186.

Brightling, C. E., Gaga, M., Inoue, H., Li, J., Maspero, J., Wenzel, S., & Bleecker, E. R. (2021). Effectiveness of fevipiprant in reducing exacerbations in patients with severe asthma (LUSTER-1 and LUSTER-2): Two phase 3 randomised controlled trials. *The Lancet Respiratory Medicine, 9*(1), 43–56.

Brunner, E., Vandemeulebroecke, M., & Mütze, T. (2021). Win odds: An adaptation of the win ratio to include ties. *Statistics in Medicine, 40*(14), 3367–3384.

Bürkner, P. C. (2018). Advanced Bayesian multilevel modeling with the R package brms. *R Journal, 10*(1), 395.

Burkoff, B., Metcalfe, P., Bartlett, J., Ruau, D. (2021). *R package dejaVu v0.3.0: Multiple Imputation for Recurrent Events*. Retrieved January 26, 2024, from https://CRAN.R-project.org/package=dejaVu

Carpenter, J. R., Roger, J. H., & Kenward, M. G. (2013). Analysis of longitudinal trials with protocol deviation: A framework for relevant, accessible assumptions, and inference via multiple imputation. *Journal of Biopharmaceutical Statistics, 23*(6), 1352–1371.

Carson, P., Teerlink, J. R., Komajda, M., et al. (2023). Comparison of investigator-reported and centrally adjudicated heart failure outcomes in the EMPEROR-reduced trial. *Heart Failure, 11*(4), 407–417.

Cook, R. J., & Lawless, J. F. (2007). *The statistical analysis of recurrent events*. Springer.

Diao, G., Liu, G. F., Zeng, D., Zhang, Y., Golm, G., Heyse, J. F., & Ibrahim, J. G. (2022). Efficient multiple imputation for sensitivity analysis of recurrent events data with informative censoring. *Statistics in Biopharmaceutical Research, 14*(2), 153–161.

European Medicine Agency. (2020). *Qualification opinion of clinically interpretable treatment effect measures based on recurrent event endpoints that allow for efficient statistical analyses*. Retrieved September 26, 2023, from https://www.ema.europa.eu/en/documents/other/qualification-opinion-clinically-interpretable-treatment-effect-measures-based-recurrent-event_en.pdf

European Medicine Agency. (2023). *Qualification of novel methodologies for medicine development*. Retrieved September 26, 2023, from https://www.ema.europa.eu/en/human-regulatory/research-development/scientific-advice-protocol-assistance/qualification-novel-methodologies-medicine-development-0

Fritsch, A., Schlömer, P., Mendolia, F., Mütze, T., Jahn-Eimermacher, A., & Recurrent Event Qualification Opinion Consortium. (2023). Efficiency comparison of analysis methods for recurrent event and time-to-first event endpoints in the presence of terminal events—Application to clinical trials in chronic Heart failure. *Statistics in Biopharmaceutical Research, 15*(2), 268–279.

Gao, F., Liu, G. F., Zeng, D., Xu, L., Lin, B., Diao, G., & Ibrahim, J. G. (2017). Control-based imputation for sensitivity analyses in informative censoring for recurrent event data. *Pharmaceutical Statistics, 16*(6), 424–432.

Gregson, J., Stone, G. W., Bhatt, D. L., Packer, M., Anker, S. D., Zeller, C., Redors, B., & Pocock, S. J. (2023). Recurrent events in cardiovascular trials: JACC state-of-the-art review. *Journal of the American College of Cardiology, 82*(14), 1445–1463.

Hauser, S. L., Bar-Or, A., Cohen, J. A., Comi, G., Correale, J., Coyle, P. K., & Kappos, L. (2020). Ofatumumab versus teriflunomide in multiple sclerosis. *New England Journal of Medicine, 383*(6), 546–557.

Huang, C. Y., & Wang, M. C. (2004). Joint modeling and estimation for recurrent event processes and failure time data. *Journal of the American Statistical Association, 99*(468), 1153–1165.

Hung, J. H. M., & Wang, S. J. (2023). Comment on "Estimands for recurrent event endpoints in the presence of a terminal event". *Statistics in Biopharmaceutical Research, 15*(2), 249–250.

International Council for Harmonisation of Technical Requirements for Pharmaceuticals for Human Use (ICH). (2019). *Addendum on estimands and sensitivity analysis in clinical trials to the guideline on statistical principles for clinical trials.* Retrieved September 26, 2023, from https://database.ich.org/sites/default/files/E9-R1_Step4_Guideline_2019_1203.pdf

International Council for Harmonisation of Technical Requirements for Pharmaceuticals for Human Use (ICH). (2021). ICH E9(R1) Estimands and Sensitivity Analysis in Clinical Trials Training Material. Retrieved January 28, 2024, from https://database.ich.org/sites/default/files/E9%28R1%29%20Training%20Material%20-%20PDF_0.pdf

Janvin, M., Young, J. G., & Stensrud, M. J. (2023a). We need subject matter expertise to choose and identify causal Estimands: Comment on "Estimands for recurrent event endpoints in the presence of a terminal event". *Statistics in Biopharmaceutical Research, 15*(2), 251–254.

Janvin, M., Young, J. G., Ryalen, P. C., & Stensrud, M. J. (2023b). Causal inference with recurrent and competing events. *Lifetime Data Analysis*, 1–60.

Keene, O. N., Jones, M. R., Lane, P. W., & Anderson, J. (2007). Analysis of exacerbation rates in asthma and chronic obstructive pulmonary disease: Example from the TRISTAN study. *Pharmaceutical Statistics, 6*(2), 89–97.

Keene, O. N., Calverley, P. M. A., Jones, P. W., Vestbo, J., & Anderson, J. A. (2008). Statistical analysis of exacerbation rates in COPD: TRISTAN and ISOLDE revisited. *European Respiratory Journal, 32*(1), 17–24.

Keene, O. N., Roger, J. H., Hartley, B. F., & Kenward, M. G. (2014). Missing data sensitivity analysis for recurrent event data using controlled imputation. *Pharmaceutical Statistics, 13*(4), 258–264.

Lasch, F., & Guizzaro, L. (2022). Estimators for handling COVID-19-related intercurrent events with a hypothetical strategy. *Pharmaceutical Statistics, 21*(6), 1258–1280.

Lawless, J. F. (1987a). Negative binomial and mixed Poisson regression. *The Canadian Journal of Statistics, 15*, 209–225.

Lawless, J. F. (1987b). Regression methods for Poisson process data. *Journal of the American Statistical Association, 82*(399), 808–815.

Lawless, J. F., & Cook, R. J. (2019). A new perspective on loss to follow-up in failure time and life history studies. *Statistics in Medicine, 38*(23), 4583–4610.

Lin, D. Y., Wei, L. J., Yang, I., & Ying, Z. (2000). Semiparametric regression for the mean and rate functions of recurrent events. *Journal of the Royal Statistical Society: Series B (Statistical Methodology), 62*(4), 711–730.

Lyu, T., Bornkamp, B., Mueller-Velten, G., & Schmidli, H. (2023). Bayesian inference for a principal stratum estimand on recurrent events truncated by death. *Biometrics, 79*(4), 3792–3802.

Mao, L. (2023). Nonparametric inference of general while-alive estimands for recurrent events. *Biometrics, 79*, 1749–1760.

National Heart, Lung, and Blood Institute. (2007). *Expert Panel Report 3: Guidelines for the Diagnosis and Management of Asthma.* Retrieved January 26, 2024, from https://www.ncbi.nlm.nih.gov/books/NBK7232/

Olarte Parra, C., Daniel, R. M., & Bartlett, J. W. (2023). Hypothetical estimands in clinical trials: A unification of causal inference and missing data methods. *Statistics in Biopharmaceutical Research, 15*(2), 421–432.

Pocock, S. J., Ariti, C. A., Collier, T. J., & Wang, D. (2012). The win ratio: A new approach to the analysis of composite endpoints in clinical trials based on clinical priorities. *European Heart Journal, 33*(2), 176–182.

Prentice, R. L., Williams, B. J., & Peterson, A. V. (1981). On the regression analysis of multivariate failure time data. *Biometrika, 68*(2), 373–379.

Rodés-Cabau, J., Horlick, E., Ibrahim, R., Cheema, A. N., Labinaz, M., Nadeem, N., & Houde, C. (2015). Effect of clopidogrel and aspirin vs aspirin alone on migraine headaches after transcatheter atrial septal defect closure: The CANOA randomized clinical trial. *JAMA, 314*(20), 2147–2154.

Roger, J. H., Bratton, D. J., Mayer, B., Abellan, J. J., & Keene, O. N. (2019). Treatment policy estimands for recurrent event data using data collected after cessation of randomised treatment. *Pharmaceutical Statistics, 18*(1), 85–95.

Rubin, D. B. (1987). *Multiple imputation for nonresponse in surveys*. John Wiley.

Schlesinger, N., Mysler, E., Lin, H. Y., De Meulemeester, M., Rovensky, J., Arulmani, U., & So, A. (2011). Canakinumab reduces the risk of acute gouty arthritis flares during initiation of allopurinol treatment: Results of a double-blind, randomised study. *Annals of the Rheumatic Diseases, 70*(7), 1264–1271.

Schmidli, H., Roger, J. H., & Akacha, M. (2023). Estimands for recurrent event endpoints in the presence of a terminal event. *Statistics in Biopharmaceutical Research, 15*(2), 238–248.

Seaman, S. R., & White, I. R. (2013). Review of inverse probability weighting for dealing with missing data. *Statistical Methods in Medical Research, 22*(3), 278–295.

Solomon, S. D., McMurray, J. J., Anand, I. S., Ge, J., Lam, C. S., Maggioni, A. P., & Lefkowitz, M. P. (2019). Angiotensin–neprilysin inhibition in heart failure with preserved ejection fraction. *New England Journal of Medicine, 381*(17), 1609–1620.

U.S. Food & Drug Administration. (2022). *Multiple endpoints in clinical trials guidance for industry*. Retrieved September 26, 2023 from https://www.fda.gov/regulatory-information/search-fda-guidance-documents/multiple-endpoints-clinical-trials-guidance-industry

Wei, L. J., Lin, D. Y., & Weissfeld, L. (1989). Regression analysis of multivariate incomplete failure time data by modeling marginal distributions. *Journal of the American Statistical Association, 84*(408), 1065–1073.

Wei, J., Mütze, T., Jahn-Eimermacher, A., & Roger, J. (2023). Properties of two while-alive estimands for recurrent events and their potential estimators. *Statistics in Biopharmaceutical Research, 15*(2), 257–267.

Chapter 18
Statistical Analysis Under the Estimand Framework: Time-to-Event Endpoints

Xin Zhang, Wentian Guo, Chen Lu, Dong Xi, Longshen Xie, and Jianfei Zheng

Abstract Time-to-event endpoints are prevalently used for efficacy analyses in clinical trials of oncology and many other diseases. This chapter reviews commonly used statistical methods of time-to-event endpoints for oncology clinical trials under the estimand framework. We focus on the considerations for properly aligning the statistical analysis to each intercurrent event strategy. We explore the complex role of censoring within the estimand framework, given its significant influence on the interpretation of treatment effects. Other aspects of the estimand, including variables, population-level summaries, and sensitivity analyses, are also discussed. A case study of a hematology clinical trial is provided at the end to illustrate the considerations to align statistical analyses to corresponding estimands.

X. Zhang (✉)
Data Sciences and Analytics, Pfizer Inc., Shanghai, China
e-mail: xin.zhang6@pfizer.com

W. Guo
Biometrics, R&D, AstraZeneca, Shanghai, China
e-mail: wentian.guo@astrazeneca.com

C. Lu
Global Biostatistical Science, Amgen, Thousand Oaks, CA, USA
e-mail: chelu@amgen.com

D. Xi
Biostatistics, Gilead Sciences Inc., Foster City, CA, USA
e-mail: dong.xi1@gilead.com

L. Xie
Department of Biometrics and Data Management, Shenyang Sunshine Pharmaceutical Co. Ltd., Shanghai, China
e-mail: xielongshen@3sbio.com

J. Zheng
Biometrics and Data Science, Fosun Pharma, Beijing, China
e-mail: zhengjianfei@fosunpharma.com

J. Wei et al. (eds.), *Estimands in Clinical Trials*, Springer Series in Pharmaceutical Statistics, https://doi.org/10.1007/978-3-032-02192-2_18

18.1 Introduction to Time-to-Event Endpoints

Time-to-event endpoints measure the time elapsed before the occurrence of clinical events of interest, such as death, appearance of a tumor, development/recurrence of a disease, and so forth. Such endpoints are used for various indications, such as oncology, Alzheimer's and Parkinson's disease, multiple sclerosis, or cardiovascular diseases. They are used not only for efficacy but also for safety and quality-of-life analyses. In time-to-event trials, some patients cannot feasibly be followed until the occurrence of clinical events of interest. This may be due to the trial reaching its planned end date or the occurrence of other events after randomization that prohibit observations for events of interest. The latter ones are intercurrent events in the estimand framework. In time-to-event analyses before the estimand framework was implemented, those participants would just be censored.

Censoring plays a crucial role in the statistical analysis of time-to-event endpoints. Various statistical methods have been developed for censored data, including:

- The Kaplan-Meier Method: to estimate survival functions for each arm.
- The Log Rank Test: to compare survival functions between arms.
- The Cox Proportional Hazards (PH) Model: to estimate the hazard ratio, which is commonly used to measure treatment effects.

In the past, intercurrent events were frequently addressed by rules defined in censoring tables. The statistical analyses may simply assume that all the censorings are non-informative, without regard to whether patients might have ended assessments because of intercurrent events. Although addressing intercurrent events via censoring is part of the estimation procedure, the clinical relevance of the implicit estimand is not clear. In addition, the non-informative censoring assumption made at an intercurrent event may not align with the estimand of interest.

There are several alternative ways to address intercurrent events under the estimand framework. When they are clinically relevant to events of interest, we could consider combining both as a composite endpoint if the combination has clinical interpretation. On the other hand, when those events are competing with events of interest, competing risk analysis should be considered. The estimand framework requires identifying relevant intercurrent events at the design stage and selecting appropriate estimand strategies. This will help precisely define the objective of a time-to-event trial and choose an appropriate statistical analysis method.

Statistical analysis of time-to-event endpoints is typically of high interest and referenced in health authority guidelines. In this chapter, we will focus on the estimand considerations for oncology clinical trials, where time-to-event endpoints are frequently considered. These considerations may not be directly applicable to other areas mentioned earlier, but they can serve as an illustration of how to apply the estimand framework to time-to-event trials.

The remainder of this chapter is structured as follows. In Sect. 18.2, we discuss different strategies for addressing intercurrent events under the estimand framework and the aligned analysis methods. In Sect. 18.3, we discuss commonly used time-to-event endpoints, as they are sometimes not consistently defined for certain trials. In Sect. 18.4, we discuss key considerations of population-level summary and the role of censoring. In Sect. 18.5, we illustrate sensitivity analysis and supplementary analysis. In Sect. 18.6, we present a real case study of a hematology clinical trial; for more examples in the oncology area with time-to-event endpoints, please refer to Chap. 7. We conclude with a discussion in Sect. 18.7.

18.2 Addressing Intercurrent Events and Missing Data

A key consideration for the estimand of a time-to-event trial is to assess whether one specific (a class of) clinical event(s) occurring after randomization is an intercurrent event or just an event leading to missing data. Both can be addressed using censoring in statistical analyses in the past.

For intercurrent events, depending on the trial objective, they can be either ignored, considered as part of a composite endpoint, or treated as competing risks, etc. Take the oncology area as an example; common intercurrent events are:

- Death
- Discontinuation of treatment
- Initiation of subsequent anticancer therapy

A common practice is to censor participants who undergo subsequent anticancer therapy for progression-free survival (PFS) analyses. The assumption implied by the censoring has an impact on the clinical question of interest. With non-informative censoring, it assumes that the risk of disease progression after starting subsequent anticancer therapy would remain the same as if a subsequent therapy had not been initiated. Thus, for participants who start a subsequent therapy, their PFS are modeled based on patients who did not start such therapy. This assumption is obviously inappropriate for the treatment policy strategy. See Sect. 18.2.1 for more discussion. Therefore, it is necessary to determine whether censoring due to intercurrent events is informative or not and apply appropriate statistical methods (Jackson et al., 2014; Zhao et al., 2014; Lu et al., 2015; Lipkovich et al., 2016; Atkinson et al., 2019).

For certain intercurrent events, there are commonly used censoring rules defined by regulatory guidelines (EMA, 2013; US FDA, 2015, 2018). In practice, they are also defined in the statistical analysis section of the study protocol and the statistical analysis plan. However, these censoring rules existed before the estimand framework and thus may not be compatible. The estimand framework requires the assessment of all potential intercurrent events at the beginning of trial design, defining appropriate strategies to address them, and discussing whether censoring is needed. If not prespecified, this may change the prespecified estimands and bias final estimates. We recommend collecting all relevant data of intercurrent events, including their causes and the investigator's assessment of their relationship to treatment.

There are also events that just lead to missing data. For example, censoring at the termination of a trial usually leads to missing data, which is non-informative. This type of missing data is commonly assumed to be missing at random. In general, we recommend recording events leading to missing data, such as terminating the trial or loss to follow-up, and only loss to follow-up for reasons unrelated to treatment can be considered as administrative censoring. For events with a potential relationship to treatment, we recommend treating them as intercurrent events and addressing them with appropriate strategies.

In summary, determining whether it is an intercurrent event or an event leading to missing data and choosing which strategy to address intercurrent events requires a thorough discussion of a trial objective and corresponding estimand. The following sections provide a detailed discussion on considerations for statistical analysis under treatment policy, hypothetical, composite, and while on treatment strategies. Statistical analysis of the principal stratum strategy is discussed in Chap. 19.

18.2.1 Treatment Policy Strategy

The treatment policy strategy ignores intercurrent events and evaluates the effect of a complete sequence of treatments beginning with randomization. When using this strategy, it is necessary to consistently follow participants even after the occurrence of intercurrent events.

Sometimes, it is challenging to follow up after the occurrence of intercurrent events in actual trials for a treatment policy strategy. For example, participants may wish to withdraw from a trial following treatment discontinuation. If these participants had stayed in a trial after treatment discontinuation, their benefit from the treatment would be different from those who received treatment throughout the trial. It is an inevitable violation of non-informative censoring (except under the null hypothesis of no treatment effect). If the proportion of such dropouts is non-negligible, missing data after dropout can be imputed, with appropriate assumptions about the behavior of patients post-censoring, using the data of the selected control group (Lu et al., 2015; Atkinson et al., 2019). If their proportion is small, we may still assume the resulting censoring is non-informative, as the impact of the assumption violation on the analysis is small. Of course, sensitivity analyses would be important to evaluate the robustness of inference when the assumption is violated.

18.2.2 Hypothetical Strategy

The hypothetical strategy considers a counterfactual scenario in which intercurrent events would not occur. For certain intercurrent events, they only exist under trial conditions. We should consider addressing them using a hypothetical strategy, as they have no clinical meaning in real-world clinical practice. One example of such intercurrent events is subsequent anticancer treatment using unapproved therapeutic drugs. On the other hand, some intercurrent events are inevitable in real-world clinical practice. Thus, it is inappropriate to apply a hypothetical strategy to assume they would not occur. One example is also for a new anticancer treatment, which is a part of standard treatment.

The censoring table for traditional time-to-event analyses in clinical trials implicitly assumes a simple hypothetical strategy. Participants are usually censored at the occurrence of intercurrent events and assume non-informative censoring. That is, the risk of events of interest for those with intercurrent events is the same as other participants after the occurrence. Under this hypothetical scenario, sensitivity analysis should be performed for the non-informative censoring assumption (Lipkovich et al., 2016).

Multiple imputation methods can be applied for statistical analyses with a hypothetical estimand when censoring is informative, although in both the literature and practice, they are often used for sensitivity analyses. Alternatively, we may consider more sophisticated causal inference methods, such as inverse probability of censoring weighting (IPCW) and rank-preserving structural failure time (RPSFT) (Watkins et al., 2013) to analyze such hypothetical estimands. These methods require strong assumptions, and they are often unverifiable. Therefore, sensitivity analyses are commonly performed. More detailed discussion of causal inference methods is in Chap. 5.

18.2.3 Composite Strategy

The composite strategy makes events of interest as composite events, including original events and intercurrent ones. For example, PFS is a composite event, including both disease progression and death. Composite strategies may be appropriate in many contexts, such as second-line treatment initiation and treatment failure. This strategy is particularly useful when intercurrent events and events of interest are positively correlated. Using a composite strategy can avoid making assumptions about data after the occurrence of intercurrent events. However, if the prevalence of intercurrent events is much higher than events of interest, the interpretation of treatment effects based on those composite events may be challenging.

18.2.4 While on Treatment Strategy

With a while on treatment strategy, the treatment effect up to the time of occurrence of intercurrent events is of interest. Anything after an intercurrent event is considered irrelevant to the clinical question of interest. The ICH E9 (R1) states, "Terminology for this strategy will depend on the intercurrent event of interest, e.g., 'while alive,' when considering death as an intercurrent event." Other examples of such intercurrent events are surgery and progression.

The implementation of a while on treatment strategy for a time-to-event trial needs to assess whether we could assume that the intercurrent event is independent of the underlying treatment effect. This also determines which statistical method (e.g., the cause-specific or sub-distribution hazard) is appropriate. See Sect. 18.4.2 for more details on these two methods. When the independent assumption is appropriate, we can consider using a cause-specific hazard model. One example is death not related to the study disease, for which we can directly apply classical survival analysis methods to censor participants at competing events. When this independence assumption is implausible, we should use sub-distribution hazard methods. Generally, the cumulative incidence function and the sub-distribution hazard model should be applied. Those methods lead to population-level summary measures different from those of traditional methods (See Sect. 18.4.2).

18.3 Variables

Regulatory agencies and academic guidelines have provided specific definitions and censoring tables for a few widely used time-to-event endpoints, such as PFS and overall survival (OS) (Eisenhauer et al., 2009; EMA, 2013; US FDA, 2015; Gourgou-Bourgade et al., 2015; Seymour et al., 2017; US FDA, 2018). Although these guidelines do not apply the estimand concept, they explicitly provide approaches to address intercurrent events through the definitions of events of interest and the censoring tables. See FDA guidance on clinical trial endpoints for the approval of non-small cell lung cancer drugs and biologics as an example (US FDA, 2015).

However, the definitions of many time-to-event endpoints are not consistent for certain trials. For example, regarding the definition of disease-free survival (DFS) for colorectal cancer, whether it includes secondary primary cancer for events of interest is not consistent across trials (Birgisson et al., 2011). Such inconsistency would implicitly lead to different estimands.

Inconsistencies in the definitions of time-to-event variables can unintentionally lead to disparate estimations of the treatment effect, a situation that should be avoided. The application of the estimand framework can facilitate more aligned and accurate definitions.

18.4 Population-Level Summary

The commonly used population-level summary for time-to-event endpoints is the hazard ratio. It is usually estimated using the Cox PH model. In addition, survival probabilities at specific timepoints, survival time quantiles (such as median), and survival curves are estimated using the Kaplan-Meier method to provide a full picture of the treatment effects of each treatment group. Another population-level summary is the restricted mean survival time (RMST); it can estimate the mean survival time restricted up to a specific timepoint. The RMST difference/ratio is widely used to measure treatment effects when the PH assumption is in question.

18.4.1 Proportional Hazard Assumption

The PH assumption requires that the ratio of hazard functions between groups remains roughly constant over time. When this assumption holds, the hazard ratio is a causal treatment effect. This is because for a hazard ratio not changing with time (denoted by λ), it is equivalent to a relative difference between two survival functions as $S_1(t) = S_0(t)^{\lambda}$. In addition, the log rank test is equivalent to the score test of the Cox PH model with the treatment term only. In this case, one could say the same method is used for both hypothesis testing and treatment effect estimation. Note that the log rank test is the uniformly most powerful test under the PH assumption (Kalbfleisch & Prentice, 2002).

There is an ongoing debate about the causal interpretation of the hazard ratio, despite its wide acceptance by regulators for quantifying a treatment effect. Some authors argue that even in randomized clinical trials, the hazard ratio at each time point has an inherent selection bias and is not a causal treatment effect (Hernan, 2010; Aalen et al., 2015; Rufibach, 2019). The selection bias arises because when T (survival time) > t ($t \neq 0$), Z (baseline variables) is not independent of X (treatment allocation). Randomized allocation can only make Z and X independent when $T = 0$. This means that as time changes, the at-risk populations for each treatment group are not comparable. This makes the hazard ratio difficult to interpret when the PH assumption does not hold.

In the case of nonproportional hazards (NPH), the weighted average hazard ratio estimated based on the Cox PH model can still be used as a population-level summary in practice. However, the weighted average hazard ratio is difficult to interpret from a clinical perspective. In addition, the estimated value depends on the distribution of censoring. Therefore, it is also impacted by the accrual and follow-up pattern (Aalen et al., 2015). Finally, when the PH assumption is explicitly violated, the power of the log rank test is reduced.

To move away from the PH assumption, we may consider those summary measures based on survival functions. For example, median survival times and survival probabilities at specific time points are commonly reported. However, they only reflect the treatment effect for a part of the survival functions. An alternative is the RMST method (Uno et al., 2014), which graphically corresponds to the area under a Kaplan-Meier curve over a specified time τ. It can be interpreted as the survival time on average when following up for τ. However, it does have the major limitation that the area under the curve is only calculated up to τ, and thus it depends on the choice of τ. To overcome this shortcoming, a data-driven truncation point is recommended by Huang and Kuan (2018) and Tian et al. (2020), similar to the way how a time window is defined for a hazard ratio and log rank test, and is shown to have desirable operating characteristics.

Overall, Kaplan-Meier curves offer a comprehensive display of treatment effect summaries. Trying to reduce these curves to a single population summary (e.g., hazard ratio, median survival times, and RMST) is challenging. Investigation and discussion are ongoing to find the appropriate summaries for PH and NPH scenarios (Pak et al., 2017; Freidin & Korn, 2019; Mukhopadhyay et al., 2022; Das et al., 2023).

18.4.2 Competing Risks

As discussed in Sect. 18.2.4, when competing events exist, we could consider using either cause-specific hazard or sub-distribution hazard methods. Two methods would lead to two sets of population-level summaries: (1) cause-specific hazard ratios and Kaplan-Meier curves; (2) sub-distribution hazard ratios and cumulative incidence functions (CIFs) (Putter et al., 2007). Cause-specific hazard is the instantaneous probability of events of interest conditional on being event-free (for both types of events). The Cox PH model is commonly used to estimate the cause-specific hazard ratio, with competing events being censored. The sub-distribution hazard is defined as the hazard of events occurring in a population, including those who had experienced any competing events. The Fine-Gray model is commonly used to estimate the sub-distribution hazard ratio, and subjects with competing events are not removed from the risk set, with their time-to-event treated as infinity.

The CIF is defined as the probability of an event occurring due to a specific cause before time t. The nonparametric Aalen-Johansen method is commonly used for estimation. It should be noted that CIF has a one-to-one correspondence with the sub-distribution hazard but not with the cause-specific hazard. Therefore, the sub-distribution hazard ratio better characterizes the differences in CIF between groups. However, it is not as intuitive as the cause-specific hazard ratio.

18.5 Sensitivity Analysis and Supplemental Analysis

For time-to-event endpoints, several additional analyses are routinely performed on key statistical assumptions. For example, additional analyses are usually performed on the PH assumption, using Schoenfeld residuals and/or log(-log(S(t))) vs log(t) plots. As such, analyses do not change the target estimand; they are sensitivity analyses under the estimand framework.

For time-to-event analyses, missing data are inevitable and commonly addressed by censoring. If missing data are unrelated to intercurrent events, such as missing visits, their censoring rules are purely part of the estimation procedure, and any changes to such rules also do not change the target estimand.

For the treatment policy strategy, it requires to systematically follow and collect data on participants after the occurrence of intercurrent events (Sect. 18.2.1). However, the missing data problem still exists; for example, when analyzing PFS data under the treatment policy, there are common intercurrent events that would lead to missing data, such as treatment discontinuation, clinical progression, or treatment modification due to unconfirmed radiological progression. We recommend summarizing the proportions of participants in the following situations after such intercurrent events to assess the appropriateness of the non-informative censoring assumption:

- Participants are still able to obtain final radiological progression.
- Participants are unable to obtain final radiological progression.
- Participants not undergoing any tumor assessment.

If observing a non-ignorable imbalance between two arms for those categories, the non-informative assumption may be questionable, and sensitivity analyses should be considered.

On some occasions, an analysis for the appropriateness of the non-informative assumption may implicitly under an estimand that differs from the one targeted by the primary analysis (Lipkovich et al., 2016); in such cases, it is considered as a supplementary analysis. Unlike a sensitivity analysis, a supplemental analysis is planned to target a supplemental estimand, which is different from the primary one by changing some attributes. It can provide additional interpretation of treatment effects. For example, supplemental analyses of certain components in composite endpoints.

18.6 Case Study

INO-VATE study (NCT01564784) (Kantarjian et al., 2016) is an open-label, two-arm, randomized, phase three trial to compare the safety and efficacy of inotuzumab ozogamicin (INO) versus standard intensive chemotherapy in adults with relapsed or refractory acute lymphoblastic leukemia (R/R ALL). Patients were randomly assigned in a 1:1 ratio to receive either inotuzumab ozogamicin or the investigator's choice of standard therapy; no crossover between arms was allowed. Stratification factors at randomization were the duration of the first remission (<12 months vs. ≥12 months), the salvage treatment line (first vs. second), and age (<55 years vs. ≥55 years). Patients who achieved complete remission could undergo stem-cell transplantation (SCT) at the investigator's discretion.

The protocol of the INO-VATE study was finalized before the release of ICH E9 (R1), and thus, it does not apply the estimand framework. For illustration purposes, we define the estimands for the primary and four supplementary analyses for overall survival (OS) in this section. The primary analysis is the traditional intent-to-treat analysis, which is similar to the analysis under a treatment policy strategy. The first supplementary analysis considers a different strategy to address subsequent therapies. The next supplementary analysis considers a summary measure not relying on the PH assumption. The last two analyses consider non-study-disease-related death, which is defined as death without prior progression or relapse of ALL, as an intercurrent event, but not an event of interest. The primary estimand is defined as follows:

(a) Population: R/R ALL Adults.
(b) Variable: OS, defined as from the time of randomization to the date of death due to any cause.
(c) Treatment: INO + subsequent therapy (standard therapy used in the control arm is not included) vs investigator's choice of standard therapy + subsequent therapy (INO is included).
(d) Intercurrent Event:

- Subsequent Therapy: treatmentpolicy, that is, the treatment effect of INO vs the investigator's choice of standard therapy, regardless of the initiation of subsequent therapy.
- Non-study-Disease-Related Death: composite, that is, it is included in the events of interest.

(e) Population-Level Summary: hazard ratio.

The event of interest is the all-cause death. The composite strategy was used for non-study-disease-related death. We use the treatment policy strategy for the subsequent therapy, including events that occurred after the initiation of subsequent therapies in the analysis. Those participants without events were censored at the last date of being known alive. The stratified Cox model was used to estimate the hazard ratio, and the Kaplan-Meier method was used to estimate the survival function for two arms.

Considering that the use of subsequent therapies would affect the survival outcome, it requires reducing the impact of those subsequent therapies that may confound the OS. Therefore, the following supplementary estimand is considered.

- Supplementary Estimand 1
  The first supplementary estimand applies a hypothetical strategy to address the subsequent therapy, and the other attributes remain the same as the primary estimand. To exclude events after the intercurrent events from the statistical analysis, participants are censored at the date of initiation of subsequent therapies. The stratified Cox model was used to estimate the hazard ratio, and the Kaplan-Meier method was used to estimate the survival function for two arms. This analysis implies that those censored participants are similar to those who do not, that is, the censoring is non-informative. To assess this assumption, a sensitivity analysis using multiple imputations could be considered.
- Supplementary Estimand 2
  In the primary analysis, the Kaplan-Meier curves of two arms crossed, indicating that the PH assumption may not hold. Thus, the hazard ratio may not be able to

capture the treatment effect. The second supplementary estimand uses the difference of RMST as the population-level summary.

- Supplementary Estimand 3 and 4
  In the INO arm, participants have higher complete remission rates, and thus more of them have received SCT. However, such transplantation might incur fatal adverse events, potentially leading to death. In addition, the INO treatment might increase the risk of sinusoidal obstruction syndrome (SOS), as shown in previous studies. This is a severe adverse event, which could lead to death. Therefore, the treatment effect of INO may be diluted by non-ignorable numbers of such deaths, which are not related to R/R ALL. In the following two estimands, we consider a while on treatment strategy for non-study-disease-related death.
- The supplementary estimand 3 uses the cause-specific hazard ratio as the population-level summary. It generally assumes that the non-study-disease-related death is uncorrelated with the death due to the study disease. The cause-specific hazard is the hazard in the risk set for all participants without any events (including competing risk). The stratified Cox model was used to estimate the cause-specific hazard ratio, and the Kaplan-Meier method was used to estimate the survival functions for death due to the disease under study for the two arms. In the analysis, patients with non-study-disease-related death are censored.
- The supplementary estimand 4 uses the sub-distribution hazard ratio as the population-level summary. The sub-distribution hazard is the hazard in the risk set for all participants without events of interest; thus, this risk set includes participants with competing risks. The stratified Fine-Gray model was used to estimate the sub-distribution hazard ratio, and the Aalen-Johansen method was used to estimate the CIF for two arms. The non-study-disease-related deaths are competing events in those analyses.

18.7 Concluding Remarks

In oncology clinical trials, time-to-event endpoints are frequently used for efficacy assessment, and corresponding statistical analyses usually involve censoring. In this chapter, we discuss the estimand considerations for statistical analyses of those time-to-event endpoints. We focus on strategies to address intercurrent events (and missing data) and other aspects of the estimand, including variables, population-level summaries, and sensitivity analyses. The estimand framework requires identifying relevant intercurrent events at the design stage and selecting appropriate estimand strategies. This will help precisely define the objective of a time-to-event trial and choose an appropriate statistical analysis method.

References

Aalen, O. O., Cook, R. J., & Røysland, K. (2015). Does Cox analysis of a randomized survival study yield a causal treatment effect? *Lifetime Data Analysis, 21*, 579–593.

Atkinson, A., Kenward, M. G., Clayton, T., & Carpenter, J. R. (2019). Reference-based sensitivity analysis for time-to-event data. *Pharmaceutical Statistics, 18*, 645–658.

Birgisson, H., Wallin, U., Holmberg, L., & Glimelius, B. (2011). Survival endpoints in colorectal cancer and the effect of second primary other cancer on disease free survival. *BMC Cancer, 11*, 438.

Das, A., Lin, T. A., Lin, C., Meirson, T., McCaw, Z. R., Tian, L., & Ludmir, E. B. (2023). Assessment of median and mean survival time in cancer clinical trials. *JAMA Network Open, 6*, e236498.

Eisenhauer, E. A., Therasse, P., Bogaerts, J., Schwartz, L. H., Sargent, D., Ford, R., Dancey, J., Arbuck, S., Gwyther, S., Mooney, M., Rubinstein, L., Shankar, L., Dodd, L., Kaplan, R., Lacombe, D., & Verweij, J. (2009). New response evaluation criteria in solid tumours: Revised RECIST guideline (version 1.1). *European Journal of Cancer, 45*, 228–247.

EMA (2013). Guideline on the evaluation of anticancer medicinal products in man. Methodological consideration for using progression-free survival (PFS) or disease-free survival (DFS) in confirmatory trials. Appendix 1.

Freidin, B., & Korn, E. L. (2019). Methods for accommodating nonproportional hazards in clinical trials: Ready for the primary analysis? *Journal of Clinical Oncology, 37*, 3455–3459.

Gourgou-Bourgade, S., Cameron, D., Poortmans, P., Asselain, B., Azria, D., Cardoso, F., A'Hern, R., Bliss, J., Bogaerts, J., Bonnefoi, H., Brain, E., Cardoso, M. J., Chibaudel, B., Coleman, R., Cufer, T., Dal Lago, L., Dalenc, F., De Azambuja, E., Debled, M., ... Dabakuyo-Yonli, T. S. (2015). Guidelines for time-to-event end point definitions in breast cancer trials: Results of the DATECAN initiative (definition for the assessment of time-to-event endpoints in cancer trials). *Annals of Oncology*, 26, 873–879.

Hernan, M. A. (2010). The hazards of hazard ratios. *Epidemiology, 21*, 13–15.

Huang, B., & Kuan, P. F. (2018). Comparison of the restricted mean survival time with the hazard ratio in superiority trials with a time-to-event end point. *Pharmaceutical Statistics, 17*(3), 202–213.

Jackson, D., White, I. R., Seaman, S., Evans, H., Baisley, K., & Carpenter, J. (2014). Relaxing the independent censoring assumption in the Cox proportional hazards model using multiple imputation. *Statistics in Medicine, 33*, 4681–4694.

Kalbfleisch, J. D., & Prentice, R. L. (2002). *The statistical analysis of failure time data*. John Wiley & Sons.

Kantarjian, H. M., DeAngelo, D. J., Stelljes, M., Martinelli, G., Liedtke, M., Stock, W., Gökbuget, N., O'Brien, S., Wang, K., Wang, T., Paccagnella, M. L., Sleight, B., Vandendries, E., & Advani, A. S. (2016). Inotuzumab Ozogamicin versus standard therapy for acute lymphoblastic leukemia. *The New England Journal of Medicine, 375*, 740–753.

Lipkovich, I., Ratitch, B., & O'Kelly, M. (2016). Sensitivity to censored-at-random assumption in the analysis of time-to-event endpoints. *Pharmaceutical Statistics, 15*, 216–229.

Lu, K., Li, D., & Koch, G. G. (2015). Comparison between two controlled multiple imputation methods for sensitivity analyses of time-to-event data with possibly informative censoring. *Statistics in Biopharmaceutical Research, 7*, 199–213.

Mukhopadhyay, P., Ye, J., Anderson, K. M., Roychoudhury, S., Rubin, E. H., Halabi, S., & Chappell, R. J. (2022). Log-rank test vs MaxCombo and difference in restricted mean survival time tests for comparing survival under nonproportional hazards in Immuno-oncology trials: A systematic review and meta-analysis. *JAMA Oncology, 8*, 1294–1300.

Pak, K., Uno, H., Kim, D. H., Tian, L., Kane, R. C., Takeuchi, M., Fu, H., Claggett, B., & Wei, L. J. (2017). Interpretability of cancer clinical trial results using restricted mean survival time as an alternative to hazard ratio. *JAMA Oncology, 3*, 1692–1696.

Putter, H., Fiocco, M., & Geskus, R. B. (2007). Tutorial in biostatistics: Competing risks and multi-state models. *Statistics in Medicine, 26*, 2389–2430.

Rufibach, K. (2019). Treatment effect quantification for time-to-event endpoints–Estimands, analysis strategies, and beyond. *Pharmaceutical Statistics, 18*, 145–165.

Seymour, L., Bogaerts, J., Perrone, A., Ford, R., Schwartz, L. H., Mandrekar, S., Lin, N. U., Litière, S., Dancey, J., Chen, A., Hodi, F. S., Therasse, P., Hoekstra, O. S., Shankar, L. K., Wolchok, J. D., Ballinger, M., Caramella, C., de Vries, E. G. E., and RECIST working group (2017). iRECIST: Guidelines for response criteria for use in trials testing immunotherapeutics. The Lancet. Oncology 18, e143–e152.

Tian, L., Jin, H., Uno, H., Lu, Y., Huang, B., Anderson, K. M., & Wei, L. J. (2020). On the empirical choice of the time window for restricted mean survival time. *Biometrics, 76*(4), 1157–1166.

Uno, H., Claggett, B., Tian, L., Inoue, E., Gallo, P., Miyata, T., Schrag, D., Takeuchi, M., Uyama, Y., Zhao, L., Skali, H., Solomon, S., Jacobus, S., Hughes, M., Packer, M., & Wei, L. J. (2014). Moving beyond the hazard ratio in quantifying the between-group difference in survival analysis. *Journal of Clinical Oncology, 32*, 2380–2385.

US FDA (2015). Clinical trial endpoints for the approval of non-small cell lung cancer drugs and biologics: Guidance for industry.

US FDA (2018). Clinical trial endpoints for the approval of cancer drugs and biologics: Guidance for industry.

Watkins, C., Huang, X., Latimer, N., Tang, Y., & Wright, E. J. (2013). Adjusting overall survival for treatment switches: Commonly used methods and practical application. *Pharmaceutical Statistics, 12*, 348–357.

Zhao, Y., Herring, A. H., Zhou, H., Ali, M. W., & Koch, G. G. (2014). A multiple imputation method for sensitivity analyses of time-to-event data with possibly informative censoring. *Journal of Biopharmaceutical Statistics, 24*, 229–253.

Chapter 19
Statistical Analysis Under the Estimand Framework: Principal Stratification

Zhiyue Huang, Longshen Xie, Wentian Guo, and Yongming Qu

Abstract Principal stratum strategy is used to address intercurrent events when the treatment effect is of interest on the subpopulation defined by a post-randomization variable, known as principal stratum. Statistical analysis for principal stratum estimand involves statistical modeling and a series of assumptions because it is impossible to directly summarize the treatment outcomes over a principal stratum. In this chapter, we will go through a few common assumptions for principal stratum strategy and the statistical analyses based on them. Sensitivity analyses are also briefly reviewed. We will also discuss the special consideration for principal stratum analysis when outcomes are time-to-event. Lastly, we listed some cases of principal stratum estimand in this book.

19.1 Introduction

The treatment effect could be of interest involving a study subpopulation defined by the occurrence of a relevant intercurrent event. For example, in a randomized placebo-controlled trial of a prophylactic human immunodeficiency virus (HIV)

Z. Huang (✉)
Quantitative Sciences and Evidence Generation, Astellas Pharma Inc., Shanghai, China
e-mail: zhiyue.huang@astellas.com

L. Xie
Department of Biometrics and Data Management, Shenyang Sunshine Pharmaceutical Co., Ltd., Shanghai, China
e-mail: xielongshen@3sbio.com

W. Guo
Biometrics, R&D, AstraZeneca, Shanghai, China
e-mail: wentian.guo@astrazeneca.com

Y. Qu
Department of Global Statistical Sciences, Eli Lilly and Company, Indianapolis, IN, USA
e-mail: qu_yongming@lilly.com

J. Wei et al. (eds.), *Estimands in Clinical Trials*, Springer Series in Pharmaceutical Statistics, https://doi.org/10.1007/978-3-032-02192-2_19

vaccine, low evidence of a lower average viral load set-point among infectees in the vaccine relative to the placebo arm may suggest clinical benefit by subsequently preventing or delaying the onset of acquired immunodeficiency syndrome (AIDS) and reducing the rate of secondary HIV transmission (Mehrotra et al., 2006).

HIV infection, which occurs after randomization, is a relevant intercurrent event because the comparison of viral load set points between arms involves a subpopulation of potential HIV infectees that cannot be identified before randomization. This necessitates the use of the principal stratum strategy to address the clinical question, as recommended by the ICH E9(R1) guideline (2019).

It is impossible to simultaneously observe the potential intercurrent event outcomes of a patient in one arm and his/her potential treatment outcomes in another, because the intercurrent events occur after randomization. Meanwhile, naively comparing summary statistics between arms of patients with (or without) the intercurrent event will likely lead to biased causal treatment effect analysis due to incomparable populations experiencing (or not experiencing) intercurrent events between arms. Therefore, implementing a principal stratum strategy requires more complex statistical methods and assumptions to predict the counterfactual treatment outcomes within principal strata.

The remainder of this section is structured as follows: In Sect. 19.2, we will introduce how to define the principal stratum using the occurrence of intercurrent events. In Sect. 19.3, we list some common assumptions to estimate the principal stratum effect. In Sect. 19.4, we briefly introduce some causal inference methods for analyzing principal stratum effects and related sensitivity analyses. Fundamental causal inference could be found in Chap. 5. Then, we discuss special considerations for the principal stratum strategy for time-to-event endpoints. Finally, we shortly summarize some cases in this book where the principal stratum strategy could be used.

19.2 Definition of the Principal Stratum

Like the potential outcomes described in Chap. 5, the potential intercurrent event variable of a patient can be defined as whether a patient will experience an intercurrent event or not. Denote by $S = 1$ occurrence and by $S = 0$ absence of a specific intercurrent event. Because the occurrence of the intercurrent event may be influenced by treatment, let $S(Z = 0)$ and $S(Z = 1)$, abbreviated as $S(0)$ and $S(1)$, be the potential intercurrent event variable under control and treatment arms, where $Z = 0$ is the assignment to the control arm and $Z = 1$ is the treatment arm.

Principal strata are population stratifications based on potential intercurrent event variables. If there are two treatment arms, we can stratify the population based on potential intercurrent event variables, as shown in Table 19.1. This is a different classification from subgroups because subgroups are classified based on baseline characteristics, which are before randomization.

Table 19.1 Principal stratum defined by the occurrence of a relevant intercurrent event

		Treatment arm	
		Occurrence of ICE $S(1) = 1$	Absence of ICE $S(1) = 0$
Control arm	Occurrence of ICE $S(0) = 1$	$S_1 = \{S(1) = 1\} \cap \{S(0) = 1\}$	$S_2 = \{S(1) = 0\} \cap \{S(0) = 1\}$
	Absence of ICE $S(0) = 0$	$S_3 = \{S(1) = 1\} \cap \{S(0) = 0\}$	$S_4 = \{S(1) = 0\} \cap \{S(0) = 0\}$

ICE intercurrent event

1. Patients in the S_1 stratum will experience the relevant intercurrent event regardless of whether they are in the treatment arm or the control arm.
2. Patients in the S_2 stratum will experience the relevant intercurrent events if in the control arm, but not if in the treatment arm.
3. Patients in the S_3 stratum will experience the relevant intercurrent events if in the treatment arm, but not if in the control arm.
4. Patients in the S_4 stratum will not experience the relevant intercurrent events regardless of whether they are in the experimental arm or the control arm.

Principal effects are causal effects within a principal stratum. We can construct corresponding principal strata according to the clinical questions of interest. For example, if we are interested in the treatment effect of the experimental drug in the subpopulation that can tolerate it and consider early treatment termination due to intolerance of the experimental drug as an intercurrent event, the corresponding principal stratum would be the union of S_2 and S_4.

19.3 Statistical Assumptions for the Principal Stratum Strategy

To estimate principal stratum effects, we need to know which principal stratum each participant belongs to. However, since the intercurrent events occur after randomization and patients cannot receive both control and treatment simultaneously, we cannot assign patients to a principal stratum directly. Therefore, to estimate the principal stratum effect, we need to make assumptions and use statistical models.

In this section, we list some common assumptions used in the principal stratum analysis, including the positivity assumption, the ignorable treatment assignment assumption, the stable unit treatment values assumption (SUTVA), the monotonicity assumption, the exclusion–restriction (ER) assumption, and the principal ignorability assumption. Not all listed assumptions are required to enable estimating principal stratum effects. The next section will discuss how these assumptions are combinedly used with the estimation methods.

19.3.1 Positivity Assumption

The positivity assumption means that the probability of a patient being in the principal stratum of interest is positive.

19.3.2 Ignorable Treatment Assignment Assumption

The ignorable treatment assignment assumption is commonly seen in causal inference. It means that, given confounding factors, the potential outcome variables and treatment assignments are conditionally independent. In a randomized trial, the ignorable treatment assumption is implicitly satisfied because of randomized treatment assignment.

19.3.3 Stable Unit Treatment Values Assumption

The SUTVA includes the following two points:

1. The potential variable of everyone does not change with the change of the intervention status of other patients. This may not always hold. For example, the probability of infection for participants receiving a placebo would ultimately be influenced by the probability of infection of those receiving the vaccine in a vaccine trial.
2. There is only one version of each intervention, i.e., the intervention of interest has been clearly defined. The second point of SUTVA implies the consistency assumption in causal inference, i.e., the observed outcome variable or the observed intercurrent event variable of everyone is consistent with his/her potential outcome variable or the potential intercurrent event variable.

Under the SUTVA for both potential outcome variable and potential intercurrent event variable, the observed outcome variable and the intercurrent event variable could be expressed as

$$Y = Y(1)Z + Y(0)(1-Z) \quad \text{and} \quad S = S(1)Z + S(0)(1-Z).$$

19.3.4 Monotonicity Assumption

Monotonicity means that if a patient experiences an intercurrent event in one arm, he/she will necessarily experience the intercurrent event in the other arm, i.e., $S(1) \geq S(0)$ or $S(0) \geq S(1)$. Monotonicity can be reasonably explained in many cases, but it is often difficult to be verified from data. For example, the principal stratum of interest is the patients who will not discontinue the drug due to poor tolerance regardless of treatment assignments, i.e., $S = 1$ if a patient discontinues the drug due to poor tolerance and $S = 0$ otherwise. Under the monotonicity assumption $S(1) \geq S(0)$, if patients are assigned to the treatment arm and do not experience this intercurrent event (i.e., treatment discontinuation due to poor tolerance), neither will they if they are assigned to the control arm. The monotonicity assumption allows estimating the proportions of certain principal strata. For example, in the previous case, due to the monotonicity assumption, patients assigned to the treatment arm and not experiencing the intercurrent event are all from the principal stratum of interest, so the proportion of the principal stratum of interest is equal to the probability of the absence of the intercurrent event in the treatment arm in a randomized controlled trial.

19.3.5 Exclusion–Restriction Assumption

The ER assumption implies that if patients have the same potential intercurrent event variables regardless of their treatment arms, then their potential outcome variables are also the same regardless of their treatment arms, i.e. $Y(0) = Y(1)$ if $S(0) = S(1)$. From a causal inference perspective, the ER assumption means that the treatment effect is realized solely through the occurrence or absence of the intercurrent event.

19.3.6 Principal Ignorability Assumption

Principal ignorability means that, given confounding factors, the potential outcome variable and the potential intercurrent event variable are conditionally independent. While we cannot simultaneously observe $S(z)$ and $Y(1 - z)$ because one patient could not be randomized into both arms, principal ignorability allows us to simplify the joint distribution of $S(z)$ and $Y(1 - z)$ through confounding factors and thus estimate the probability of principal stratum membership of each patient.

In summary, the use of the principal stratum strategy to address intercurrent events requires multiple assumptions. The positivity assumption, the SUTVA, and the ignorable treatment assignment assumption are required by most of the statistical methods to estimate principal stratum effects. With other additional assumptions, researchers can estimate principal stratum effects to provide more detailed insights into the relationships between treatments, intercurrent events, and variables. It is important to carefully consider these assumptions in the specific context of each study and understand their implications for the validity of causal estimates.

19.4 Analysis Methods and Sensitivity Analysis

In this section, we will briefly introduce some statistical methods to estimate the principal stratum effect. The assumptions needed to implement these methods have been introduced in the previous section. However, most of the discussed assumptions cannot be tested. Thus, sensitivity analysis for these assumptions is also essential for principal stratum analysis. A detailed review could be found in Lipkovich et al. (2022).

Traditional instrumental variable methods rely on the SUTVA, the ER assumption, the monotonicity assumption, and the positivity assumption (Angrist et al., 1996; Baiocchi et al., 2014). It is often interested in the principal stratum effect on the principal stratum S_3 and the calculation is based on expanding the average treatment effect on the overall population with the average treatment effect on each stratum by the conditional expectation formula. Under the ER assumption and the monotonicity assumption, the principal stratum effect on S_3 is identifiable.

The ER assumption implies no treatment effect in principal strata $S_1 = \{S(1) = 1\} \cap \{S(0) = 1\}$ and $S_4 = \{S(1) = 0\} \cap \{S(0) = 0\}$. This often makes the ER assumption unreasonable in a clinical trial. To relax the ER assumption, we can consider parametrically modeling the stratum-specific treatment effects. For example, a logit parameter was used with a Bayesian prior to model the stratum-specific probabilities of an outcome variable under different arms in Magnusson et al. (2019). Similarly, a sensitivity parameter, which is treated as fixed and known in a single analysis, in the stratum-specific probability modeling could relax the monotonicity assumption (Gilbert et al., 2003; Lu et al., 2013).

Without the ER assumption, one also could estimate principal stratum effects using a crude difference in an outcome variable between arms among those who experienced or did not experience a specific intercurrent event and then subtracting a sensitivity analysis parameter (Chiba & VanderWeele, 2011). The sensitivity analysis parameter is set by the investigator according to what is thought plausible. By adjusting the sensitivity analysis parameter values, sensitivity analysis can be conducted for the principal stratum effect. The bounds of principal stratum effects could also be estimated as described in Richardson et al. (2014).

Other than instrumental variable methods, we can also predict potential outcome variables in the principal strata using statistical models with covariates and estimate the principal stratum effects using the predicted potential outcome variables (Jo et al. 2009; Ding & Lu, 2017). Meanwhile, we can appropriately relax the ER assumption and monotonicity assumption, but the principal ignorability assumption will be required (this assumption relies on all confounding factors affecting potential intercurrent event variables and potential outcome variables being included in the model). When the principal ignorability assumption is not satisfied, tipping point analysis can be conducted for the statistical models used (Bornkamp et al., 2021), or sensitivity analysis can be performed assuming the presence of possible unmeasured confounders (Schwartz et al., 2012).

Additionally, since unobserved potential outcome variables and potential intercurrent event variables can be treated as missing data, the information from covariates can be used for multiple imputations, and the estimation results of each complete dataset can be combined based on Rubin's rule (Luo et al., 2022), or the maximum likelihood estimation of parameters and Markov chain Monte Carlo methods can be employed using the Expectation-Maximization algorithm (Ding & Lu, 2017).

Bayesian analysis could provide unified inferential frameworks for principal stratum analysis through enabling imputation of all missing potential outcome and intercurrent event variables. The Bayesian approach allows us to simulate the joint distribution of the stratum-specific treatment effect, the missing outcome, and intercurrent event variables by iteratively imputing missing variables given the stratum-specific treatment effect and updating the posterior of the principal stratum effect given the imputed missing outcome and intercurrent event variables (Li et al. 2023). Applications could be found in Baccini et al. (2017) and Lyu et al. (2023). With a different prior selection, the analysis assumptions could also be relaxed. For example, a prior probability very close to zero can be assigned to a certain potential principal stratum, which is a relatively mild monotonicity assumption (Bornkamp et al., 2021). Sensitivity analysis can generally be conducted by changing prior distributions or their parameters.

19.5 Special Considerations for Time-to-Event Endpoints

For time-to-event endpoints, special attention is needed because, in some cases, the intercurrent events may be competing or semi-competing events to the outcome event. Ignoring the competing risk while directly using the occurrence (or nonoccurrence) of intercurrent events to define principal strata will lead to bias in causal treatment effect estimation.

Semi-competing risks (Fine et al., 2001) occur in trials where observation of a nonterminal event (e.g., progression) may be pre-empted by a terminal event (e.g., death), but not vice versa. For example, in a randomized and placebo-controlled Phase II trial for recurrent glioma patients (Xu et al., 2022), the occurrence of cerebellar progression is precluded by the occurrence of an intercurrent event (e.g., death), and the estimand of interest is a time-varying treatment effect on time to progression in patients who would survive regardless of treatments. To estimate principal stratum effects under such a setting, Bayesian nonparametric models (Xu et al., 2022) and parametric frailty models (Comment et al., 2019) were proposed for modeling the joint distribution of observed data with different assumptions.

Terminal time-to-event outcomes (e.g., death) could preclude the occurrence of an intercurrent event such as treatment switching. Because such type of intercurrent event could either never occur or happen in continuous time with the presence of the terminal time-to-event outcomes, the potential intercurrent event variable is semi-continuous. It makes the principal stratification with respect to the intercurrent event consists of a continuum of principal strata such that each principal stratum comparises patients with the same time to intercurrent event. In Mattei et al. (2025), a flexible Bayesian parametric approach was proposed, including flexible parametric models for modeling the intercurrent event status (occurrence vs. absence) and the time-to-terminal event outcomes, and the Weibull distribution for the potential time to intercurrent event and the potential time-to-terminal event.

19.6 Cases Where the Principal Stratum Estimand Is Implemented

Several cases where the principal stratum estimand could be implemented are described in this book. This section provides a short summary of each case. Details of estimand considerations can be found in the corresponding sections.

Sect. 6.5 provides a scenario where the principal stratum strategy could be used to answer a patient's question that "If I can adhere to the treatment as prescribed, what effect will it have on my disease?" Because the treatment adherence occurs post-randomization, the treatment effect on those patients who would adhere to the treatment is of interest.

Sect. 9.2.5 describes the principal stratum estimand for a specific question, "whether the treatment effect would also be present in patients who do not experience relapses in secondary progressive multiple sclerosis?". This question is from the placebo-controlled randomized trial EXPAND (NCT01665144, Kappos et al., 2018) of siponimod in patients with secondary progressive multiple sclerosis. As relapses after randomization are intercurrent events, we are interested in the population that does not experience relapses after randomization. The population is defined as patients who would not experience relapses in both the treatment and control arms. The endpoint of interest is whether patients are assessed as having disability progression before a specific time point. The risk ratio is chosen as the population-level summary. The main analysis uses a Bayesian approach for the principal stratum effects.

Sect. 10.5 introduces a few common intercurrent events, such as not completing the vaccine regimen, acquisition of disease being targeted prior to the disease endpoint case surveillance period, and experiencing events that could affect the efficacy assessments in preventive vaccine trials. They are dealt with principal stratum strategy because subjects potentially with these intercurrent events are not in the population where evaluating a preventive vaccine efficacy is of interest.

19.7 Concluding Remarks

The principal stratum strategy is one of the four intercurrent event strategies introduced in ICH E9 (R1). It describes the clinical questions where the principal stratum effect is of interest. Given that it is impossible to simultaneously observe both the outcomes and their counterfactual on such a subpopulation, statistical modeling and related assumptions are necessary to estimate the principal stratum effect, whether using a frequentist or Bayesian approach. Consequently, sensitivity analysis plays an important role in assessing the robustness of these results.

Applying the principal stratum strategy to analyze time-to-event data adds another layer of complexity due to the (semi-)competing risk posed by intercurrent events and outcome events. This book provides numerous examples of principal stratum estimands for readers' reference, illustrating how to navigate these complexities effectively.

References

Angrist, J. D., Imbens, G. W., & Rubin, D. B. (1996). Identification of causal effects using instrumental variables. *Journal of the American Statistical Association, 91*, 444–455.

Baccini, M., Mattei, A., & Mealli, F. (2017). Bayesian inference for causal mechanisms with application to a randomized study for postoperative pain control. *Biostatistics, 18*, 605–617.

Baiocchi, M., Cheng, J., & Small, D. S. (2014). Instrumental variable methods for causal inference. *Statistics in Medicine, 33*, 2297–2340.

Bornkamp, B., Rufibach, K., Lin, J., Liu, Y., Mehrotra, D. V., Roychoudhury, S., Schmidli, H., Shentu, Y., & Wolbers, M. (2021). Principal stratum strategy: Potential role in drug development. *Pharmaceutical Statistics, 20*, 737–751.

Chiba, Y., & VanderWeele, T. J. (2011). A simple method for principal strata effects when the outcome has been truncated due to death. *American Journal of Epidemiology, 173*, 745–751.

Comment, L., Mealli, F., Haneuse, S., & Zigler, C. (2019). Survivor average causal effects for continuous time: A principal stratification approach to causal inference with semicompeting risks. *arXiv*. preprint arXiv:1902.09304.

Ding, P., & Lu, J. (2017). Principal stratification analysis using principal scores. *Journal of the Royal Statistical Society: Series B (Statistical Methodology), 79*, 757–777.

Fine, J. P., Jiang, H., & Chappell, R. (2001). On semi-competing risks data. *Biometrika, 88*, 907–919.

Gilbert, P. B., Bosch, R. J., & Hudgens, M. G. (2003). Sensitivity analysis for the assessment of causal vaccine effects on viral load in HIV vaccine trials. *Biometrics, 59*, 531–541.

Jo, B., & Stuart, E. A. (2009). On the use of propensity scores in principal causal effect estimation. *Statistics in Medicine, 28*(23), 2857–2875. https://doi.org/10.1002/sim.3669. PMID: 19610131; PMCID: PMC2757143

Kappos, L., Bar-Or, A., Cree, B. A., Fox, R. J., Giovannoni, G., Gold, R., & Kaida, K. (2018). Siponimod versus placebo in secondary progressive multiple sclerosis (EXPAND): A double-blind, randomised, phase 3 study. *The Lancet, 391*, 1263–1273.

Li, F., Ding, P., & Mealli, F. (2023). Bayesian causal inference: A critical review. *Philosophical Transactions of the Royal Society A, 381*, 20220153.

Lipkovich, I., Ratitch, B., Qu, Y., Zhang, X., Shan, M., & Mallinckrodt, C. (2022). Using principal stratification in analysis of clinical trials. *Statistics in Medicine, 41*, 3837–3877.

Lu, X., Mehrotra, D. V., & Shepherd, B. E. (2013). Rank-based principal stratum sensitivity analyses. *Statistics in Medicine, 32*, 4526–4539.

Luo, J., Ruberg, S. J., & Qu, Y. (2022). Estimating the treatment effect for adherers using multiple imputation. *Pharmaceutical Statistics, 21*, 525–534.

Lyu, T., Bornkamp, B., Mueller-Velten, G., & Schmidli, H. (2023). Bayesian inference for a principal stratum estimand on recurrent events truncated by death. *Biometrics, 79*, 3792–3802.

Magnusson, B., Schmidli, H., Rouyrre, N., & Scharfstein, D. (2019). Bayesian inference for a principal stratum estimand to assess the treatment effect in a subgroup characterized by post-randomization events. *Statistics in Medicine, 38*, 4761–4771.

Mattei, A., Ding, P., Ballerini, V., & Mealli, F. (2025). Assessing Causal Effects in the Presence of Treatment Switching Through Principal Stratification. *Bayesian Analysis, 20*, 851–878.

Mehrotra, D. V., Li, X., & Gilbert, P. B. (2006). A comparison of eight methods for the dual-endpoint evaluation of efficacy in a proof-of-concept HIV vaccine trial. *Biometrics, 62*, 893–900.

Richardson, A., Hudgens, M. G., Gilbert, P. B., & Fine, J. P. (2014). Nonparametric bounds and sensitivity analysis of treatment effects. *Statistical Science: A Review Journal of the Institute of Mathematical Statistics, 29*, 596.

Schwartz, S., Fan, L., & Reiter, J. P. (2012). Sensitivity analysis for unmeasured confounding in principal stratification settings with binary variables. *Statistics in Medicine, 31*, 949–962.

Stuart, E. A., & Jo, B. (2015). Assessing the sensitivity of methods for estimating principal causal effects. *Statistical Methods in Medical Research, 24*, 657–674.

Xu, Y., Scharfstein, D., Müller, P., & Daniels, M. (2022). A Bayesian nonparametric approach for evaluating the causal effect of treatment in randomized trials with semi-competing risks. *Biostatistics, 23*, 34–49.

Chapter 20
Statistical Analysis Under the Estimand Framework: Covariate Adjustment

Kelly Van Lancker, Marlena Bannick, and Ting Ye

Abstract This chapter explores the role of covariate adjustment in randomized clinical trials under the estimand framework. In recent years, there has been growing interest in this technique, particularly with the US Food and Drug Administration issuing guidance that underscores the need to differentiate between conditional and unconditional treatment effects. While these effects may be the same in linear models, they generally differ in other contexts—a distinction often overlooked in clinical trial practice. This chapter examines when and how to implement covariate adjustment in randomized controlled trials, focusing mainly on unconditional effects and emphasizing its role in increasing precision and statistical power by accounting for baseline covariates in the analysis. Various statistical methods, including analysis of covariance (ANCOVA), inverse probability weighting, and g-computation, are discussed. Practical considerations, such as handling missing data, managing small sample sizes, and available software, are also addressed.

20.1 Background

20.1.1 Introduction to Covariate Adjustment

Adjusting for baseline covariates in randomized clinical trials has a long history and rich statistical literature. Over the years, it has gained recognition as a strategy to improve the reliability and efficiency of treatment effect evaluation. Baseline

K. Van Lancker (✉)
Department of Mathematics, Computer Science and Statistics, Ghent University, Ghent, Belgium
e-mail: kelly.vanlancker@ugent.be

M. Bannick · T. Ye
Department of Biostatistics, University of Washington, Seattle, WA, USA
e-mail: mnorwood@uw.edu; tingye1@uw.edu

J. Wei et al. (eds.), *Estimands in Clinical Trials*, Springer Series in Pharmaceutical Statistics, https://doi.org/10.1007/978-3-032-02192-2_20

covariates may be accounted for at the design and/or statistical analysis stage of a clinical trial.

At the design stage, covariate-adaptive randomization such as stratified permuted block randomization (Matts & Lachin, 1988) and minimization (Taves, 1974) has become the standard practice for its ability to balance the number of patients in each treatment arm across baseline prognostic factors, strengthening the credibility of the results. From 1989 to 2008, more than 500 randomized clinical trials (RCTs) used minimization (Taves, 2010). In 2009 and 2014, 237 out of nearly 300 trials published in these two years utilized covariate-adaptive randomization (Ciolino et al., 2019). However, it is important to note that covariate-adaptive randomization generates a dependent sequence of treatment assignments, which one needs to account for in subsequent statistical analysis, particularly when estimating the variance of the treatment effect (EMA, 2015; FDA, 2023; Ye et al., 2022; Shao et al., 2010). Often, a stratified analysis is used to accommodate this, which may target a treatment effect conditional on stratification factors (i.e., conditional effect; see Sect. 20.2) rather than a population-average treatment effect (i.e., unconditional/marginal effect; see Sect. 20.2). While the conditional treatment effect focuses on specific subgroups (here defined by stratification factors) within the population, the unconditional treatment effect provides a general assessment of the treatment effect across the entire population, without conditioning on any specific factors. We will later discuss approaches that take into account the covariate-adaptive randomization but can also target unconditional estimands.

At the analysis stage, covariate adjustment refers to the technique of using prespecified variables collected at baseline (e.g., in a regression model) when estimating the target parameter. This target parameter can focus on a stratum-specific effect (i.e., conditional effect) or on the entire population (i.e., unconditional effect). It is important that such an approach relies on minimal statistical assumptions similar to those for unadjusted estimation (especially when estimating an unconditional effect). When targeting an unconditional effect, a key reason to account for baseline covariates at the analysis stage is to increase statistical efficiency. Specifically, for unconditional treatment effects, adjusted estimators have been shown to be more efficient than unadjusted estimators. It is, however, important to note that a covariate-adjusted estimate of a conditional effect may not always be more efficient than an unadjusted estimate of an unconditional effect (Daniel et al., 2021). Additionally, adjusting for baseline variables can reduce conditional bias due to chance imbalance in those variables across treatment arms (where one conditions on the imbalance). Importantly, while chance imbalance should decrease with increasing sample size, it remains a concern in large studies (Senn, 1989). Therefore, the improvements in statistical efficiency by adjusting for baseline prognostic variables are realized at any sample size. In this chapter, we will focus on adjusting for covariates at the analysis stage; we will discuss its rich history and link with the ICH E9(R1) guideline further in the following sections.

Intuitively, whether we gain precision from adjustment depends on the randomization strategy. Even if a categorical variable is perfectly balanced in a particular trial that uses simple randomization, this balance is by chance. Further adjusting for that variable can therefore still lead to a precision gain (Proschan et al., 2005). However, if we instead use stratified permuted block randomization by the categorical variable, each realized trial will have (near)-perfect balance in that covariate. In general, adjusting for that variable will not gain us much precision, as we have already reduced the variance due to that variable at the design stage. Specifically, further adjusting for that variable will asymptotically lead to the same variance as not adjusting for it. This result reflects the duality of design and analysis in covariate adjustment (Ye et al., 2022), which says that for categorical covariates, a full adjustment with a linear model achieves the same asymptotic efficiency as stratifying with those covariates during randomization (provided that the correct variance estimator is used). Yet, in small samples, there may be a slight advantage. Nonetheless, even if adjustment is not imperative, the variance estimator should appropriately factor in stratification, leading to the widespread practice of adjusting for stratification factors in treatment effect estimation. Specifically, an unadjusted analysis will lead to too wide confidence intervals, too low Type I error rates, and reduced power (Kahan & Morris, 2012).

Of course, we cannot stratify randomization based on a continuous variable. Therefore, it is often the case that covariate-adaptive randomization is performed using categorical versions of prognostic, continuous variables. One can then still achieve further variance reduction by including the continuous version of that variable at the analysis stage.

20.1.2 Regulatory Guidelines on Covariate Adjustment

Given its rich history of statistical innovations, whether and how to perform covariate adjustment in RCTs has been debated extensively. One central point of contention has consistently been the worry that it affords researchers the chance to "cheat" by conducting several analyses and selectively presenting only those that showcase the most favorable results (Kahan & Morris, 2012). Motivated by the need to establish consistent practices across industry, several regulatory agencies have released guidance on covariate adjustment.

20.1.2.1 ICH E9 (R1) Guideline

The ICH E9 (R1) guideline emphasizes the need for a precise description of the treatment effect (referred to as estimand) that directly pertains to the clinical question raised by the specific clinical trial objective(s) (ICH, 2019). This states the essence of first defining the estimand before making decisions on whether and how to implement covariate adjustment (see Fig. 20.1).

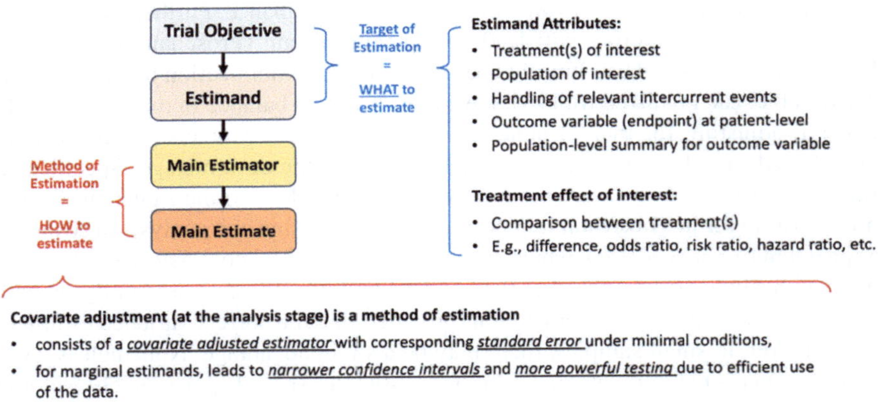

Fig. 20.1 Interpretation of estimand framework with covariate adjustment as a method of estimation. This figure is an adaptation of a figure from the ICH E9(R1) training material (ICH, 2021), modified by adding the explanatory text to the right and bottom

20.1.2.2 FDA and EMA Guidelines on Covariate Adjustment

The European Medicines Agency (EMA) released guidelines in 2015 on adjusting for baseline covariates in clinical trials (EMA, 2015). Until recently, there was no set standard for covariate adjustment for industry sponsors seeking approval within the US from the US Food and Drug Administration (FDA). However, in 2023, the FDA released comprehensive guidelines on performing covariate adjustment to increase statistical efficiency in randomized clinical trials (FDA, 2023).

These guidance documents, along with the ICH E9 (R1) guideline, highlight the importance of critically thinking about estimands in clinical research (see Fig. 20.1). The most clinically relevant target of estimation should guide the choice of statistical estimators. In particular, the FDA guidance highlights the difference between unconditional treatment effects and conditional treatment effects. We will discuss this distinction further in Sect. 20.2.

Both guidance documents encourage the use of covariate adjustment to improve statistical efficiency when prognostic baseline variables are available. The EMA guidance additionally stresses that baseline values of continuous outcome variables should be included as covariates at the analysis stage. The EMA also provides specific guidance on treatment-by-covariate interactions: if interactions are suspected, one should stratify randomization based on those covariates, and one should provide treatment effect estimates separately by covariate subgroup. Historically, practitioners have required correct model specification when targeting subgroup effects through interactions. However, in the following sections, we discuss how we can leverage interactions to improve efficiency in estimating the unconditional treatment effect as well, without making assumptions about model specification. Most importantly, both documents emphasize that any type of covariate adjustment should be prespecified in trial protocols.

20.2 Clinical Trial Objectives and Estimands

All clinical trials should have an objective and an associated target of estimation: the estimand. Covariate adjustment must be tailored to the estimand. In other words, determining the estimand comes before deciding whether and how to perform covariate adjustment. If we perform covariate adjustment for population-average/unconditional/marginal treatment effects, we still want to target the same inference regardless of whether the analysis is adjusted for covariates or not. We can think of estimands in two stages.

The first is making a choice regarding the targeted quantity specific to a treatment arm, like the mean of the outcome variable. In this stage, we need to consider whether we are interested in unconditional quantities or conditional quantities. Let Y be the outcome variable, Z be the treatment assignment labels with $Z = 1$ if a patient is assigned to the treatment of interest and $Z = 0$ if assigned to the control, and X be baseline covariates. In addition, let Y^z denote the potential/counterfactual outcome that would have been observed had someone been assigned to treatment $Z = z$ (see also Chap. 3). An example of a conditional estimand is $E(Y^z | X = x)$, that is, the expected potential outcome under treatment z for someone with covariate profile x. An unconditional estimand $E(Y^z)$ averages over the possible covariate profiles with respect to some distribution. With unconditional estimands, we are not interested in how the expected outcome differs by levels of the covariate; we are interested in the overall mean over the distribution of X. We include these examples in Fig. 20.2.

The second stage is choosing a summary measure to make between-arm comparisons, using the arm-specific quantities we have discussed. Consider an example. If the objective of a trial is to establish whether a treatment reduces blood pressure, the estimand could be the difference in the change in blood pressure between baseline and follow-up between the treatment and control arms. We have chosen an

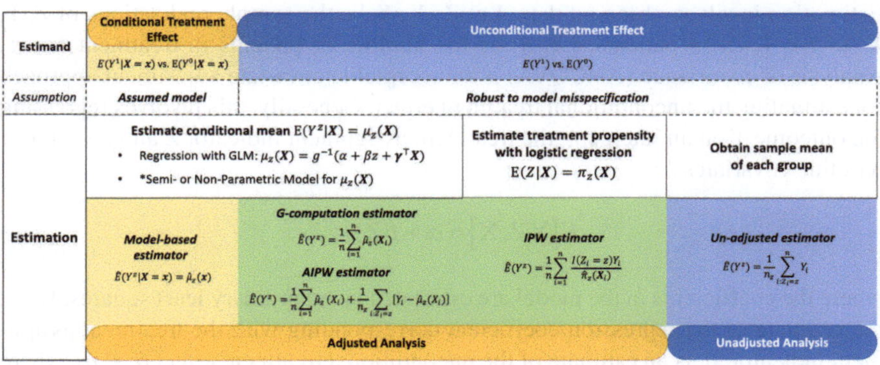

Fig. 20.2 Comparison of conditional and unconditional estimands, and adjusted and unadjusted approaches to estimation. *Cross-fitting may be required if data-adaptive methods are used to estimate the conditional mean

unconditional estimand for the first stage and a difference in means as our summary for the second stage. One may prefer other summary measures for different types of endpoints. For binary and ordinal endpoints, we may consider risk differences, relative risks, odds ratios, or the Mann–Whitney estimand. For time-to-event data, we may consider differences in restricted mean survival times, differences in survival probabilities at a particular time, and relative cumulative risks up to a particular time point. We can compute any of these summary measures using unconditional or conditional quantities. If one is willing to make an assumption of proportional hazards, hazard ratios can also be considered.

It is worth noting that the magnitude of some effect measures may change upon conditioning on an additional baseline covariate (that is independent of treatment) whenever that covariate is associated with the outcome. That is, the unconditional treatment effect may not lie within the range of any of the conditional treatment effects. This phenomenon is called non-collapsibility (Agresti, 2002; Daniel et al., 2021). Odds ratios and hazard ratios are non-collapsible, while mean differences, risk differences, and relative risks are collapsible. Given the subtleties involved, we encourage the interested reader to explore Sjölander et al. (2016) and Daniel et al. (2021) for additional insights, see also Chap. 16.

In this chapter, we do not seek to involve ourselves in the discussion about whether to report unconditional or conditional effects. Moreover, even though we discuss conditional estimands, our primary focus will be on estimating unconditional effect estimands, acknowledging the recent emphasis on covariate adjustment for unconditional estimands (FDA, 2023).

20.3 Estimation of Unconditional Estimands

20.3.1 Linear

Estimation involves observed data. Let Z_i, Y_i, X_i be the sample realizations of Z, Y, X for i = 1, …, n patients. Let n_z be the number of patients in treatment arm z. Analysis of covariance (ANCOVA) is an acceptable covariate adjustment approach for estimating the unconditional treatment effect. Generally, this involves regressing the outcome Y on an intercept, the treatment assignment indicator Z and a vector of baseline covariates X:

$$E\left[\mathrm{Y}|\mathrm{Z},\mathrm{X}\right]=\alpha+\beta Z+\gamma X$$

where the coefficients in the model are estimated using ordinary least squares. Here, the estimate of the regression coefficient corresponding with the treatment assignment indicator, β, is an estimate of the unconditional treatment effect $\theta_1 - \theta_0$, where $\theta_z = E[Y^z]$. This estimator is even consistent when the linear regression model is mis-specified, that is, fails to accurately capture the (true) relationships between the outcome, baseline covariates, and treatment (Yang & Tsiatis, 2001). Nevertheless, as the power of hypothesis tests and the accuracy of estimates typically increase when the model more accurately approximates the true relationships, one should be motivated to consider a model that captures the true relationship reasonably well.

In general, when no treatment-by-covariate interactions are included, we can perform inference by using robust standard errors such as the Huber–White sandwich standard error (Rosenblum & van der Laan, 2009; Lin, 2013; FDA, 2023) or a nonparametric bootstrap procedure. Note that for two-arm trials with 1:1 randomization, model-based standard errors will provide valid inference, even if the model is mis-specified (Wang et al., 2023).

The model above assumes that there are no treatment-by-covariates interactions. This statistical assumption, which is not implied by randomization, might be incorrect in many cases, as it is often reasonable that patients with different baseline characteristics experience different benefits when receiving the same treatment.

With the aim of fitting a model that closely captures the true relationship, it is therefore reasonable to consider a model that includes treatment-by-covariate interactions:

$$E\left[\mathrm{Y|Z,X}\right] = \alpha + \beta Z + \gamma X + \delta ZX$$

This approach, also known as ANCOVA2, has a long history in the statistics literature (Yang & Tsiatis, 2001; Tsiatis et al., 2008; Cassel et al., 1976). By including this interaction term in the model, β and δ typically lose their marginal/unconditional interpretation, unless the baseline covariates X are sample-centered (the added noise due to the centering step cannot be ignored when calculating the robust standard error). We refer to the latter approach, where the baseline covariates are sample-centered, as the ANalysis of HEterogeneous COVAriance (ANHECOVA) (Ye et al., 2022). ANHECOVA enjoys several desirable properties, including consistency under mis-specified models, guaranteed efficiency gain (in large samples) over the estimator without using any covariates, and universal applicability to simple randomization and commonly used covariate-adaptive randomization schemes (such as the stratified permuted block randomization) when all the covariates used in covariate-adaptive randomization are included in ANHECOVA. We can obtain valid inference by using a robust standard error (Ye et al., 2022). In general, linear adjustment can still be used to improve efficiency when the estimand is defined by an estimation equation (Zhang et al., 2008).

Alternatively, we can perform estimation of an unconditional treatment effect using linear working models by averaging across the whole observed distribution of baseline covariates. Specifically, let $\hat{\mu}_z(x)$ be some estimate of the conditional mean $E[Y|Z = z, X = x]$. Then we can estimate $E[Y^z]$ as the mean of the model-based predictions $\hat{\mu}_z(X_i)$ over the distribution of baseline covariates x_i of all patients in the trial:

$$\hat{\theta}_z = \frac{1}{n}\sum_{i=1}^{n}\hat{\mu}_z(X_i)$$

This method is known as g-computation or standardization (Robins, 1986; Vansteelandt & Keiding, 2011; Hernán & Robins, 2023) and allows us to perform covariate adjustment for continuous outcomes while also accounting for potential treatment-by-covariate interactions. This estimator, along with several other estimators in this section, has been previously introduced in Chap. 3. In the linear case, the g-computation estimator for $\theta_1 - \theta_0$, leads to

$$\frac{1}{n}\sum_{i=1}^{n}\left(\hat{\alpha}+\hat{\beta}+\hat{\gamma}X_i\right)-\frac{1}{n}\sum_{i=1}^{n}\left(\hat{\alpha}+\hat{\gamma}X_i\right)=\hat{\beta}$$

for $[Y|Z, X] = \alpha + \beta Z + \gamma X$, and

$$\frac{1}{n}\sum_{i=1}^{n}\left(\hat{\alpha}+\hat{\beta}+\hat{\gamma}X_i+\hat{\delta}X_i\right)-\frac{1}{n}\sum_{i=1}^{n}\left(\hat{\alpha}+\hat{\gamma}X_i\right)=\frac{1}{n}\sum_{i=1}^{n}\left(\hat{\beta}+\hat{\delta}X_i\right)$$

for $E[Y|Z, X] = \alpha + \beta Z + \gamma X + \delta ZX$. Here, the coefficients in the model are estimated using ordinary least squares. We can obtain a correct variance estimate via a sandwich estimator using the Delta method (Tsiatis et al., 2008). Note that, if X_i are centered, the last equation reduces to $\hat{\beta}$. This also shows why ANHECOVA for continuous outcomes targets an unconditional treatment effect.

Another alternative is inverse probability of treatment weighting (IPW; Hernán & Robins, 2023; Williamson et al., 2014). This involves fitting a model for the probability of being randomized to the experimental treatment arm given measured baseline covariates, $e(X) = P(Z = 1|X)$. This model is referred to as the propensity score model. Once the propensity score has been estimated, we can fit a simple linear model contrasting the experimental treatment and control arm, weighting the individuals in the treatment arm by $1/e(X)$ and patients in the control arm by $1/[1 - e(X)]$. By doing so, a pseudo-population through a weighted trial sample is created, ensuring that both trial arms exhibit an identical distribution of observed covariate values. For two-arm trials, Shen et al. (2014) showed that fitting the propensity score using most parametric families leads to a consistent IPW estimator of the average treatment effect. In particular, the IPW estimator based on the logistic propensity score model is asymptotically equivalent to the ANHECOVA estimator. Nonetheless, the regression adjustment framework (e.g., g-computation and augmented inverse probability weighting (AIPW) estimators) is more general than the current IPW framework in handling multiple arms and nonlinear adjustment.

20.3.2 Nonlinear: Binary, Ordinal, and Count Endpoints

Estimation methods for binary and ordinal endpoints are generally analogous to estimation methods for continuous outcomes. The difference is that with these nonlinear outcomes, estimation requires outcome models with a nonlinear link function, that is, $\hat{\alpha}_z$ is some nonlinear function.

Generalized linear models (GLMs) are a framework through which to think of modeling noncontinuous outcomes. Therefore, we frequently specify $\hat{\mu}_z(x) = g^{-1}\left(\hat{\alpha} + \hat{\beta}z + \hat{\gamma}x\right)$ where g is the canonical link function for a generalized linear model (Rosenblum & van der Laan, 2009; Van Lancker et al., 2024), and $\left(\hat{\alpha}, \hat{\beta}, \hat{\gamma}\right)$ are estimated via maximum likelihood. As such, the linear case is a special case of the nonlinear case, with g^{-1} being the identity function. We show various approaches to estimation and how it relates to the estimand of interest in Fig. 20.2. Importantly, note that to estimate $\hat{\theta}_z$ we need to marginalize over the entire distribution of covariates, not just the covariates within treatment arm z. This is a fundamental concept in g-computation.

It is important to use a correct variance estimator for g-computation (Bannick et al., 2023). An initial thought may be to obtain a sandwich variance estimate for the estimated coefficients, and then use the Delta method with the function g^{-1}. However, this is an incorrect approach when g is nonlinear. There is not only uncertainty in the estimated coefficients but also in the summation over the observed variables X_i. See, for example, Ye et al. (2023b) for correct variance estimators in the case where g is the link function for a logistic regression model.

A major benefit of using g-computation in randomized clinical trials is that it is robust to model misspecification if a prediction unbiasedness condition holds:

$$\frac{1}{n_a} \sum_{i:Z_i=z} \hat{\mu}_z(X_i) = \frac{1}{n_a} \sum_{i:Z_i=z} Y_i$$

In other words, the average of the predicted means within a treatment arm should match the average of the outcome variables within that treatment arm. Due to the empirical score equations from maximum likelihood estimation, this holds true for g-computation with nonlinear outcomes using canonical link functions. For noncanonical link functions, there is no guarantee that prediction unbiasedness holds. In this case, augmented inverse probability weighting (AIPW) methods can be employed instead to restore model robustness (Robins et al., 1994):

$$\hat{\theta}_z = \frac{1}{n} \sum_{i=1}^{n} \hat{\mu}_z(X_i) + \left\{ \frac{1}{n_z} \sum_{i:Z_i=z} Y_i - \frac{1}{n_z} \sum_{i:Z_i=z} \hat{\mu}_z(X_i) \right\}$$

We can then use the estimated mean $\hat{\theta}_z$ to construct arbitrary treatment contrasts. This estimation approach can be seen as a combination of g-computation and IPW. Specifically, it uses a g-computation estimator (first summation) with an additional correction term (the weighted sum of discrepancies between the predicted and observed outcomes), which comes from a weighting model. Also note that (regular) IPW, as described in Sect. 20.3.1, can still be used for noncontinuous endpoints.

Data-adaptive approaches, including stepwise regression and machine learning, can be used with this strategy, https://doi.org/10.48550/arXiv.2404.11150. Alternatively, targeted maximum likelihood estimation (TMLE) offers a framework that accommodates these techniques as well (Van Der Laan & Rose, 2011; Moore

& van der Laan, 2009; Díaz et al., 2016; Williams et al., 2022). TMLE can be viewed as an extension of g-computation and AIPW methods with nonparametric models for the conditional mean. Instead of relying on a generalized linear model to estimate $\hat{\mu}_z(x)$, machine learning algorithms can be applied, with predictions updated in a targeted manner to ensure prediction unbiasedness. We can also employ this for continuous outcomes. Classically, machine learning methods must satisfy certain conditions to ensure valid behavior, including rates of convergence of the estimator to the true parameter and limits of the complexity of function classes. Some of these conditions can be modified or relaxed using a technique called "cross-fitting" (Chernozhukov et al., 2017). However, under model misspecification or using flexible methods to estimate the conditional mean, g-computation and AIPW are not guaranteed to be more efficient than an unadjusted estimator of the treatment effect. To address this, recent work has proposed a general strategy to restore guaranteed efficiency gain asymptotically in a two-stage modeling approach (Cohen & Fogarty, 2024; Bannick et al., 2023). In this approach, we use generalized linear models or flexible nonparametric and machine learning methods to "impute" the counterfactual outcomes for everyone under all treatment arms and use those imputed counterfactual outcomes as derived covariates in a linear regression.

20.3.3 Time-To-Event Endpoints

Analyzing time-to-event endpoints is complex due to censoring and the variety of common approaches used to summarize the unconditional distribution of these endpoints, such as hazard, restricted mean survival time, median survival time, and survival probability at a fixed timepoint.

We start with nonparametric testing methods. The log-rank test is a commonly used method to analyze time-to-event endpoints. It tests the null hypothesis that the unconditional hazard (or survival) functions in two treatment arms are equal, assuming independence of censoring and failure time conditional on treatment arm. The log-rank test does not adjust for covariates and is conservative under stratified randomization (Ye & Shao, 2020). To adjust for covariates, Ye et al. (2023c) proposed a covariate-adjusted log-rank test that first obtains a particular "derived outcome" from linearizing the log-rank test and then applies ANHECOVA for covariate adjustment (Ye et al., 2023c). Importantly, this covariate-adjusted log-rank test not only tests the same null hypothesis under the same assumptions as the log-rank test but also enjoys a guaranteed efficiency gain over it, as well as universal applicability (i.e., the test is asymptotically size alpha under different covariate-adaptive randomization schemes) due to ANHECOVA. Another popular method is the stratified log-rank test, which tests the null hypothesis that the stratified hazard (or survival) functions in two treatment arms are equal, assuming independence of censoring and failure time conditional on the treatment arms and stratification factor. As proved in Ye and Shao (2020), the stratified log-rank test enjoys universal applicability.

Furthermore, Ye et al. (2023c) also proposed a covariate-adjusted stratified log-rank test that can further adjust for continuous covariates.

Beyond testing, it is often of interest to estimate and construct a confidence interval for the magnitude of the treatment effect. The hazard ratio is traditionally used to summarize the treatment effect under the additional Cox proportional hazard model assumption:

$$\lambda(t|z) = \lambda_0(t)e^{\beta z}$$

Commonly, this model is fitted using the partial likelihood approach to estimate the unconditional hazard ratio β without adjusting for covariates, assuming independence of censoring and failure time conditional on treatment arm. Under the same assumption on censoring, one can calculate the covariate-adjusted estimator of β using the method proposed by Lu and Tsiatis (2008) for simple randomization and by Ye et al. (2023c) for covariate-adaptive randomization. This approach can be extended to the stratified Cox proportional hazards model:

$$\lambda(t|z,s) = \lambda_{0s}(t)e^{\beta z}$$

where $\lambda(t|z, s)$ denotes the hazard function in treatment arm z and stratum s, $\lambda_{0s}(t)$ is the baseline hazard function in stratum s, and β is the hazard ratio for every stratum. Under this stratified Cox model, a covariate-adjusted method to estimate and make inferences about β has been developed in Ye et al. (2023c). Relatedly, Daniel et al. (2021) proposed a simulation-based g-computation estimator for the unconditional causal hazard ratio. They hereby estimate unconditional causal survivor functions following the fitting of a conditional Cox model, which they then use to estimate a unconditional causal hazard ratio.

Although hazard ratios are routinely used for summarizing treatment effects, they require the additional (stratified) Cox proportional hazard model assumption and are not straightforward to interpret (Hernán, 2010; Uno et al., 2014). Therefore, there is growing interest and development in alternative estimands that are well-defined nonparametrically and easily interpretable. Along this line, Zhang (2015) proposed a covariate-adjusted Kaplan-Meier estimator of the survival function, and Díaz et al. (2019) proposed a covariate-adjusted estimator of the restricted mean survival time (RMST) (Zhang, 2015; Díaz et al., 2019).

20.4 Estimation and Testing of Conditional Estimands

Conditional treatment effects are also widely used, particularly for discrete and time-to-event endpoints. Estimating these effects typically involves fitting regression models. For example, logistic regression is often used to estimate the conditional odds ratio, and the Cox proportional hazards regression is often used to estimate the conditional hazard ratio.

It is important to note that the correct estimation of the conditional treatment effect requires correctly specified models. Specifically, if the model is mis-specified (e.g., an important quadratic term is missing), the estimated treatment effect may be biased. If a model without treatment-by-covariates interactions (which is often considered in practice) reflects the truth, then the conditional treatment effect is constant across different levels of the covariate values. If the model is mis-specified and the treatment effect varies substantially across different covariate levels, interpreting the results can be challenging. Considering this, the FDA emphasizes that sponsors "should discuss any planned assessment of model assumptions" (FDA, 2023). As mentioned in Sect. 20.1.2.2, the EMA also provides specific guidance on treatment-by-covariate interactions. Specifically, if interactions are suspected, they recommend stratifying randomization based on those covariates and providing treatment estimates separately by covariate subgroup (EMA, 2015). Furthermore, the interpretation of the conditional treatment effect should be done within the context of the conditional expected outcome under control, which should not be confused with the unconditional expected outcome under control. Understanding the conditional baseline level is essential for proper interpretation. Lastly, it is worth noting that the interpretation of the conditional treatment effect depends on which covariates are adjusted for in the analysis. The inclusion or exclusion of certain covariates can influence the observed treatment effect (e.g., due to non-collapsibility). This also complicates cross-trial comparisons of conditional effects, as different trials may be reporting conditional effects conditioned on different sets of covariates.

Testing the null hypothesis that the conditional treatment effect is equal to zero can sometimes be done robustly in the sense that the test remains valid even when the model is mis-specified. Several examples include the stratified log-rank test, which tests for equality of hazard ratios across all strata; the robust score test based on the Cox proportional hazards model, which tests the conditional hazard ratio being one (Ye et al., 2023c); and the test based on the generalized linear model, which tests for conditional independence between the outcome and treatment given covariates (Gail et al., 1988).

Although for non-collapsible measures the conditional estimand is at least as far from the null as the unconditional estimand (Daniel et al., 2021), there exist equally powerful estimators for both estimands. Specifically, for generalized linear models with canonical link and without interactions, $g\{E(Y|Z, X)\} = \alpha + \beta Z + \gamma X$, it moreover holds that a Wald test based on $\hat{\beta}$ (estimated via maximum likelihood) and g-computation based on this model (without interactions) both control the Type I error rate (asymptotically) and are equally powerful in large samples (Rosenblum & Steingrimsson, 2016). To robustly test the null hypothesis, we typically need robust standard errors. It is important to note that the null hypothesis of no conditional treatment effect is more restrictive than the null hypothesis of no unconditional treatment effect because the former implies the latter. Furthermore, after conducting the test, it is often still of interest to report the effect size of the treatment effect. Hence, the considerations and interpretations discussed earlier in this section still apply.

20.5 Practical Considerations

20.5.1 Missing Data

Despite making efforts to collect the data required for estimation, some data may still be missing. In randomized controlled trials, it is common to observe missing data in covariates, prompting a significant question: how do we handle the adjustment of covariates that have missing values?

Provided that the treatment allocation remains unrelated to the initial covariates and the mechanism for missing data—an assumption anticipated to be valid due to randomization—simple techniques like single imputation and the missingness indicator approach can be utilized when targeting an unconditional treatment effect. As covariate adjustment remains valid regardless of the prespecified covariates used, the reliability of this method is guaranteed. However, less accurate imputations can lead to reduced efficiency gains due to diminished prognostic value of the covariates.

While more complex imputation methods can be utilized, it is important to ensure the imputation model does not depend on treatment and outcome to maintain the independence of treatment and covariates in the imputed data. Recent investigations by Zhao and Ding (2022) and Song et al. (2024) delved into these approaches for handling missing covariate information and demonstrated their potential to enhance efficiency.

Benkeser et al. (2020) recommend excluding baseline covariates with extensive missing data from the analysis to safeguard precision. Excluding patients rather than imputing or excluding missing covariates ensures randomization can still estimate a causal effect, but this has two drawbacks: a reduced sample size, which lowers statistical power, and the ability to generalize the treatment effect only to a population with non-missing baseline covariates.

Unlike for missing baseline covariates, it becomes necessary to make assumptions to handle the missing outcome data in the statistical analysis (ICH, 2019). As stated in the ICH E9(R1) addendum, handling of missing data should be based on clinically plausible assumptions and, where possible, guided by the strategies employed in the description of the estimand.

Using an adaptation of the covariate adjustment techniques discussed in previous sections, one can make the assumption that the outcomes are missing at random conditional on treatment and covariates, rather than the stronger missing at random conditional on treatment only, which is made by unadjusted estimators. The former implies that missingness should be independent of the outcomes given treatment and covariates. For example, one can then tweak the aforementioned standardization procedure to make predictions for all patients in the dataset, rather than just for the complete cases. This is also known as regression imputation or single imputation (Little & Rubin, 2019). Unlike the setting without missing outcome data, the validity of the resulting treatment effect estimator now relies on a correctly specified outcome model. Multiple imputation offers an alternative method that depends on similar modeling assumptions (Rubin, 2004; Schafer, 1997) and employs "Rubin's Rules" to manage the uncertainty in the imputations.

If both outcome and covariate data are missing, mean imputation and missing indicator strategies for covariates may become inadequate since the missing at random assumption may not hold for these imputed covariates. Determining the best approach in such situations is an ongoing area of research.

20.5.2 Multiple Treatment Arms

Multiple treatment arms, which usually include a placebo arm or active control and different doses (or regimes) of the investigational treatment, are common in clinical trials (Juszczak et al., 2019). In some applications, the primary analysis may focus on comparing just two treatments. A simple way to compare the two treatment arms is to subset data from the two arms of interest and apply statistical analyses. Without covariate adjustment, this approach does not incur efficiency loss due to the exclusion of data from other treatment arms. Yet, when considering covariate adjustment, this approach does lose efficiency since it fails to fully capitalize on covariate information available from other treatment arms (Ye et al., 2022). Therefore, using data from all arms is recommended in covariate adjustment. Ye and colleagues recommend a general model-assisted estimator that can study multiple arms as well as arbitrary functions of response means (including linear contrasts, ratios, and odds ratios), with guaranteed efficiency gain and universal applicability.

20.5.3 Sample Size Calculations

In trials incorporating covariate adjustment, the determination of sample size and statistical power can stem from either adjusted or unadjusted approaches (FDA, 2023). The adjusted method evaluates the potential increase in precision achievable through external (trial) data when computing sample size (Li et al., 2023). An incorrect projection of a covariate's prognostic value, however, may still lead to an over- or underpowered future trial. The unadjusted method takes a conservative stance, assuming that covariate adjustment will not enhance precision. In this case, any gains in precision would boost power.

Alternatively, one can choose to combine covariate adjustment with an information adaptive design, also recognized as information monitoring (Tsiatis & Davidian, 2022; Van Lancker et al., 2025). This approach involves continuous monitoring of statistical information (closely tied to the actual precision improvement) throughout the trial to ascertain the optimal timing for conducting the analysis. Compared to the more standard sample size calculations, this ensures a correctly powered trial. In case a covariate-adjusted estimator is more efficient than an unadjusted estimator, the sample size and duration of the trial will be automatically adapted to the faster accrual of information. Specifically, covariate adjustment will then lead to shorter trials.

20.5.4 Small Samples

This chapter focuses on asymptotic results, which are applicable with a large sample size and a small number of covariates. However, some clinical trials may have a relatively small sample size (which may occur for earlier phase trials or rare diseases) and/or a relatively large number of covariates (e.g., when attempting to adjust for all sites). In such situations, covariate adjustment should be applied with caution.

For g-computation with models fitted separately in each arm, a potential approach is to multiply robust variance estimators by a small-sample correction factor (Tsiatis et al., 2008):

$$\frac{(n_0 - p_0 - 1)^{-1} + (n_1 - p_1 - 1)^{-1}}{(n_0 - p_0)^{-1} + (n_1 - p_1)^{-1}}.$$

Here, n_z is the number of patients used to fit the outcome working model in arm z (i.e., the number of patients in arm z), and p_z the numbers of parameters fitted in these models, exclusive of intercepts. Although employing small-sample adjustment to robust variance estimators can improve performance, there is no guarantee of good statistical performance.

Another approach to statistical inference is through randomization or permutation tests, which is particularly useful in small sample sizes because it can make exact inference rather than asymptotic inference (Lin, 2013; Guo & Basse, 2023). Randomization tests can also be easily applied to covariate-adaptive randomization schemes by resampling treatment assignments according to the design (Shao et al., 2010; Simon & Simon, 2011; Bugni et al., 2018). However, it is important to note that these finite-sample guarantees are achieved when testing more restrictive null hypotheses, such as the treatment does not change the outcome distribution (not only its expectation) (Simon & Simon, 2011), and Fisher's sharp null hypothesis that the treatment has no effect on any patients (Zhao & Ding, 2022).

20.5.5 Convergence of the Algorithm

The different estimation approaches discussed in this chapter (e.g., g-computation, ANHECOVA, IPW, and AIPW for unconditional estimands, and direct adjustment for conditional estimands) all rely on algorithms to estimate the working models and parameters. Morris et al. (2022) caution against choosing a procedure that may not converge, highlighting convergence as a crucial requirement for the chosen analysis procedure. In the analysis of randomized trials, non-convergence typically arises from two primary causes. First, issues may arise with specific models, such as generalized linear models with binomial outcome distribution and identity- or log-link functions. Second, non-convergence can result from incorporating an excessive number of parameters relative to the effective sample size.

Van Lancker et al. (2024) also advised keeping the number of covariates small relative to the sample size to avoid inflated Type I error. In line with regulatory guidelines, a conservative approach would be to include a small number of key covariates (EMA, 2015; FDA, 2023). As choosing a canonical link function enhances the likelihood of convergence, IPW, g-computation (using GLMs with a canonical link), AIPW (using GLMs with a canonical link), and ANHECOVA appear to be reliable methods with respect to achieving convergence. Direct adjustment targeting a conditional estimand is more vulnerable to this issue (Morris et al., 2022).

20.5.6 Software

In this section, we provide a brief and informal overview of open-source software in R that trial statisticians and researchers can easily access (Table 20.1).

Table 20.1 Overview of R packages for covariate adjustment of unconditional estimands

R-package	Approaches	Endpoints	Pros
RobinCar (Ye et al., 2023a)	g-computation and ANHECOVA	Continuous, binary, ordinal, and time-to-event	Allows for machine learning, as well as the combination with covariate-adaptive randomization
AIPW (Zhong et al., 2021)	AIPW and TMLE	Continuous and binary	Allows for machine learning using cross-fitting
speff2trial (Juraska et al., 2022)	AIPW	Continuous, binary, and time-to-event	Allows for model selection
Adjrct (Díaz & Williams, 2021)	TMLE	Time-to-event and ordinal	Allows for machine learning, as well as violations of proportional hazards and odds assumption
survtmle (Benkeser & Hejazi, 2017)	TMLE	Time-to-event	Allows for machine learning, as well as incorporation of competing risks
drord (Benkeser, 2021)	TMLE	Ordinal	Allows for machine learning
PSW	IPW	Continuous and binary	Also considers average treatment effect of the treated and of the controls

20.6 Concluding Remarks

The focus of this chapter was on the application of covariate adjustment in randomized controlled trials to enhance precision—a crucial aspect given the evolving regulatory landscape (ICH, 2019; FDA, 2023). We highlighted the difference between conditional and unconditional estimands, stressing the necessity of aligning statistical analysis methods with the chosen estimand. We also shared practical considerations for clinical trialists to bear in mind regarding covariate adjustment. Numerous choices exist for adjusting for covariates in estimating unconditional treatment effects, creating a challenge for the trialist in selecting the most suitable approach for the data upfront. It is crucial to note that the competing estimators covered in this chapter can be considered as part of a broader class of estimators (Van Lancker et al., 2024). With larger sample sizes, g-computation and similar approaches are simple to explain and allow a flexible choice of working model for the outcome. A well-chosen model gives the best chance of variance reduction. With small sample sizes and when convergence issues are a concern, methods like ANHECOVA with efficiency guarantees (relative to the unadjusted estimator) may be preferred. Further investigation is needed to determine the most suitable covariate adjustment approaches for specific settings.

Acknowledgments The authors would like to thank Xin Zhang for comments on an earlier draft of the chapter.

References

Agresti, A. (2002). Describing contingency tables. In *Categorical data analysis* (pp. 36–69). John Wiley & Sons, Ltd. https://doi.org/10.1002/0471249688.ch2

Bannick, M. S., Shao, J., Liu, J., Du, Y., Yi, Y., & Ye, T. (2023). A general form of covariate adjustment in randomized clinical trials (arXiv:2306.10213). arXiv. https://doi.org/10.48550/arXiv.2306.10213.

Benkeser, D. (2021). drord: Doubly-robust estimators for ordinal outcomes (1.0.1). *Computer software*, https://cran.r-project.org/web/packages/drord/index.html

Benkeser, D., & Hejazi, N. (2017). Survtmle: Compute targeted minimum loss-based estimates in right-censored survival settings (1.0.0). *Computer Software*. https://CRAN.R-project.org/package=survtmle

Benkeser, D., Díaz, I., Luedtke, A., Segal, J., Scharfstein, D., & Rosenblum, M. (2020). Improving precision and power in randomized trials for COVID-19 treatments using covariate adjustment, for binary, ordinal, and time-to-event outcomes. *Biometrics*. https://doi.org/10.1111/biom.13377

Bugni, F. A., Canay, I. A., & Shaikh, A. M. (2018). Inference under covariate-adaptive randomization. *Journal of the American Statistical Association, 113*(524), 1784–1796.

Cassel, C. M., Sarndal, C. E., & Wretman, J. H. (1976). Some results on generalized difference estimation and generalized regression estimation for finite populations. *Biometrika, 63*(3), 615–620. https://doi.org/10.2307/2335742

Chernozhukov, V., Chetverikov, D., Demirer, M., Duflo, E., Hansen, C., Newey, W., & Robins, J. (2017). Double/Debiased Machine Learning for Treatment and Causal Parameters. arXiv. http://arxiv.org/abs/1608.00060

Ciolino, J. D., Palac, H. L., Yang, A., Vaca, M., & Belli, H. M. (2019). Ideal vs. real: A systematic review on handling covariates in randomized controlled trials. *BMC Medical Research Methodology, 19*(1), 136. https://doi.org/10.1186/s12874-019-0787-8

Cohen, P. L., & Fogarty, C. B. (2024). No-harm calibration for generalized Oaxaca–Blinder estimators. *Biometrika, 111*(1), 331–338. https://doi.org/10.1093/biomet/asad036

Daniel, R., Zhang, J., & Farewell, D. (2021). Making apples from oranges: Comparing noncollapsible effect estimators and their standard errors after adjustment for different covariate sets. *Biometrical Journal, 63*(3), 528–557. https://doi.org/10.1002/bimj.201900297

Díaz, I., & Williams, N. (2021). adjrct: Efficient estimators for survival and ordinal outcomes in RCTs without proportional hazards and odds assumptions (0.1.0). *Computer Software*. https://github.com/nt-williams/adjrct

Díaz, I., Colantuoni, E., & Rosenblum, M. (2016). Enhanced precision in the analysis of randomized trials with ordinal outcomes. *Biometrics, 72*(2), 422–431. https://doi.org/10.1111/biom.12450

Díaz, I., Colantuoni, E., Hanley, D. F., & Rosenblum, M. (2019). Improved precision in the analysis of randomized trials with survival outcomes, without assuming proportional hazards. *Lifetime Data Analysis, 25*(3), 439–468. https://doi.org/10.1007/s10985-018-9428-5

EMA. (2015). Guideline on adjustment for baseline covariates in clinical trials.

FDA. (2023). Adjusting for covariates in randomized clinical trials for drugs and biological products. https://www.fda.gov/regulatory-information/search-fda-guidance-documents/adjusting-covariates-randomized-clinical-trials-drugs-and-biological-products

Gail, M. H., Tan, W. Y., & Piantadosi, S. (1988). Tests for no treatment effect in randomized clinical trials. *Biometrika, 75*(1), 57–64. https://doi.org/10.1093/biomet/75.1.57

Guo, K., & Basse, G. (2023). The generalized oaxaca-blinder estimator. *Journal of the American Statistical Association, 118*(541), 524–536.

Hernán, M. A. (2010). The hazards of hazard ratios. *Epidemiology, 21*(1), 13–15.

Hernán, M. A., & Robins, J. M. (2023). *Causal Inference*. CRC Press.

ICH. (2019). ICH E9(R1) addendum on estimands and sensitivity analysis in clinical tri-als to the guideline on statistical principles for clinical trials. Step 4 document available at www.ich.org.

ICH. (2021). E9(R1) training material. Available at www.ich.org

Juraska, M., Gilbert, with contributions from P. B., Lu, X., Zhang, M., Davidian, M., & Tsiatis, A. A. (2022). speff2trial: Semiparametric efficient estimation for a two-sample treatment effect (1.0.5) *Computer software*, https://cran.r-project.org/web/packages/speff2trial/index.html

Juszczak, E., Altman, D. G., Hopewell, S., & Schulz, K. (2019). Reporting of multiarm parallel-group randomized trials: Extension of the consort 2010 statement. *Journal of the American Medical Association, 321*(16), 1610–1620.

Kahan, B. C., & Morris, T. P. (2012). Improper analysis of trials randomised using stratified blocks or minimisation. *Statistics in Medicine, 31*(4), 328–340.

Li, X., Li, S., & Luedtke, A. (2023). Estimating the efficiency gain of covariate-adjusted analyses in future clinical trials using external data. *Journal of the Royal Statistical Society Series B: Statistical Methodology, 85*(2), 356–377.

Lin, W. (2013). Agnostic notes on regression adjustments to experimental data: Reexamining Freedman's critique. *The Annals of Applied Statistics, 7*(1), 295–318. https://doi.org/10.1214/12-AOAS583

Little, R. J., & Rubin, D. B. (2019). *Statistical analysis with missing data*. John Wiley & Sons.

Lu, X., & Tsiatis, A. A. (2008). Improving the efficiency of the log-rank test using auxiliary covariates. *Biometrika, 95*(3), 679–694.

Matts, J. P., & Lachin, J. M. (1988). Properties of permuted-block randomization in clinical trials. *Controlled Clinical Trials, 9*(4), 327–344.

Moore, K. L., & van der Laan, M. J. (2009). Increasing power in randomized trials with right censored outcomes through covariate adjustment. *Journal of Biopharmaceutical Statistics, 19*(6), 1099–1131. https://doi.org/10.1080/10543400903243017
Morris, T. P., Walker, A. S., Williamson, E. J., & White, I. R. (2022). Planning a method for covariate adjustment in individually randomised trials: A practical guide. *Trials, 23*(1), 328.
Proschan, M. A., Leifer, E., & Liu, Q. (2005). Adaptive regression. *Journal of Biopharmaceutical statistics, 15*(4), 593–603.
Robins, J. (1986). A new approach to causal inference in mortality studies with a sustained exposure period—Application to control of the healthy worker survivor effect. *Mathematical Modelling, 7*(9), 1393–1512. https://doi.org/10.1016/0270-0255(86)90088-6
Robins, J. M., Rotnitzky, A., & Zhao, L. P. (1994). Estimation of regression coefficients when some regressors are not always observed. *Journal of the American Statistical Association, 89*(427), 846–866. https://doi.org/10.2307/2290910
Rosenblum, M., & Steingrimsson, J. (2016). *Matching the efficiency gains of the logistic regression estimator while avoiding its interpretability problems, in randomized trials*. Johns Hopkins University, Dept. of Biostatistics Working Papers. https://biostats.bepress.com/jhubiostat/paper281
Rosenblum, M., & van der Laan, M. J. (2009). Using regression models to analyze randomized trials: Asymptotically valid hypothesis tests despite incorrectly specified models. *Biometrics, 65*(3), 937–945. https://doi.org/10.1111/j.1541-0420.2008.01177.x
Rubin, D. B. (2004). *Multiple imputation for nonresponse in surveys* (Vol. 81). John Wiley & Sons, Ltd.
Schafer, J. L. (1997). *Analysis of incomplete multivariate data*. CRC Press.
Senn, S. J. (1989). Covariate imbalance and random allocation in clinical trials. *Statistics in Medicine, 8*(4), 467–475.
Shao, J., Yu, X., & Zhong, B. (2010). A theory for testing hypotheses under covariate-adaptive randomization. *Biometrika, 97*(2), 347–360. https://doi.org/10.1093/biomet/asq014
Shen, C., Li, X., & Li, L. (2014). Inverse probability weighting for covariate adjustment in randomized studies. *Statistics in Medicine, 33*(4), 555–568.
Simon, R., & Simon, N. R. (2011). Using randomization tests to preserve type I error with response-adaptive and covariate-adaptive randomization. *Statistics and Probability Letters, 81*(7), 767–772.
Sjölander, A., Dahlqwist, E., & Zetterqvist, J. (2016). A note on the noncollapsibility of rate differences and rate ratios. *Epidemiology, 27*(3), 356–359.
Song, Y., Hughes, J. P., & Ye, T. (2024). Adjusting for incomplete baseline covariates in randomized controlled trials: a crossworld imputation framework. *Biometrics, 80*(3). https://doi.org/10.1093/biomtc/ujae094
Taves, D. R. (1974). Minimization: A new method of assigning patients to treatment and control groups. *Clinical Pharmacology & Therapeutics, 15*(5), 443–453. https://doi.org/10.1002/cpt1974155443
Taves, D. R. (2010). The use of minimization in clinical trials. *Contemporary Clinical Trials, 31*(2), 180–184. https://doi.org/10.1016/j.cct.2009.12.005
Tsiatis, A. A., & Davidian, M. (2022). Group sequential methods for interim monitoring of randomized clinical trials with timelagged outcome. Statistics in Medicine, 41(28), 5517–5536. https://doi.org/10.1002/sim.9580
Tsiatis, A. A., Davidian, M., Zhang, M., & Lu, X. (2008). Covariate adjustment for two-sample treatment comparisons in randomized clinical trials: A principled yet flexible approach. *Statistics in Medicine, 27*(23), 4658–4677. https://doi.org/10.1002/sim.3113
Uno, H., Claggett, B., Tian, L., Inoue, E., Gallo, P., Miyata, T., et al. (2014). Moving beyond the hazard ratio in quantifying the between-group difference in survival analysis. *Journal of Clinical Oncology, 32*(22), 2380.
Van Der Laan, M. J., & Rose, S. (2011). *Targeted learning: Causal inference for observational and experimental data*. Springer. https://doi.org/10.1007/978-1-4419-9782-1

Van Lancker, K., Betz, J. F., & Rosenblum, M. (2025). Combining covariate adjustment with group sequential, informationadaptive designs to improve randomized trial efficiency. *Biometrics, 81*(1). https://doi.org/10.1093/biomtc/ujaf020

Van Lancker, K., Bretz, F., & Dukes, O. (2024). Covariate adjustment in randomized controlled trials: General concepts and practical considerations. *Clinical Trials, 21*(4), 399–411.

Van Lancker, K., Díaz, I., & Vansteelandt, S. (2024). Automated, efficient and model-free inference for randomized clinical trials via data-driven covariate adjustment. arXiv preprint arXiv:2404.11150.

Vansteelandt, S., & Keiding, N. (2011). Invited commentary: G-computation–lost in translation? *American Journal of Epidemiology, 173*(7), 739–742.

Wang, B., Susukida, R., Mojtabai, R., Amin-Esmaeili, M., & Rosenblum, M. (2023). Model-robust inference for clinical trials that improve precision by stratified randomization and covariate adjustment. *Journal of the American Statistical Association, 118*(542), 1152–1163.

Williams, N., Rosenblum, M., & Díaz, I. (2022). Optimising precision and power by machine learning in randomised trials with ordinal and time-to-event outcomes with an application to COVID-19. *Journal of the Royal Statistical Society. Series A, (Statistics in Society).* https://doi.org/10.1111/rssa.12915

Williamson, E. J., Forbes, A., & White, I. R. (2014). Variance reduction in randomised trials by inverse probability weighting using the propensity score. *Statistics in Medicine, 33*(5), 721–737.

Yang, L., & Tsiatis, A. A. (2001). Efficiency study of estimators for a treatment effect in a pretest-posttest trial. *The American Statistician, 55*(4), 314–321.

Ye, T., & Shao, J. (2020). Robust tests for treatment effect in survival analysis under covariate-adaptive randomization. *Journal of the Royal Statistical Society: Series B (Statistical Methodology), 82*(5), 1301–1323. https://doi.org/10.1111/rssb.12392

Ye, T., Shao, J., Yi, Y., & Zhao, Q. (2022). Toward better practice of covariate adjustment in analyzing randomized clinical trials. *Journal of the American Statistical Association*, 1–13. https://doi.org/10.1080/01621459.2022.2049278

Ye, T., Bannick, M., Yi, Y., & Bian, F. (2023a). RobinCar: Robust estimation and inference for covariate-adaptive randomization (0.1.0) [R]. https://doi.org/10.5281/zenodo.8216051.

Ye, T., Bannick, M., Yi, Y., & Shao, J. (2023b). Robust variance estimation for covariate-adjusted unconditional treatment effect in randomized clinical trials with binary outcomes. *Statistical Theory and Related Fields, 7*(2), 159–163. https://doi.org/10.1080/24754269.2023.2205802

Ye, T., Shao, J., & Yi, Y. (2023c). Covariate-adjusted log-rank test: Guaranteed efficiency gain and universal applicability. *Biometrika, asad045*. https://doi.org/10.1093/biomet/asad045

Zhang, M. (2015). Robust methods to improve efficiency and reduce bias in estimating survival curves in randomized clinical trials. *Lifetime Data Analysis, 21*(1), 119–137. https://doi.org/10.1007/s10985-014-9291-y

Zhang, M., Tsiatis, A. A., & Davidian, M. (2008). Improving efficiency of inferences in randomized clinical trials using auxiliary covariates. *Biometrics, 64*(3), 707–715. https://doi.org/10.1111/j.1541-0420.2007.00976.x

Zhao, A., & Ding, P. (2022). To adjust or not to adjust? Estimating the average treatment effect in randomized experiments with missing covariates. *Journal of the American Statistical Association*, 1–11. https://doi.org/10.1080/01621459.2022.2123814

Zhong, Y., Kennedy, E. H., Bodnar, L. M., & Naimi, A. I. (2021). AIPW: An R package for augmented inverse probability–weighted estimation of average causal effects. *American Journal of Epidemiology, 190*(12), 2690–2699. https://doi.org/10.1093/aje/kwab207

Part V
Leveraging the Estimand Framework in Diverse Clinical Trial Settings

The final part of this book explores the application of the estimand framework across a range of clinical trial settings. It begins with an introduction to integrated evidence planning, including its use in early-phase development and its relevance for safety and benefit–risk assessments. The discussion further demonstrates the role of estimands in observational studies and the generation of real-world evidence. This part also discusses the relationship between the estimand framework and the patient, intervention, comparison, outcome (PICO) framework commonly used in health technology assessments when defining research questions related to the effectiveness, costs, and the broader impact of health care interventions. Moreover, this part of the book discusses the implementation of estimands in varied trial designs, including non-inferiority and equivalence trials, complex innovative designs, multiregional clinical trials, complex treatment regimens, and decentralized clinical trials. The final chapter presents strategies for handling disruptions to clinical trials, illustrating the flexibility and adaptability of the estimand framework in response to unexpected events, such as the COVID-19 pandemic.

Chapter 21
Leveraging the Estimand Framework for Integrated Evidence Planning

Wentian Guo, Lisa V. Hampson, Rima Izem, Alice Wang, Na Yang, Qiong Du, Chen Lu, and Jonathan M. Siegel

Abstract This chapter explores the application of the estimand framework beyond single-trial efficacy assessments, emphasizing its potential role in integrated evidence planning for drug marketing evaluations, which involves various types of clinical data from various development phases as well as real-world data. By doing so, it aims to enhance the integration of evidence across development programs and inform health authority decisions on benefits and risks. Particularly, the chapter discusses the challenges and benefits of using the estimand framework to formalize clinical questions in early-phase exploratory studies, safety evaluations, and real-world evidence studies. To this end, the chapter is structured into sections focusing on early drug development, safety and benefit-risk assessments, observational studies and real-world evidence, and comparisons between estimands and the population, intervention, control, or comparator, and outcome (PICO) framework.

W. Guo (✉) · A. Wang
Biometrics, R&D, AstraZeneca, Shanghai, China
e-mail: wentian.guo@astrazeneca.com; alice.wang2@astrazeneca.com

L. V. Hampson · R. Izem
Advanced Methodology and Data Sciences/Statistical Methodology, Novartis Pharma AG, Basel, Switzerland
e-mail: lisa.hampson@novartis.com; rima.izem@novartis.com

N. Yang
Evidence Generation and Decision Sciences, Sanofi, Beijing, China
e-mail: na3.yang@sanofi.com

Q. Du
China Biometrics, ClinChoice, Shanghai, China
e-mail: Qiong.Du@ClinChoice.com

C. Lu
Global Biostatistical Science, Amgen, Thousand Oaks, CA, USA
e-mail: chelu@amgen.com

J. M. Siegel
Clinical Statistics, Bayer US LLC, Whippany, NJ, USA
e-mail: Jonathan.siegel@bayer.com

J. Wei et al. (eds.), *Estimands in Clinical Trials*, Springer Series in Pharmaceutical Statistics, https://doi.org/10.1007/978-3-032-02192-2_21

21.1 Introduction

The chapters in Part 2–4 focus on efficacy assessments within one trial under the estimand framework. However, a drug marketing evaluation will be based on the totality of evidence accumulated on benefits and risks rather than the demonstration of efficacy in a single or even multiple studies. Potential sources of evidence include clinical data from different development phases, including early-phase studies, and real-world data relevant to the experimental drug, the standard of care, and/or the natural history of the intended indication. Applying the estimand framework more broadly and using it to formalize clinical questions other than the efficacy objectives of confirmatory trials is less straightforward, and there is a lack of guidelines, publications, and applications to inform practice. However, utilizing this framework can enhance the thinking process in these settings, enabling users to formalize clinical questions in early-phase exploratory studies or safety evaluations and streamline efficacy objectives in real-world evidence studies. Therefore, the use of the estimand framework can further facilitate the integration of evidence across the development program and better inform health authority decision-making on benefits and risks. In this chapter, we introduce the concepts, possibilities, and obstacles of applying the estimand framework in these settings.

The chapter is structured as follows. Section 21.2 focuses on estimand considerations in early drug development. Section 21.3 discusses the unique points to be considered for safety estimands beyond what has already been discussed for efficacy evaluations, including extensions to benefit-risk assessments based on integrated efficacy and safety data. Section 21.4 discusses the application of the estimand framework for evidence generation in non-randomized studies such as observational studies or single-arm studies with external control arms, which often involve real-world data. The target trial framework for real-world evidence generation and its link to the estimand framework are also discussed in Sect. 21.4. Section 21.5 gives a concise comparison between the estimand framework and the population, intervention, control or comparator, and outcome (PICO) framework, which is proposed for the construction of clinical questions in the field of evidence-based medicine. Finally, Section 21.6 concludes this chapter with additional remarks.

21.2 Early Drug Development

21.2.1 Background

Clinical drug development generally consists of four stages, often referred to as Phases I through IV. Phase I clinical trials constitute the preliminary stage where the investigational product is first administered to humans. These trials primarily aim to explore safety and toxicity, tolerability, pharmacokinetics (PK), pharmacodynamics

(PD), as well as early evaluation of drug mechanism. The scope of these trials encompasses safety (especially in first-in-human trials), drug-drug interactions, food effects, proof of mechanism, as well as considerations for special populations, etc. Trial design is typically flexible and may include open-label with dose escalation, open-label, baseline-controlled, randomized, and double-blind designs, as well as parallel or crossover designs.

Clinical research in Phase II primarily focuses on the efficacy of treatment (Phase IIa) and dose finding (Phase IIb) in the specified patient population. The primary objective of a Phase IIa study is to evaluate the efficacy of the drug as well as its safety; it aims to provide an initial understanding of how effectively the drug works. Phase IIb studies aim to determine the drug's dose-effect relationship for the target indication (ICH, 1994). Trial designs can vary in complexity and "range from simple parallel group designs to more complex variants" (ICH, 2021). Complex designs include randomized, placebo-controlled studies; adaptive designs; master protocols; or platform designs to evaluate the efficacy and safety of drug treatment for specific indications.

The clinical drug development stages presented in this section are not necessarily absolute or set in stone. As stated in ICH (2021): "Although clinical drug development is often described as consisting of four temporal phases (Phases I–IV), it is important to appreciate that the phase concept is a description and not a requirement, and that the phases of drug development may overlap or be combined." For example, due to the irreversible toxicity associated with oncology drugs, first-in-human trials will begin with dose escalation within the target population and then continue with further exploration of dose safety and efficacy using expansion cohorts.

This section mainly focuses on the estimand considerations in phase I and II clinical trials. Relative to their application in confirmatory trials, the integration of the estimand framework in early development is still a developing field. The upcoming subsection will summarize current considerations pertinent to this usage.

21.2.2 Estimand Considerations

In early exploratory PK/PD studies, the recommended trial population is healthy subjects if drug toxicity permits. The primary analysis population is either the PK or PK/PD population, which includes all randomized/enrolled and treated participants with evaluable PK results (PK population) or at least one post-baseline PD measurement in the PK population (PK/PD population). Potential intercurrent events could include dose adjustments, noncompliance with the protocol, or treatment discontinuation.

Akacha et al. (2021) suggested that the estimand framework can be utilized in early-phase clinical trials, especially in clinical studies aiming at building PK/PD models. They have recommended several strategies to address specific intercurrent events that align with the scientific questions being asked. For instance, if intercurrent events such as noncompliance with the protocol result in altered drug concentrations, the hypothetical strategy can be applied. This strategy aims to determine what the outcomes would have been had all subjects adhered to the trial protocol. To evaluate the robustness of results, sensitivity analyses can be conducted with varying assumptions. Different strategies may be more appropriate for addressing other types of intercurrent events, tailored to meet specific scientific questions of interest and the needs of stakeholders like sponsors or regulatory authorities. For example, if the regulatory authority is considering a new dose adjustment scheme for approval, a treatment policy strategy may be appropriate for the intercurrent event of dose adjustment. This strategy would incorporate intercurrent events as a part of the treatment attribute.

Given the characteristics of phase I trials, such as short clinical trial durations, small sample sizes, and a low frequency of intercurrent events, it is advisable to maintain proactive communication with regulatory authorities to discuss the impact of intercurrent events and the appropriateness and methodology for constructing estimands in such scenarios.

In the context of Phase II clinical trials, particularly during the preliminary exploration of target indications, it is recommended to incorporate the estimand framework into the protocol for constructing both the primary and sensitivity analyses. This allows for a thorough exploration of the clinical questions of interest, enabling the selection of appropriate estimands. Collecting data on potential intercurrent events during early-stage trials is crucial for estimating the types, causes, and frequencies of these events. It also facilitates the assessment of each intercurrent event's impact on the interpretation of results, which can inform the design and analysis plans for subsequent clinical trials.

The strategies for addressing intercurrent events in Phase IIa/IIb studies may differ from those applied in later-phase studies, depending on the clinical question of interest. When the focus is on the "pure" treatment effect or the therapeutic effect due to exposure in early development, hypothetical strategies may be more appropriate. Additionally, supplementary analyses may explore other intercurrent event strategies that could be relevant for future confirmatory trials, such as treatment policy strategies. This early exploration of different estimands provides robust support for the development of estimands for subsequent Phase III clinical trials. In the field of oncology, particularly in early clinical development, Phase Ib or Phase II non-randomized open-label single-arm clinical trials may serve as the basis for registration. Englert et al. (2023) have provided further discussion on the application of the estimand framework within this context.

21.3 Safety and Benefit-Risk Assessments

21.3.1 Background

Assessing a medical product's safety in a development lifecycle is multifactorial, with a broad set of clinical questions. Safety outcomes include but are not limited to adverse events (AEs), laboratory test results, vital signs, physical examinations, electrocardiogram (ECG) data, and quality of life data. Also important for safety evaluations are study medication doses and duration, study medication interruption and discontinuation, and concomitant medications (Council for International Organizations of Medical Sciences, 2005). Each safety outcome has several dimensions, including frequency, severity, and seriousness; it can be classified as known, anticipated, expected, or unexpected. Safety assessments never end but are integrated as information accrues, with, for example, signal detection informing signal evaluation, and assessments on biomarkers informing whether future assessment of downstream clinical outcomes is warranted. While the ICH E9(R1) guideline did not reduce the scope of application of the estimand framework to efficacy, the breadth of the safety clinical questions of interest calls into question whether the estimand framework should be used or would be relevant in safety.

This section will discuss the application of the estimand framework in safety in situations where its application is not currently common practice but could shed new light on existing challenges. These situations include clinical studies primarily focused on other (e.g., efficacy) objectives. Therefore, studies with a main specific safety objective are out of scope because there is no ambiguity that the estimand framework principles apply in that situation. Moreover, because safety is not the main design driver of sample size, it is important not only to consider the estimand but also the estimation and testing properties. For example, some studies will not be powered to detect or rule out a risk for some safety estimands, and targeting some estimators may be practically infeasible with rare events or short trials.

While some considerations in this section apply broadly to all safety objectives, the case studies and the benefit-risk subsections will focus on the safety outcomes in confirmatory studies that are critical to the benefit-risk evaluation at marketing authorization (e.g., safety event of special interest or adverse event of special interest (AESI)). Thus, safety signal detection objectives are out of scope of Sect. 21.3.3 and 21.3.4, because they are nonspecific.

Each of the following subsections will share considerations not only on the safety estimand but also on its estimation. Because the current practice of collecting and reporting on safety does not explicitly state the target estimands and focuses on estimation, reflecting on the implications of a specific estimand choice as compared to current practice (estimators) can help bridge the gap from current to future practice and illustrate potential new estimands and estimators in safety.

21.3.2 Estimand Considerations

Despite the complexity of safety evaluation, the estimand thinking process is still relevant. In current practice, safety estimands are not explicitly stated in protocols and analysis plans. Thus, the following subsections discuss considerations for each attribute of the safety estimand as well as its estimation and, where relevant, compare the safety estimand with the efficacy estimand driving the trial design. Also, relevant considerations of currently used safety estimators are discussed with respect to each estimand attribute. While we discuss these attributes separately for simplicity, some of the concepts overlap and, regardless of how considerations are raised, serve the ultimate goal of refining the question of interest.

21.3.2.1 Population

In general, we expect the population attribute for each safety estimand to be the same as the efficacy estimand driving the trial because we typically want a trial to evaluate risks and benefits of the experimental intervention in the same population. Nevertheless, as for the efficacy estimand, the definition of the population attribute for each safety estimand should ultimately reflect the clinical question that needs to be answered. In addition, intercurrent event strategies can impact the definition of population, which will be further discussed in Sect. 21.3.2.4.

21.3.2.2 Treatment

The treatment attribute of the safety estimand defines the main comparison of interest and would also be generally expected to be the same as for the main efficacy estimand. As for the population attribute, different strategies of intercurrent events, for example, different strategies to address nonstart of treatment or a change in therapy, could further refine the treatment attribute in a comparison and introduce differences between efficacy and safety evaluations. This will be illustrated in Sect. 21.3.2.4.

21.3.2.3 Variable

The variable attribute will be specific to each safety objective and will typically differ from the variable attribute in efficacy. The variable attribute in safety would ideally include not only the safety outcome but also the time of assessment. For example, the variable of interest evaluating an AESI endpoint during a timeframe of interest post-study entry can be the occurrence or nonoccurrence of the event, time to the first event, or number of events within a patient if the event is recurring.

Similarly, for laboratory data, the variable of interest can be changed from baseline at a certain posttreatment time, maximum change from baseline during the trial, or an indicator of whether the laboratory value ever exceeded a prespecified range during the trial.

As we discuss in Sects. 21.3.2.4 and 21.3.2.6, the choice of the timeframe of interest is sometimes implicit, and different intercurrent event strategies would lead to different design strategies for follow-up in a given clinical trial.

21.3.2.4 Intercurrent Events

The terminology of intercurrent events is not commonly used in safety. Nevertheless, current practice in safety monitoring in clinical trials implicitly emphasizes the intercurrent event of treatment initiation and either treatment discontinuation or end of exposure for all safety outcomes.

More broadly, when applying the estimand thinking to safety questions of interest, the list of potential intercurrent events for safety shares commonalities with those for efficacy. This list would include nonstart of treatment, treatment discontinuation, exposure to rescue medication or exposure to concomitant medication, and/or death. However, for the same intercurrent event, the adopted strategy may differ in safety and efficacy. The strategy will have implications for the design and duration of assessment of safety outcomes as well as analyses, estimation, and interpretation. There is no one-size-fits-all strategy for addressing intercurrent events, and it is best to select a fit-for-purpose strategy that reflects each clinical question of interest. As with efficacy, the choice of intercurrent event strategy can help refine earlier attributes of the estimand, such as population, treatment, and variable.

For example, the treatment policy strategy may be meaningful for the use of rescue medication as an intercurrent event when this medication is considered part of the treatment regimen along with the test drug in clinical practice. Similarly, if the treatment attribute includes any delay between assignment to the regimen and exposure to the test drug, then using a treatment policy to address nonstart of treatment may be meaningful. Conversely, a treatment policy strategy may be harder to justify for treatment discontinuation or the nonstart of treatment if the causal association between exposure and outcome is of primary clinical interest and unexposed patients are not at risk for the safety outcome. In such cases, we may only be interested in those who actually initiate the drug for safety evaluations and adopt a principal stratum strategy for the nonstart of treatment with the population defined as the stratum of patients who would actually take the assigned drug under both experimental and control arms (Kahan et al., 2023). See also Chap. 19 for principal stratification.

In addition, the composite strategy can be a meaningful way to address the intercurrent event of death for several safety objectives, thereby changing the variable from the safety variable alone to a composite of the safety variable and death. The while alive strategy, or, alternatively, considering the principal stratum of those who would be alive regardless of treatment received, may also be reasonable if the clinical question regards the safety evaluation while patients are alive, and death is a priori unrelated to treatment.

The latency of the safety outcome relative to the initial or the cumulative exposure can guide the choice between the while on treatment, hypothetical, and treatment policy strategies. For example, for AEs with short latency, which are expected to occur shortly after initial exposure (e.g., prophylaxis), a while on treatment strategy would be meaningful. Conversely, for long-latency AEs, the treatment policy strategy may be a better fit, as it considers a longer time period for the causal effect to be observed. The trial design to align with this latter strategy requires monitoring the AE beyond the end of treatment. Finally, a hypothetical strategy would be meaningful to investigate long-term safety outcomes beyond the intercurrent event had the intercurrent event not occurred. This strategy may require assumptions about patterns of variation over time of the variable and any potential association between the intercurrent event and the outcome of interest.

21.3.2.5 Population-Level Summary

Different population-level summaries can also result in different estimands even for a specific variable and intercurrent event strategy. For example, for the incidence of the AE variable, the population-level summary for each treatment arm can be the proportion of AE occurrence (or crude incidence rate) or exposure-adjusted incidence rate (EAIR) (Zhou et al., 2015). For the comparison of two treatments, the population-level summary can be the difference of proportions, the odds ratio, the relative risk, or the hazard ratio. Deciding among different between-arm population-level summaries is not so important when the (background) incidence rate of a safety event is low. That is because for rare safety events, the odds ratio, rate ratio, and hazard ratio are asymptotically equivalent measures, and the tests based on those estimates will also be asymptotically the same.

While the difference of proportions and the odds ratio do not adjust for the follow-up time, the relative risk and hazard ratio do. Therefore, when addressing treatment discontinuation using the while on treatment strategy, using the proportion of AE occurrence as the summary measure may be challenging to interpret if the time to treatment discontinuation differs between treatment arms. Similarly, the use of relative risk may be challenging to interpret when the hazard is not constant, and the use of hazard ratio is challenging when the hazard ratio is not constant or there are important competing risks. As mentioned in the intercurrent events subsection, the while alive strategy may sometimes be reasonable for death. In this situation, if the risk of death differs between arms, we can regard death as an important competing event and use estimators from multistate/competing risk models for a better fit-for-purpose interpretation (Unkel et al., 2019; Rufibach, 2019; Siegel et al., 2022). See also Chap. 18 for a discussion of time-to-event endpoints.

21.3.2.6 Estimation

As with the efficacy estimands, estimation methods should be aligned with the target safety estimands with reasonable assumptions. In current practice, the safety analysis set typically includes all exposed rather than all randomized patients and therefore could lead to a mismatch between the analysis sets for safety and efficacy if some randomized patients do not initiate the therapy they were randomized to, although the mismatch generally remains minimal (Wang et al., 2023). As mentioned in Kahan et al. (2023), the estimator that excludes nonstarters of treatment from the safety set is unbiased for a principal stratum estimand under the assumption that the nonstart of treatment is not affected by the assigned treatment arm, that is, patients who initiate treatment in one arm would also do so in the other arm (i.e., if someone began the investigational arm, they would also have begun the control arm, and vice versa).

Current safety estimates are not described using the estimand framework but rather reported as either "on-treatment," if events are assessed from treatment initiation to the end of exposure, or as "on-study" if events are assessed from treatment initiation to the end of the assessment period for all patients in the trial (Duke-Margolis FDA workshop, 2022). For example, for the summary measure of hazard ratio, the on-treatment analysis censors follow-up at the end of exposure without any adjustments for censoring. This analysis implicitly targets either the while on treatment strategy or the hypothetical strategy for the intercurrent event of the end of exposure. Nevertheless, because the on-treatment analysis is often linked to short-term follow-up, the implicit target estimand is more closely aligned with the while on treatment strategy than the hypothetical strategy. In contrast, the on-study analysis does not censor follow-up at the end of exposure and implicitly targets the treatment policy strategy for the intercurrent event of treatment discontinuation. Whether the on-treatment or the on-study analyses are more clinically meaningful in safety is a source of debate. For example, Yang et al. (2019) warned about the limitations of on-treatment analyses, while DeMets and Cook (2019) argued for the use of on-study analyses in comparative randomized clinical trials. They illustrated these opinions with several examples that we will summarize in Sect. 21.3.3.

21.3.3 Case Study

In this section, we illustrate the debate between on-study and on-treatment estimates with two published case studies. While we discuss estimation rather than estimands in this section, these debates are helpful to consider when defining a meaningful clinical estimand in safety.

The randomized clinical trial (SAVOR) results reported in Yang et al. (2019) illustrated a case where on-treatment analyses indicated higher harm to survival than on-study analyses. This trial was a 1:1 randomized clinical trial in Type 2 diabetes mellitus comparing the cardiovascular risk of saxagliptin to placebo. This was an event-driven trial, and patients were followed for an average of 3 years. The on-treatment periods varied in mean duration between the arms, with the placebo arm having more treatment discontinuation early due to the occurrence of life-threatening events. Because of the depletion of those susceptible to experiencing death in the placebo arm compared with the saxagliptin arm, an on-treatment comparison showed higher mortality on saxagliptin, with the hazard ratio exceeding 1.18 when the treatment period included 30 days beyond treatment and a larger hazard ratio for shorter gaps. However, the hazard ratio from an on-study analysis, which included the off-placebo and on-rescue period for those who discontinued the placebo arm as well as the off-treatment period for those who discontinued the saxagliptin arm did not show an excess risk for saxagliptin. The two estimators were targeting different estimands, so it is not surprising that they differ. Yet, under the null hypothesis of no excess risk, whether short-term or long-term, both hazard ratios should be close to one. The reason they are not may have more to do with differential treatment discontinuation and how to account for the use of rescue therapy in the comparison than with excess risk in one arm.

On-treatment and on-study analyses of mortality in the APPROVE trial of rofecoxib versus placebo for cancer prevention, discussed in DeMets and Cook (2019), not only differed but also showed a different pattern of change in risk over time. The clinical trial had originally stopped monitoring adverse events 14 days after treatment discontinuation. The on-treatment analyses of mortality showed the risk of rofecoxib kicked in only beyond 18 months posttreatment initiation. Adding survival information from off-treatment periods and up to a year in on-study analyses showed an increased risk of rofecoxib that kicked in immediately after randomization without a delay of 18 months. In this example also, the two analyses were targeting different estimands. However, the longer-term on-study assessment changed the interpretation of the findings for the shorter-term risk. Therefore, describing one estimand, while on treatment, as more suitable for short-term evaluation and another estimand, treatment policy, as more suitable for long-term evaluation, as we did in Sect. 21.3.2.4, is a simplification.

Moreover, the anturane reinfarction trial results reported in DeMets and Cook (2019) led to different conclusions depending on whether on-treatment or on-study analyses were used, making it difficult to assess the benefit of sulfinpyrazone relative to placebo for preventing recurrence of a myocardial infarction in those who experienced a recent myocardial infarction.

As both publications pointed out, the choice of estimand can have consequences on the design of when safety outcomes are collected. Therefore, if the target estimand corresponds to a while on treatment strategy, then safety outcomes may not be collected after a prespecified interval following treatment discontinuation, which would make estimating the on-study estimate impossible after the trial is completed. Although the Type 2 diabetes trial SAVOR had planned on an on-treatment analysis, following events past treatment discontinuation allowed the sponsor to discover a potential depletion of susceptibles issue in interpreting the on-study estimate and informed post hoc analyses targeting other estimands. Similarly, amendments to the APPROVE trial protocol and additional data collections were needed to evaluate the longer-term risk of rofecoxib that changed the results observed for shorter time periods.

21.3.4 Benefit-Risk Estimands

The initial marketing approval, as well as post-marketing regulatory and payer decisions, relies on an evaluation of the benefit-risk profile of the medicine. We focus in this section on the evaluation of benefit-risk by the sponsor when submitting a new or supplemental drug or biologic application for regulatory approval.

There are two possible approaches for evaluating benefit-risk (Wang et al., 2023). The first and most common approach, the population-based benefit-risk assessment, evaluates multiple target estimands, one for each benefit or each risk question of interest, and reports the resulting estimates separately. For example, the label for rivaroxaban, an antiplatelet therapy, shows results for stroke prevention (an efficacy outcome) as well as bleeding risk (a safety outcome) separately. These analyses considered the first event that occurred, with the occurrence of one event censoring follow-up for the other event.

The choice of estimand attribute is tailored to the benefit or risk question, although the more similar the choice of attribute, the easier it is to compare benefits and risks side-by-side. For example, the attributes of population and treatment are typically defined similarly for benefits and risks in population-level benefit-risk assessments. Some intercurrent events (e.g., end of exposure) are also relevant for both efficacy and safety variables, and one can choose to address them similarly in population-level benefit-risk assessments. Nevertheless, because efficacy and safety outcomes rely on different variable attributes with potentially different assessment timings, the list of intercurrent events can differ between safety and efficacy. Also, the cause or the consequence of an intercurrent event may have different implications for safety than efficacy (e.g., taking a concomitant medication to mitigate a safety outcome). Therefore, on the one hand, restricting the list of intercurrent events and how to address them to be the same for safety as efficacy may be overly restrictive and limit the interpretation of each estimand. On the other hand, using different strategies for efficacy and safety may impair the interpretability of the comparison of one with the other. Thus, one has to balance tailoring the estimand to the safety question with comparability to the efficacy estimand for a meaningful population-based benefit-risk assessment.

The second approach, the patient-level benefit-risk assessment, evaluates the multivariate distribution of benefit and risk and summarizes this distribution at the patient level. These types of analyses answer the question of "what is the effect of the drug on those patients who can tolerate it?" and "What are the long-term safety effects on those patients who continue taking the drug because it is effective?" In these approaches, the multivariate distribution could be summarized, and the benefit-risk evaluation could focus on the proportion of those patients who benefit without harm (Chuang-Stein, 1994). In this summary, all benefits are considered together, and all harms are considered together. The method can give equal weight to benefits and harms or weigh them differently. Alternatively, one can use win-ratio-type statistics (Dong et al., 2018), considering a sequence of benefit and harm outcomes after pairing patients in the treatment arm with those in the control arm to determine winners and losers in each pair relative to the benefit-risk consideration. In practice, prioritizing outcomes, including both benefits and risks, in a sequence and handling ties may be challenging in the win ratio (Brunner et al., 2021). In these analyses, the attributes of the estimand and more particularly the type of intercurrent events and how to address them need to consider the list of all benefits and risk outcomes for each patient.

21.3.5 Summary

This section discusses the status quo of safety estimators, consideration of safety estimands, and the connection between the estimands and the currently used estimators. The difference between the safety and efficacy estimands driving the trial design is also discussed extensively. The estimand framework while not currently used is clearly applicable to safety planning and reporting. Using the estimand framework in safety will not resolve the common debates in safety around what variables to focus on, what timeframe of interest to consider, or what summary measure to use in comparative analyses. However, explicit elicitation of each attribute through the estimand framework clarifies the target of inference and aligns safety monitoring and estimation to that target. This is achieved by considering the specificity of the intercurrent event, the duration of exposure, the latency of these events, and the expected shape of the incidence function.

Therefore, we recommend following the estimand framework for a more comprehensive assessment of each attribute of the estimand, and specifically intercurrent events and how to address them. The benefits include ensuring that safety monitoring in the trial encompasses the timeframe of interest identified in the variable attribute; ensuring that intercurrent events are collected in the case report form and may be mitigated by design; and establishing that the analytical strategy is not a moving target but is justified.

In addition, safety evaluations need to consider integrating evidence from multiple sources. The product development life cycle involves multiple data sources (Ball et al., 2020), including preclinical data, clinical data, spontaneous adverse event reports, and real-world data after approval. How to define a proper safety estimand for aggregating different sources of information remains a challenging topic. More discussions about such estimands for real-world data can be found in Sect. 21.4.

21.4 Observational Studies and Real-World Evidence

21.4.1 Background

Real-world evidence studies (RWS) have received much recent attention due to their potential to accelerate the clinical drug development process and advance patient access to effective and safe medicines. Several health authorities have released guidelines related to real-world data (RWD), real-world evidence (RWE), and RWS design; see Sect. 14.3 for references to these. Generally speaking, RWD sources take the form of "nonexperimental data" (Franklin & Schneeweiss, 2017) that are either generated with the intention of addressing prespecified research question(s); or that are captured originally with one objective in mind (often to inform insurance billing or to document patient care) but which are then repurposed to address a research question (Franklin & Schneeweiss, 2017; Levenson et al., 2023). In this section, we will adopt the nomenclature of the European Medicines Agency (EMA) Data Quality Framework to refer to these two types of RWD as "primary-use" and "secondary-use," respectively (EMA, 2023). Note that the re-evaluation of secondary-use data can be preplanned (as it would be in a pragmatic randomized controlled trial) or can occur at a later time point to answer a post hoc clinical question.

There are many potential applications of RWE in both the pre- and post-approval settings. For example, RWE can be used to inform the design of drug development programs, as well as the design, conduct, and analysis methods of individual clinical trials through an improved understanding of disease epidemiology and natural history and of patient treatment journeys. Use cases that can impact multiple development programs include the identification and/or validation of surrogate outcomes, prognostic factors, or effect modifiers. At the level of an individual trial, RWE can be used to verify the assumptions underpinning a sample size calculation. One application that has generated much interest is the use of RWE to address causal questions about treatment efficacy or safety. The resulting RWE may be used by sponsors to inform internal decisions, such as whether or not to launch the next clinical trial in a drug development program, or by health authorities to support decisions on approval or reimbursement.

Several workflows have been proposed for guiding trial design, analysis, and reportage, which begin with clarifying the question of interest; see, for example, the Causal Roadmap (Dang et al., 2023, and references therein), the PRINCIPLED process (Desai et al., 2024), and the estimand framework outlined in the ICH E9(R1) guideline (ICH, 2019). Planning an RWS should therefore start with this step. Chen et al. (2024) presented a framework for defining the estimand(s) for an RWS, characterizing these through the five attributes described in ICH E9(R1). Those authors highlighted that more varied treatment strategies and complex patient journeys are typically expected in RWS, and these should be reflected in the estimand. To limit complexity, however, it may be necessary to restrict attention to a (high-impact) subset of intercurrent events if several are expected (Chen et al., 2024; Hampson et al., 2023). For an RWS aiming to answer a causal question, Canada's Drug and Health Technology Agency (CADTH) Guidance for Reporting Real-World Evidence (CADTH, 2023) recommended first articulating the clinical question to be addressed via the Population, Intervention, Comparator, Outcome, Timing and Setting (PICOTS) framework and then specifying the RWS design and analysis plan to emulate the "target trial" that would address it. See Sect. 21.5 for more information on the PICO framework (Richardson et al., 1995) and its variations. Hernán and Robins (2016) proposed the target trial framework with a view to mitigating the potential biases that may otherwise damage the validity of causal inferences drawn from a non-randomized trial. For example, most RWS do not feature randomization, meaning estimates of causal treatment effects may be biased due to confounding if not adjusted properly.

In slight contrast to other authors (Hernán & Robins, 2016; Hernán et al., 2022), in this section, we consider the target trial framework to comprise three main steps:

1. Specification of the randomized target trial by defining (at a high level) important parts of the protocol of this study.
2. Planning the emulation of the target trial based on fit-for-purpose data and methods.
3. Execution of the emulation and interpretation of the results.

In Step 1, the key sections of the target trial protocol that should be outlined are: eligibility criteria, treatment strategies, method of treatment assignment, outcomes, start and end of follow-up, the causal contrast, and statistical analysis plan (Hernán, 2021). It is important to note that the target trial is a thought experiment; that is, it is a hypothetical study and represents the randomized trial one would perform to obtain an unbiased and consistent estimate of the causal estimand of interest.

There are several constraints on which causal estimands can be formulated within the target trial framework. Firstly, using RWD, it will typically only be possible to target those estimands that could be estimated from open-label, pragmatic, active-controlled randomized trials (Hernán, 2021; Hernán et al., 2022). This is because in routine clinical practice, doctors and patients will be aware of the treatment they are prescribing and receiving, respectively. Secondly, it must be possible to directly estimate the causal estimand through a randomized trial. For example, principal stratum effects, such as the causal effect of treatment in patients who would not experience an adverse event irrespective of treatment assignment, cannot be directly estimated from a randomized experiment (Stensrud & Dukes, 2022) and therefore cannot be considered within the target trial framework. For those causal estimands that could be estimated via a randomized trial, specification of the target trial protocol will result in a clear characterization of the quantity of interest.

For studies based on secondary-use RWD, prior to commencing Step 2 of the target trial framework, investigators will need to identify RWD source(s) that can emulate (at the very least) critical features of the target trial and may access outcome-blind summaries of the data that can inform the design of the emulation. Within Step 2, limitations in the available RWD and other operational or ethical constraints on the RWS design and conduct may result in differences between the target trial and its emulation that must then either be bridged with assumptions or mitigated via sensitivity analyses aligned with the estimand. If a "causal gap" is identified, that is, there are no plausible assumptions under which the "statistical estimand" (a contrast of moments of the observed outcome distributions) will equal the "causal estimand" (a contrast of moments of potential outcome distributions) (Dang et al., 2023), then this may prompt the feasibility of the RWS to be reevaluated. Such identification challenges may also lead investigators to refocus the RWS around a different estimand (Chen et al., 2024).

While the target trial framework was proposed in the setting of observational research and the estimand framework was proposed to align the "planning, design, conduct, analysis and interpretation" (ICH, 2019) of randomized clinical trials, there are many similarities between these two approaches. As noted above, Step 1 of the target trial framework culminates in a detailed definition of the causal quantity of interest, with the target trial protocol capturing, at least to some degree, several of the estimand attributes outlined in the ICH E9(R1) guideline. Intercurrent events and their strategies, however, are not listed in a dedicated section of the target trial protocol, assuming that these will be reflected in other attributes, such as treatment strategies (Hernán & Scharfstein, 2018), population, or outcomes. In practice, however, it may be helpful to broaden the scope of the target trial protocol to feature a component that would detail any intercurrent events and their strategies that cannot be clearly reflected in other attributes (Hampson et al., 2023). On the other hand, there are components of the target trial protocol that go beyond the five estimand attributes defined in ICH E9(R1), such as the time of start of follow-up (commonly referred to as "time zero"). The definition of time zero, that is, the baseline for the outcome variable, brings clarity on an estimand attribute that is critical for RWS (Hernán et al., 2016). However, this attribute would not be explicitly defined within the estimand framework (Hampson et al., 2023) since for randomized controlled trials, time zero is tacitly defined as time of randomization (Hampson et al., 2024). With these potential limitations of the target trial and estimand frameworks in mind, several authors (Hampson et al., 2024; Polito et al., 2024) have considered applying them in tandem to RWS, leveraging clinical trials and secondary-use RWD to draw causal inferences.

Below, we outline a five-step workflow (WF) using the estimand and target trial frameworks to plan the design and analysis of a non-randomized RWS intended to support causal inferences. There are several commonalities between this workflow and those proposed by other authors (for example, Desai et al., 2024; Mishra-Kalyani et al., 2022; Polito et al., 2024). The scope of our proposed workflow could cover the use of a registry to perform a retrospective cohort study (see Sect. 12.7 for more information) or the use of patient-level RWD to contextualize a single-arm trial.

- WF1: Identify the evidence gap and consider how RWE will add value for addressing the clinical question.
- WF2: Carefully and completely characterize the causal effect using the ICH E9(R1) estimand and target trial frameworks.

- WF3: Identify suitable RWD source(s).
- WF4: Formulate the design of the RWS through emulation of the target trial.
- WF5: Devise an analysis plan, with the aim of mitigating potential biases through analyses aligned with the estimand.

As one can see, the workflow starts by defining the clinical question. The estimand is then specified by first defining the estimand attributes per ICH E9(R1); the estimand definition is then further refined by outlining the protocol of the corresponding target trial (articulating "other intercurrent events" not reflected elsewhere in a separate protocol section). This, in turn, is used to drive RWD selection and the design and analysis plan of the RWS by means of a careful emulation of the target trial. In cases where RWD are leveraged for an externally controlled trial, critical elements of the emulation include: (1) how to select the external controls by appropriately defining and applying the target trial eligibility criteria; (2) how to match time of randomization, fulfillment of eligibility criteria, and start of follow-up; and (3) how to plan the RWS analysis so as to emulate randomization. Achieving these will mitigate the risk of confounding and selection bias. Two single-arm studies with external controls are described in the next section to further illustrate the considerations and challenges inherent in applying the target trial and estimand frameworks to generate RWE for causal effects.

21.4.2 RWE Case Studies

This section introduces three case studies of real-world evidence (RWE), which will be the focus of the discussion in Sect. 21.4.3. Due to space limitations, these examples are only briefly described here. For more detailed information, please refer to the references provided in this chapter.

Case Study 1 A hypothetical retrospective RWS to "estimate the effect of postmenopausal hormone therapy on the 5-year risk of breast cancer" (Hernán & Robins, 2016). The data source for this hypothetical study was imagined to be a medical claims database, and the primary objective was to compare the 5-year risk of a breast cancer diagnosis between two treatment strategies: (1) starting and adhering to "estrogen plus progestin hormone therapy" (Hernán & Robins, 2016), with certain exceptions permitted, versus (2) abstaining from hormone therapy. The population of the target trial was "postmenopausal women within 5 years of menopause between the years 2005 and 2010 and with no history of cancer and no use of hormone therapy in the past 2 years" (Hernán & Robins, 2016). This case study was used by Hernán and Robins (2016) to illustrate the considerations and potential challenges one might encounter when emulating a target trial.

Case Study 2 An RWD-based external control arm was retrospectively created in support of the New Drug Application (NDA) for Selinexor for late-line "patients with relapsed/refractory multiple myeloma" (FDA, 2019). The Flatiron Health

Analytics Database (FHAD), containing information derived from electronic health records, was used to obtain patient-level external controls for a single-arm trial (STORM Part 2; Chari et al., 2019). The primary objective was to compare these two cohorts with respect to overall survival. No documentation for this indirect comparison (such as the analysis plan) was shared with the U.S. Food and Drug Administration (FDA) ahead of time, as mentioned by their multidisciplinary review document (FDA, 2019). FDA's review examines the data and statistical methods used by the sponsor and highlights concerns with the FHAD selection criteria and time zero definition. These will be elaborated on in the next subsection.

Case Study 3 Tisagenlecleucel is a chimeric antigen receptor (CAR)-T cell therapy considered for heavily pretreated patients with relapsed/refractory follicular lymphoma. ELARA was planned as a confirmatory Phase II single-arm clinical trial to support the regulatory submission of tisagenlecleucel for this indication, with complete response (was this achieved, yes/no) as the primary outcome and progression-free survival and overall survival as secondary outcomes (Fowler et al., 2022). A health authority rapporteur reviewing the ELARA trial protocol noted that patient-level external controls would be useful to contextualize this study, should there be a submission (Hampson et al., 2024). Two sources of RWD were identified: 1) FHAD and 2) ReCORD-FL (Salles et al., 2022a, b), a retrospective chart review study. Eligible patients from these two data sources were not pooled. Instead, each RWD source was used to create a different external control arm (Hampson et al., 2024; Hao et al., 2023). The protocol and statistical analysis plan for each indirect comparison (ELARA vs external control arm) were prespecified before outcome data on the external controls were revealed. The estimand and target trial frameworks were applied in tandem to describe the estimand for each indirect comparison and to align the design and analysis of each comparison with that.

In Sect. 21.4.3, we use these three case studies to illustrate some reflections on the 5-step workflow proposed in the previous section. In particular, we focus on Step 2 of the workflow (WF2), where we first specify the estimand following the estimand framework and then translate and add additional granularity to the estimand definition by defining the target trial through important features of its protocol. As part of this discussion, we consider the mapping between the five estimand attributes defined in ICH E9(R1) and elements of the target trial protocol. As argued in Sect. 21.4.1, we claim that both steps are necessary to adequately articulate an RWS estimand.

21.4.3 Specification of the Target Trial by Describing Key Features of Its Protocol

Important features of the target trial protocol (Hernán & Robins, 2016; Hernán, 2021) are listed below. As mentioned in the previous section, while the target trial protocol covers many of the attributes of the estimand framework, it does not explicitly mention the addressing of intercurrent events, and we propose listing other intercurrent events not captured elsewhere in a dedicated protocol section. Accounting for important intercurrent events is essential for exactly defining the causal effect of interest. Of course, since many RWS are based on secondary-use data, sometimes the desired intercurrent event strategy cannot be fully supported by the available data, and researchers must carefully evaluate the impact of this for answering the clinical question and the feasibility of the RWS.

21.4.3.1 Eligibility Criteria

When translating estimand attributes to define the target trial, the population attribute can be mapped to the target trial eligibility criteria. This follows because the target trial is a thought experiment: in the 5-step workflow proposed in Sect. 21.4.1, it is the randomized trial that would support reliable estimation of the estimand, and, therefore, the eligibility criteria of this hypothetical study should be closely aligned with the estimand population attribute. We distinguish, however, the target trial from its eventual emulation, where these two may differ with regard to their eligibility criteria either due to limitations in the RWD or because these differences are intentional. To illustrate the latter case, we first note that in a drug development setting, it is common for the population attribute of the estimand to be broader than the population defined by the clinical trial inclusion/exclusion criteria. This is because the former typically represents the population the sponsor would propose for inclusion in the label should the drug be approved. However, the eligibility criteria of the clinical trial may capture only a subgroup of this wider population for scientific reasons or due to ethical and/or feasibility constraints. Should the clinical trial results be positive, the sponsor may then need to provide a rationale to justify inclusion of the broader population in the label. A similar situation may occur if an RWS is performed to support a regulatory submission. When we come to emulate the target trial, it may be desirable or necessary to design the RWS with inclusion/exclusion criteria that are more restrictive than the target trial eligibility criteria. If this is the case, the assumptions needed to transport findings from the RWS to the population of interest would need to be listed and justified.

In other scenarios, it is more natural that there should be a close mapping between the population targeted by the clinical question and the RWS population. In Case Study 1, the population targeted by the comparative efficacy question is "postmenopausal women within 5 years of menopause between the years 2005 and 2010 and with no history of cancer and no use of hormone therapy in the past 2 years" (Hernán & Robins, 2016). As a second example, consider an externally controlled trial with patient-level controls drawn from RWD. For such a study, it is common to define the primary estimand as the average effect of treatment on the treated (ATT), so that the population targeted by the scientific question is those who would meet the inclusion/exclusion criteria of the single-arm trial. This population, therefore, should also be reflected in the eligibility criteria of the target trial. Failure to emulate critical elements of these criteria would be regarded as a severe limitation, increasing the risk of bias due to confounding.

When emulating a target trial, it may be infeasible to "retrofit" important target trial eligibility criteria to existing RWD. For example, in Case Study 2, a necessary criterion for participation in the STORM Part 2 trial is an expected survival of at least four months, but this cannot be applied at time zero to select external controls from the FHAD because no such assessment was made for real-world patients. This limitation in the emulation may introduce selection bias (FDA multidiscipline review 2019).

In cases where the target trial eligibility criteria cannot be emulated in the RWS, we must reflect on whether to refine the clinical question so as to address a different objective or whether to abandon the RWS altogether. To illustrate this, in Case Study 1, Hernán and Robins (2016) imagined the scenario that the question is refocused toward a more targeted population who, in addition to meeting the original eligibility criteria, would also have no breast calcification detected via a mammography at time zero. To evaluate whether targeting such a patient population would be feasible, first, we would need to consider whether the RWD includes mammography results. The imagined data in Case Study 1 are from a medical claims system, which typically only records the payment information for mammographies but not the medical results themselves, meaning emulating this exclusion criterion would not be possible. Hernán and Robins (2016) noted that in light of this consideration, we would need to reassess whether the initial research question, which aims to evaluate the effectiveness of hormone therapy in women regardless of whether breast calcifications are detected at time zero, retains its clinical relevance.

21.4.3.2 Treatment Strategies

The treatment attribute of the estimand can be directly mapped to this section of the target trial protocol. RWS are well placed to address questions about treatment strategies that reflect the constraints and practicalities of usual clinical care. This is in contrast to "explanatory" clinical trials, where patients are typically closely followed and their adherence to a precisely defined treatment protocol is carefully recorded (Thorpe et al., 2009). With this in mind, the treatment attribute of the estimand for an RWS should stipulate clinically meaningful treatment regimens that reflect approaches for addressing intercurrent events that are likely to occur in a real-world setting (Hernán & Scharfstein, 2018). To mitigate selection bias, a patient's treatment should also generally be classified based on the medication they are following at time zero (Hernán & Robins, 2016). One important advantage of having clearly defined treatment strategies in place is that it enables patterns of nonadherence to be identified during execution of the target trial emulation (Hernán & Scharfstein, 2018). This is critical if the RWS objective is to estimate a hypothetical estimand (e.g., the causal effect of a novel treatment strategy versus its comparator if nonadherence is not permitted), in which case methods of causal inference will be used to statistically correct for nonadherence in the RWS analysis.

21.4.3.3 Assignment Procedures

This is a unique and essential element of the target trial protocol. While there is no estimand attribute that directly corresponds to the treatment assignment component, its definition is implied by the causal interpretation of the estimand. The ICH E9(R1) guideline defines a treatment effect as "how the outcome of treatment compares to what would have happened to the same subjects under alternative treatment …" (ICH, 2019). Since the target trial framework is intended to facilitate causal inferences, the target trial will be defined by the randomization of treatments to patients.

To emulate such a trial with non-randomized data, statistical techniques are needed to balance baseline prognostic factors and effect modifiers between treatment cohorts. Common approaches include propensity score-based methods (matching or weighting strategies are particularly popular in practice) or doubly robust inference (Webster-Clark et al., 2021; Hernán & Robins, 2016). Diagnostics that evaluate the similarity of treatment arms with respect to measured confounders at time zero before and after propensity score matching or weighting (Austin and Stuart 2015) can be used to evaluate the success of our emulation of randomization. However, many analysis methods, including propensity score-based approaches, rely on an assumption of "no unmeasured confounders." However, this assumption cannot be verified from observed data. Negative controls (Lipsitch et al., 2010) could be used to pressure test our control of confounding and inform decisions on the feasibility of the RWS (McGrath et al., 2020). Sensitivity analyses could also be planned to evaluate the robustness of findings to the presence and magnitude of unmeasured confounding; see Ding et al. (2023) for a review of methods. Alternatively, analytical approaches that do not necessarily require unmeasured confounding, such as instrumental variable approaches (Maciejewski & Brookhart, 2019), could be used.

21.4.3.4 Outcomes

The variable attribute of the estimand can be mapped to this element of the target trial protocol, which specifies the outcome to be measured and the timing of the assessment. Investigators may encounter several challenges when trying to emulate this aspect of the target trial within an RWS. In Case Study 3, the conventionally defined progression-free survival (PFS) outcome was missing for many real-world patients; therefore, starting a new anticancer therapy was regarded as a PFS event for all patients to avoid introducing bias into the comparison (Hampson et al., 2024). An additional complication is that a response may be defined according to different criteria in the real world versus the clinical trial setting. For example, in an oncology setting, complete response and progression are often evaluated using "real-world" versions of the criteria applied in trials.

21.4.3.5 Time Zero and Follow-Up Period

The follow-up period of the target trial is specified by the start and end of patient monitoring. Different outcomes may necessitate different lengths of follow-up so that, at a minimum, follow-up should be long enough to measure the primary and important secondary outcomes. Time zero in a randomized trial is defined as the time of randomization. Adequate emulation of this important feature, while not straightforward using RWD, is key to mitigating immortal time bias (Hernán et al., 2016). As previously mentioned, time zero is not explicitly captured in the estimand attributes. However, the length of follow-up may be captured indirectly through the variable attribute if this defines the time of measurement of the outcome.

To illustrate the complexities associated with emulating time zero of a target trial using RWD, consider Case Study 2, where the sponsor initially proposed to define time zero for STORM Part 2 patients and external controls as the time of failure of their most recent line of therapy (i.e., disease progression). However, this approach introduced immortal time bias (favoring STORM) because, by construction, there could be no deaths among STORM patients from the time of this failure until starting the STORM trial intervention, whereas the external controls were immediately at risk of death (FDA multidiscipline review 2019). To eliminate this source of bias, the FDA proposed defining time zero as the time at which the STORM Part 2 intervention was commenced (FDA multidiscipline review 2019).

When emulating the target trial in Case Study 1, a patient could potentially meet all the target trial eligibility criteria at all timepoints between 2005 and 2010 (i.e., assuming a woman started menopause at the end of 2004). Time zero, therefore, could be defined in a variety of ways, and it is necessary to consider which time point(s) should be regarded as each patient's start of follow-up.

In the context of Case Study 3, while the ELARA single-arm trial followed patients across several lines of therapy, the primary outcome (complete response) evaluated a patient's response to the first line of therapy received after enrollment. However, follow-up across a longer horizon was available for the external controls. This raised the question of how to define a baseline for an external control. Case Study 3 adopted a propensity score method whereby for each external control, one first estimates a propensity score (for participation in the single-arm trial) at the start of each eligible line of therapy and then selects as their time zero the time at which they started the line corresponding to their highest estimated propensity score (Hampson et al., 2024).

More generally, common approaches for defining time zero for patients who meet the RWS eligibility criteria at more than one timepoint include the following (Hernán & Robins, 2016; Backenroth, 2021):

1. Use the first time at which a patient meets all inclusion and exclusion criteria.
2. Randomly select an eligible timepoint.
3. Choose a timepoint that makes the control and treatment arms' population characteristics as similar as possible. The propensity score method used in Case Study 3 can be considered in this category.
4. Consider all applicable timepoints.

Method 4 typically yields the greatest precision (Hernán & Robins, 2016). Nonparametric bootstrap, for example, could be used to calculate the variance of the treatment effect estimate derived using this approach, accounting for the correlation created by using a patient's data several times (Hernán & Robins, 2016). Moreover, Backenroth (2021) used plasmode simulation to show that for the case of an externally controlled single-arm trial, Method 2 may produce biased estimates, while Method 4 can mitigate selection bias.

21.4.3.6 Causal Contrast(S) of Interest

This specifies which contrast(s) of the moments of distributions of potential outcomes are of interest (Hernán, 2021). There is, therefore, some link, in principle, between the population-level summary attribute of the estimand, which defines how summaries of observed outcomes on different treatment strategies will be compared, and this section of the target trial protocol. However, there is incomplete alignment between these two features since definitions of the target trial specification tend to focus this element around outlining the different strategies that will be used to address intercurrent events related to treatment adherence and the causal effects these correspond to, namely the "intention-to-treat" or "per-protocol" effects (Hernán & Robins, 2016).

21.4.3.7 Analysis Plan

The estimand framework also connects the estimand to the primary estimator and sensitivity analyses, as well as supplementary analyses that target different, but clinically relevant, quantities.

21.4.4 Discussion

It is worth noting that sometimes the target trial is not entirely consistent with the RWS that can be executed, especially in studies comparing a single-arm trial cohort with real-world controls. If the external controls are sourced from secondary-use RWD, it is possible that these two cohorts may differ in several ways, including, for example, with respect to how outcomes and covariates are measured, the distribution of prognostic factors at baseline, and patient follow-up (FDA, 2023). However, even so, the estimand and target trial frameworks can still assist in the planning, implementation, and communication of RWS.

21.5 Estimands and the PICO Framework

Evidence-based medicine (EBM) refers to the process of combining the best available clinical evidence with clinical expertise and patient values and preferences to inform medical decisions (Masic et al., 2008). Clinical evidence regarding the efficacy and/or safety of interventions can be derived from systematic searches, evaluations, and clinical studies of various designs. In general, the quality and reliability of evidence range from high to low for the following designs (listed in order): systematic review and meta-analysis of randomized controlled trials or n-of-1 trials; individual randomized controlled trial; non-randomized controlled cohort study; case-control study or case series; animal experiments; laboratory research supporting mechanism-based reasoning, etc. (OCEBM Levels of Evidence Working Group, 2011). The evidence strength/level may be graded down or up on the basis of study quality or effect size, etc. A systematic review identifies, appraises, and synthesizes the evidence that meets prespecified eligibility criteria to answer a given clinical or research question. It is commonly used in medical and public health research and is a core methodology for health technology assessment (HTA). In order to obtain the best current clinical evidence, it is necessary to accurately and precisely retrieve relevant research literature. To achieve this, it is crucial to construct (state) relevant clinical (scientific) questions and define the inclusion/exclusion criteria for the review ahead of time (McKenzie et al., 2019).

The PICO framework constructs treatment-related clinical questions from the following four aspects: population, intervention, control or comparator, and outcome (Huang et al., 2006). For different types of studies, PICO can help clarify research questions more accurately and efficiently and facilitate searches for high-quality evidence, thereby contributing to evidence-based decision-making.

The broader PICOT (PICO plus timing), PICOS (PICO plus study type or setting), or PICOTS (PICO plus timing and study type or setting) frameworks include one or two components in addition to the standard PICO ones (Samson & Schoelles, 2012). Timing refers to the timing of the outcome assessment and thus may be incorporated as part of the outcomes or as part of the intervention. Setting defines the setting (primary, specialty, inpatient, nursing homes, or other long-term care

Table 21.1 Comparison of PICO and estimand frameworks

Estimand Framework	PICO Framework
Population	P (Population)
Treatment strategies	I (Intervention) C (Control or Comparator)
Variable (or endpoint)	O (Outcome)
Other intercurrent events[a]	–
Population-level summary	–

[a]For those intercurrent events not addressed by precise specifications of population, treatment, and variable

setting) where the study is performed and the relevance of the study setting to real-world use. This element may be incorporated as part of the population or intervention. Therefore, here we prefer to focus on comparing the PICO framework with the estimand framework.

Both the PICO framework and the estimand framework are useful for precisely defining the scientific question. As shown in Table 21.1, the PICO components partially overlap with the estimand attributes. Both frameworks include "population," the "intervention," and "control." PICO components correspond to the "treatment" attribute of an estimand. Meanwhile, the "outcome" PICO component corresponds to the "variable" attribute of an estimand. However, the estimand framework goes further than the PICO framework by specifying how the treatment effect is summarized and highlighting the importance of addressing intercurrent events to ensure a clear summary of treatment effects (Lawrance et al., 2020; Keene et al., 2023).

In general, the two frameworks are applied in different scenarios and can complement each other when necessary. In evidence-based medicine, the PICO framework is well-known and widely used. With the increasingly extensive and in-depth application of estimands in different types of trials, the estimand framework may play an important role in the field of evidence-based medicine in the future. Remiro-Azócar (2022) proposed extending the PICO framework to PICOSI by adding S (summary measure) and I (intercurrent events), which enables users to translate estimands to the PICO language and therefore may promote the implementation of estimands in evidence-based medicine.

21.6 Concluding Remarks

In recent discussions, the application of the estimand framework has gained prominence in clinical research. However, certain areas, such as early-phase trials, safety outcomes, and real-world studies (RWS), still lack comprehensive utilization of this framework. While some domains, like RWS, have clearer roadmaps and more extensive discussions in recent literature, others remain in the conceptual stage.

This chapter delves into the current status of these areas, highlighting their uniqueness and the challenges associated with the implementation of the estimand framework in these contexts. By bridging the gap between existing practices and the estimand framework, we aim to foster a deeper understanding of this evolving field. We also anticipate significant developments in the near future as researchers continue to explore and refine the use of estimands in these areas.

References

Akacha, M., Bartels, C., Bornkamp, B., Bretz, F., Coello, N., Dumortier, T., et al. (2021). Estimands—What they are and why they are important for pharmacometricians. *CPT: Pharmacometrics & Systems Pharmacology, 10*(4), 279.

Austin, P. C., & Stuart, E. A. (2015). Moving towards best practice when using inverse probability of treatment weighting (IPTW) using the propensity score to estimate causal treatment effects in observational studies. *Statistics in medicine, 34*(28), 3661–3679.

Backenroth, D. (2021). How to choose a time zero for patients in external control arms. *Pharmaceutical Statistics, 20*(4), 783–792.

Ball, G., Reblin, T., Buchanan, J., Hendrickson, B. A., Lewis, E., Schnell, P. M., & Rockhold, F. W. (2020). A framework for safety evaluation throughout the product development life-cycle. *Therapeutic Innovation & Regulatory Science, 54*(4), 821–830. https://doi.org/10.1007/s43441-019-00021-5

Brunner, E., Vandemeulebroecke, M., & Mütze, T. (2021). Win odds: An adaptation of the win ratio to include ties. *Statistics in Medicine, 40*(14), 3367–3384.

CADTH (2023). CADTH methods and guidelines. Guidance for reporting real-world evidence. Available at: https://www.cadth.ca/guidance-reporting-real-world-evidence

Chari, A., Vogl, D. T., Gavriatopoulou, M., Nooka, A. K., Yee, A. J., Huff, C. A., et al. (2019). Oral Selinexor-dexamethasone for triple class refractory multiple myeloma. *New England Journal of Medicine, 381*, 727–738.

Chen, J., Scharfstein, D., Wang, H., Yu, B., Song, Y., He, W., et al. (2024). Estimands in real-world evidence studies. *Statistics in Biopharmaceutical Research, 16*(2), 257–269.

Chuang-Stein, C. (1994). A new proposal for benefit-less-risk analysis in clinical trials. *Controlled Clinical Trials, 15*(1), 30–43.

Council for International Organizations of Medical Sciences. (2005). Management of safety information from clinical trials: report of CIOMS Working Group VI. In *Management of safety information from clinical trials: report of CIOMS Working Group VI.*

Dang, L. E., Gruber, S., Lee, H., Dahabreh, I. J., Stuart, E. A., Williamson, B. D., et al. (2023). A causal roadmap for generating high-quality real-world evidence. *Journal of Clinical and Translational Science, 7*(1), e212.

DeMets, D. L., & Cook, T. (2019). Challenges of non–intention-to-treat analyses. *JAMA, 321*(2), 145–146.

Desai, R. J., Wang, S. V., Sreedhara, S. K., Zabotka, L., Khosrow-Khavar, F., Nelson, J. C., et al. (2024). Process guide for inferential studies using healthcare data from routine clinical practice to evaluate causal effects of drugs (PRINCIPLED): Considerations from the FDA Sentinel Innovation Center. *BMJ, 384*.

Ding, P., Fang, Y., Faries, D., Gruber, S., Lee, H., Lee, J. Y., et al. (2023). Sensitivity analysis for unmeasured confounding in medical product development and evaluation using real world evidence. *arXiv. preprint arXiv:2307.07442*.

Dong, G., Qiu, J., Wang, D., & Vandemeulebroecke, M. (2018). The stratified win ratio. *Journal of Biopharmaceutical Statistics, 28*(4), 778–796.

Duke-Margolis FDA Workshop: Advancing Premarket Safety Analytics. (2022). Final slide deck available at https://healthpolicy.duke.edu/events/advancing-premarket-safety-analytics

EMA (2023). Data quality framework for EU medicines regulation. Available at: https://www.ema.europa.eu/en/documents/regulatory-procedural-guideline/data-quality-framework-eu-medicines-regulation_en.pdf

Englert, S., Mercier, F., Pilling, E. A., Homer, V., Habermehl, C., Zimmermann, S., & Kan-Dobrosky, N. (2023). Defining estimands for efficacy assessment in single arm phase 1b or phase 2 clinical trials in oncology early development. *Pharmaceutical Statistics, 22*(5), 921–937.

FDA. (2019). NDA/BLA Multi-disciplinary review and evaluation of XPOVIO (Selinexor). Available at: https://www.accessdata.fda.gov/drugsatfda_docs/nda/2019/212306Orig1s000MultidisciplineR.pdf

FDA. (2023). *Considerations for the design and conduct of externally controlled trials for drug and biological products*. Guidance for Industry. Available at: https://www.fda.gov/media/164960/download

Fowler, N. H., Dickinson, M., Dreyling, M., Martinez-Lopez, J., Kolstad, A., Butler, J., et al. (2022). Tisagenlecleucel in adult relapsed or refractory follicular lymphoma: The phase 2 ELARA trial. *Nature Medicine, 28*, 325–332.

Franklin, J. M., & Schneeweiss, S. (2017). When and how can real world data analyses substitute for randomized controlled trials? *Clinical Pharmacology and Therapeutics, 102*, 924–933.

Hampson, L. V., Degtyarev, E., Tang, R., Lin, J., Rufibach, K., & Zheng, C. (2023). Comment on "biostatistical considerations when using RWD and RWE in clinical studies for regulatory purposes: A landscape assessment". *Statistics in Biopharmaceutical Research, 15*(1), 23–26.

Hampson, L. V., Chu, J., Zia, A., Zhang, J., Hsu, W. C., Parzynski, C. S., et al. (2024). Combining the target trial and estimand frameworks to define the causal estimand: An application using real-world data to contextualize a single-arm trial. *Statistics in Biopharmaceutical Research, 16*(1), 1–10.

Hao, Y., Hsu, W. C., Parzynski, C. S., Degtyarev, E., Hampson, L. V., Masood, A., & Wu, W. H. (2023). Effectiveness of tisagenlecleucel versus real-world standard of care in relapsed/refractory follicular lymphoma. *Journal of Comparative Effectiveness Research, 12*(7), e220173.

Hernán, M. A. (2021). Methods of public health research—Strengthening causal inference from observational data. *New England Journal of Medicine, 385*(15), 1345–1348.

Hernán, M. A., & Robins, J. M. (2016). Using big data to emulate a target trial when a randomized trial is not available. *American Journal of Epidemiology, 183*(8), 758–764.

Hernán, M. A., & Scharfstein, D. (2018). Cautions as regulators move to end exclusive reliance on intention to treat. *Annals of Internal Medicine, 168*(7), 515–516.

Hernán, M. A., Sauer, B. C., Hernández-Díaz, S., Platt, R., & Shrier, I. (2016). Specifying a target trial prevents immortal time bias and other self-inflicted injuries in observational analyses. *Journal of Clinical Epidemiology, 79*, 70–75.

Hernán, M. A., Wang, W., & Leaf, D. E. (2022). Target trial emulation: A framework for causal inference from observational data. *JAMA, 328*(24), 2446–2447.

Huang, X., Lin, J., & Demner-Fushman, D. (2006). Evaluation of PICO as a knowledge representation for clinical questions. *American Medical Informatics Association Annual Symposium Proceedings*, 359–363.

ICH. (1994). E4 dose-response information to support drug registration. Step 4 document available at www.ich.org

ICH. (2019). E9(R1) addendum on estimands and sensitivity analysis in clinical trials to the guideline on statistical principles for clinical trials. Step 4 document available at www.ich.org

ICH. (2021). E8(R1) general considerations for clinical studies. Step 4 document available at www.ich.org

Kahan, B. C., White, I. R., Edwards, M., & Harhay, M. O. (2023). Using modified intention-to-treat as a principal stratum estimator for failure to initiate treatment. *Clinical Trials, 20*(3), 269–275.

Keene, O. N., Lynggaard, H., Englert, S., Lanius, V., & Wright, D. (2023). Why estimands are needed to define treatment effects in clinical trials. *BMC Medicine, 21*(1), 276.

Lawrance, R., Degtyarev, E., Griffiths, P., Trask, P., Lau, H., D'Alessio, D., et al. (2020). What is an estimand & how does it relate to quantifying the effect of treatment on patient-reported quality of life outcomes in clinical trials? *Journal of Patient-Reported Outcomes, 4*(1), 1–8.

Levenson, M., He, W., Chen, J., Fang, Y., Faries, D., Goldstein, B. A., et al. (2023). Biostatistical considerations when using RWD and RWE in clinical studies for regulatory purposes: A landscape assessment. *Statistics in Biopharmaceutical Research, 15*(1), 3–13.

Lipsitch, M., Tchetgen, E. T., & Cohen, T. (2010). Negative controls: A tool for detecting confounding and bias in observational studies. *Epidemiology, 21*(3), 383–388.

Maciejewski, M. L., & Brookhart, M. A. (2019). Using instrumental variables to address bias from unobserved confounders. *JAMA, 321*(21), 2124–2125.

Masic, I., Miokovic, M., & Muhamedagic, B. (2008). Evidence based medicine–new approaches and challenges. *Acta Informatica Medica, 16*(4), 219.

McGrath, L. J., Spangler, L., Curtis, J. R., Ehrenstein, V., Sørensen, H. T., Saul, B., et al. (2020). Using negative control outcomes to assess the comparability of treatment groups among women with osteoporosis in the United States. *Pharmacoepidemiology and Drug Safety, 29*(8), 854–863.

McKenzie, J. E., Brennan, S. E., Ryan, R. E., Thomson, H. J., Johnston, R. V., & Thomas, J. (2019). Defining the criteria for including studies and how they will be grouped for the synthesis. *Cochrane Handbook for Systematic Reviews of Interventions*, 33–65.

Mishra-Kalyani, P. S., Amiri Kordestani, L., Rivera, D. R., Ibrahim, A., DeClaro, R. A., Shen, Y., et al. (2022). External control arms in oncology: Current use and future directions. *Annals of Oncology, 33*(4), 376–383.

OCEBM Levels of Evidence Working Group* (2011). "The Oxford 2011 Levels of Evidence". Available at: https://www.cebm.ox.ac.uk/files/levels-of-evidence/cebm-levels-of-evidence-2-1.pdf. *Oxford Centre for Evidence-Based Medicine*. http://www.cebm.net/index.aspx?o=5653.

Polito, L., Liang, Q., Pal, N., Mpofu, P., Sawas, A., Humblet, O., et al. (2024). Applying the Estimand and target trial frameworks to external control analyses using observational data: A case study in the solid tumor setting. *Frontiers in Pharmacology, 15*, 1223858.

Remiro-Azócar, A. (2022). Some considerations on target estimands for health technology assessment. *Statistics in Medicine, 41*(28), 5592.

Richardson, W. S., Wilson, M. C., Nishikawa, J., & Hayward, R. S. (1995). The well-built clinical question: A key to evidence-based decisions. *ACP Journal Club, 123*(3), A12–AA3.

Rufibach, K. (2019). Treatment effect quantification for time-to-event endpoints–Estimands, analysis strategies, and beyond. *Pharmaceutical Statistics, 18*(2), 145–165.

Salles, G., Schuster, S. J., Fischer, L., Kuruvilla, J., Patten, P. E. M., von Tresckow, B., et al. (2022a). A retrospective cohort study of treatment outcomes of adult patients with relapsed or refractory follicular lymphoma (ReCORD-FL). *HemaSphere, 6*(7), e745.

Salles, G., Schuster, S. J., Dreyling, M., Fischer, L., Kuruvilla, J., et al. (2022b). Efficacy comparison of tisagenlecleucel vs usual care in patients with relapsed or refractory follicular lymphoma. *Blood Advances, 6*(22), 5835–5843.

Samson, D., & Schoelles, K. M. (2012). Chapter 2: Medical tests guidance (2) developing the topic and structuring systematic reviews of medical tests: Utility of PICOTS, analytic frameworks, decision trees, and other frameworks. *Journal of General Internal Medicine, 27*, 11–19.

Siegel, J., Weber, H. J., Englert, S., & Liu, F. (2022). Time-to-event estimands and loss to follow-up in oncology in light of the estimands framework. *arXiv preprint arXiv:2203.01781*.

Stensrud, M. J., & Dukes, O. (2022). Translating questions to estimands in randomized clinical trials with intercurrent events. *Statistics in Medicine, 41*(16), 3211–3228.

Thorpe, K. E., Zwarenstein, M., Oxman, A. D., Treweek, S., Furberg, C. D., Altman, D. G., et al. (2009). A pragmatic–explanatory continuum indicator summary (PRECIS): A tool to help trial designers. *Journal of Clinical Epidemiology, 62*(5), 464–475.

Unkel, S., Amiri, M., Benda, N., Beyersmann, J., Knoerzer, D., Kupas, K., et al. (2019). On estimands and the analysis of adverse events in the presence of varying follow-up times within the benefit assessment of therapies. *Pharmaceutical Statistics, 18*(2), 166–183.

Wang, X., Yang, P., Yuan, S. S., & Wang, W. W. (2023). Application of estimand framework in ICH E9 (R1) to safety evaluation. *Journal of Biopharmaceutical Statistics, 33*(4), 476–487.

Webster-Clark, M., Stürmer, T., Wang, T., Man, K., Marinac-Dabic, D., Rothman, K. J., et al. (2021). Using propensity scores to estimate effects of treatment initiation decisions: State of the science. *Statistics in Medicine, 40*(7), 1718–1735.

Yang, F., Wittes, J., & Pitt, B. (2019). Beware of on-treatment safety analyses. *Clinical Trials, 16*(1), 63–70.

Zhou, Y., Ke, C., Jiang, Q., Shahin, S., & Snapinn, S. (2015). Choosing appropriate metrics to evaluate adverse events in safety evaluation. *Therapeutic Innovation & Regulatory Science, 49*(3), 398–404.

Chapter 22
Leveraging the Estimand Framework Across Trial Designs

Zhiwei Jiang, Zhiyue Huang, Rima Izem, Wenting Li, Xue Vang, Frank Bretz, Wentian Guo, Eva Hua, Juliane Manitz, Na Vang, and Xin Zhang

Z. Jiang (✉)
KeyTech Consulting, Beijing, China
e-mail: zhi.wei.jiang@ktstat.com

Z. Huang
Quantitive Sciences and Evidence Generation, Astellas Pharma Inc., Shanghai, China
e-mail: Zhiyue.huang@astellas.com

R. Izem
Statitical Methodology, Novartis Pharma AG, Basel, Switzerland
e-mail: rima.izem@novartis.com

W. Li
Biostatistics, dMed Biopharmaceutical Co., Ltd, Shanghai, China
e-mail: wenting.li@caidya.com

X. Vang
Statistics and Decision Sciences, Johnson & Johnson Inovative Medicine, R&D, Shanghai, China
e-mail: xyang36@its.jnj.com

F. Bretz
Advanced Methodology and Data Sciences/Statistical Methodology, Novartis Pharma AG, Basel, Switzerland
e-mail: frank.bretz@novartis.com

W. Guo
Biometrics, AstraZeneca Global R&D(China) Co., Ltd, Shanghai, China
e-mail: Wentian.guo@astrazeneca.com

E. Hua
Advanced Quantitative Sciences/Immunology statistics, Novartis Institutes for Biomedical Research Co., Shanghai, China
e-mail: eva.hua@novartis.com

J. Manitz
Chelsea, MA, USA
e-mail: Juliane@manitz.org

J. Wei et al. (eds.), *Estimands in Clinical Trials*, Springer Series in Pharmaceutical Statistics, https://doi.org/10.1007/978-3-032-02192-2_22

N. Vang
Evidence Generation and Decision Science - Asia Pacific Statistics, Sanofi, Beijing, China
e-mail: Na3.yang@sanofi.com

X. Zhang
Global Biometrics & Data Management, Pfizer Inc., Shanghai, China
e-mail: xin.zhang6@pfizer.com

Abstract This chapter reviews the implications of the estimand framework on various clinical trial designs. It details the unique estimand considerations for non-inferiority and equivalence trials, focusing on strategies for addressing intercurrent events. It also explores the application of the estimand framework in adaptive and master protocol designs, highlighting the need for careful planning and consideration of treatment-related and population-specific intercurrent events. In multiregional clinical trials, the estimand framework formalizes the treatment effect assessment in the overall population and the specific regional populations. This chapter also discusses different strategies addressing treatment switching in oncology trials for estimating overall survival benefits. Finally, this chapter reviews decentralized clinical trials, emphasizing the impact of decentralization on estimands and the estimator's properties, along with the potential for targeting novel estimands through patient-centric measures. Different case studies illustrate practical applications of the estimand framework in various trial designs, demonstrating its flexibility and utility. This chapter concludes by highlighting the evolving nature of clinical trial designs and the importance of the estimand framework in improving trial design, conduct, and analysis.

22.1 Introduction

An estimand describes the quantity to be estimated to address the specific trial objective. It includes a definition of a population-level effect measure of a specific treatment that is applicable to all patients in the target population, including those who may experience certain post-randomization events known as intercurrent events during the trial (Ratitch et al., 2020). The ICH E9(R1) guideline aims to define and structure a proper scientific approach where the objectives and estimands drive the trial design and analysis, rather than the other way around (ICH, 2019). Successful implementation of the ICH E9(R1) guideline can potentially help improve trial design, conduct, and analysis.

This chapter discusses estimand considerations under specific trial designs. Non-inferiority and equivalence trials are two common trial designs with distinctive features leading to different estimand considerations, as discussed in Sect. 22.2. Section 22.3 explores estimand considerations in complex innovative design, including adaptive design and master protocol designs (i.e., basket, umbrella, and platform trial designs). Multiregional clinical trials have become increasingly common as a mean to accelerate global drug development. In such trials, consistency across regions is an important concern, in addition to evaluating the overall treatment effect, and related estimand considerations are reviewed in Sect. 22.4. Section 22.5 discusses four different estimands under various scenarios for trial designs with treatment switching. Finally, estimand considerations in decentralized trials are introduced in Section 22.6.

22.2 Estimands in Non-Inferiority and Equivalence Trials

22.2.1 Background

The ICH E9 guideline (1998b) provides guidance on statistical considerations in clinical trials, including non-inferiority and equivalence trials. Estimand considerations in non-inferiority and equivalence trials are different from those in superiority trials, particularly from a regulatory perspective (ICH, 2021).

The objective of a non-inferiority trial is to demonstrate that the difference between treatment and active control is within an acceptable range. Assay sensitivity, which is the ability of the trial to detect a difference between treatments of a specified size, ensures the reliability of the non-inferiority conclusion (FDA, 2016). The determination of a non-inferiority margin is based on comparing the treatment effect of the active control and placebo in historical studies. The "95–95" method is a widely used approach for establishing this margin (FDA, 2016). However, differences in trial designs between the designing non-inferiority trial and historical trials, as well as the variation of trial results, need to be considered.

The objective of an equivalence trial is to confirm the similarity of a treatment and a control when their difference falls within predefined lower and upper bounds. Equivalence designs are often utilized in bioequivalence and biosimilarity studies. Specifying the equivalence margin in the trial protocol is vital, with assay sensitivity playing a crucial role in this assessment.

22.2.2 Estimand Considerations

Common intercurrent events in non-inferiority trials, as well as superiority trials, include the use of rescue medication and discontinuation of study treatment for various reasons. The choice of strategy to address these intercurrent events should be guided by the specific clinical question of interest. The ICH E9(R1) guideline introduces five strategies to address intercurrent events: treatment policy, hypothetical, composite, while-one-treatment, and principal stratum. These strategies are applicable in non-inferiority and equivalence trials as well, based on the underlying clinical context.

In a superiority trial, a treatment policy strategy is often considered for some intercurrent events, such as the use of rescue medications after randomization (Polverejan & Dragalin, 2020). In this context, the clinical question of interest is to compare, for example, "treatment, plus rescue medication as needed" and "control, plus rescue medication as needed." However, considerations for constructing an estimand in a non-inferiority trial may differ from those in a superiority trial because the clinical question of interest is to confirm the investigational treatment's efficacy by demonstrating that the treatment is not worse than the active control.

In non-inferiority trials, the hypothetical strategy may be considered in the primary estimand to handle the intercurrent events when the treatment effect without the intercurrent event is of interest (Nauta, 2024; Rehal et al., 2023). As an additional estimand to the primary estimand, the intercurrent events can also be addressed using a treatment policy strategy to determine the treatment effect, including all outcomes, no matter whether the events occur (Rehal et al., 2023).

Morgan et al. (2023) introduced the concept of trial-specific intercurrent events, which are defined as intercurrent events that occur in a specific trial setting but would not occur in clinical practice, and the following recommendations were made for a non-inferiority trial.

- A single primary estimand should be chosen based on clinical considerations, as in other trial designs, if trial-specific intercurrent events do not occur.
- A single primary estimand should be defined, in which trial-specific intercurrent events are addressed using a hypothetical strategy, and others are addressed based on clinical considerations if trial-specific intercurrent events do occur and can be identified.
- If trial-specific intercurrent events do occur but cannot be identified, two estimands should be identified: (i) the first one assumes there is no trial-specific intercurrent event and is chosen based on clinical considerations and (ii) the second one uses a hypothetical strategy for intercurrent events that may be trial-specific. Both estimands should be evaluated to determine non-inferiority.

A principal stratum strategy is another option for addressing intercurrent events in a non-inferiority trial when the clinical question of interest is to evaluate the efficacy in patients who are potentially compliant (Lou et al., 2019a, b). This strategy differs from a per-protocol (PP) analysis, which has commonly been used in non-inferiority trials (Keene, 2023; Mo et al., 2020). In a PP analysis, non-compliers are excluded, which may introduce bias due to post-baseline exclusions (Matilde Sanchez & Chen, 2006; Brittain & Lin, 2005). However, the principal stratum estimand targets patients who are potentially compliant and aims to estimate the causal effect (Lou et al., 2019a, b). Sensitivity analyses are recommended to explore the potential selection bias and evaluate the robustness of results from the principal stratification (Wiens & Lipkovich, 2020). More details on the principal stratum estimand can be found in Chap. 19.

Furthermore, the determination of a non-inferiority margin depends on the strategies to address intercurrent events in the historical studies. For example, a conservative difference between active control and placebo leads to a narrower margin when a treatment policy strategy is considered. It is important to ensure that the strategies utilized in the historical studies are consistent with the ones in the new trial so that the non-inferiority margin and control response determined from historical studies are appropriate for the new trial (Rehal et al., 2023). This may be challenging because it is often unclear what the intended estimand was for trials conducted before the estimand framework was established.

Recently, Lynggaard et al. (2024) examined what clinical questions of interest can be formulated in the context of non-inferiority trials and argued why it is sensible to describe an estimand as "conservative." Moreover, the authors discuss the impact of the estimand framework on key considerations in non-inferiority trials, such as whether trials should have more than one primary estimand, the choice of non-inferiority margin, assay sensitivity, switching from non-inferiority to superiority, and estimation.

The clinical questions of interest between non-inferiority and equivalence trials may differ. Equivalence trials, which aim to detect differences between treatments (e.g., biosimilars) (NMPA, 2018), are likely to require different estimands compared to non-inferiority trials that aim to quantify evidence of efficacy. Estimands can be constructed to prioritize sensitivity to detect differences if this is important for decision making (ICH, 2021).

22.2.3 Case Study

22.2.3.1 Trial Objective and Design

The four-month moxifloxacin-based regimens for treatment-sensitive tuberculosis (REMoxTB) were a three-arm, double-blinded, randomized, phase III trial to test the non-inferiority of two moxifloxacin-containing four-month regimens compared to the standard six-month regimen (Gillespie et al., 2014). A total of 1931 eligible patients were randomly assigned in a balanced manner to one of the following three daily regimens: A control regimen, which consisted of isoniazid, rifampicin, pyrazinamide, and ethambutol for 8 weeks, followed by 18 weeks of isoniazid and rifampicin (control group); a regimen where moxifloxacin was replaced by ethambutol for 17 weeks, followed by 9 weeks of placebo (isoniazid group); and a regimen where moxifloxacin was replaced by isoniazid for 17 weeks, followed by 9 weeks of placebo (ethambutol group).

Patients were requested to attend clinic visits every week for the first 8 weeks, and then at weeks 12, 17, 22, 26, 38, 52, 65, and 78. At each visit, at least one sputum sample was taken and sent to a laboratory to test for the presence/absence of Mycobacterium tuberculosis. Contaminated results were considered as missing data. The primary efficacy outcome was the proportion of patients who had bacteriologically or clinically defined failure or relapse within 18 months after randomization. Non-inferiority would be declared if the upper boundary of the two-sided

97.5% confidence interval for the between-group difference was less than six percentage points, with a Bonferroni correction for multiplicity.

REMoxTB was completed in 2014 (Gillespie et al., 2014) and subsequently reviewed under the estimand framework as follows (Rehal et al., 2023).

22.2.3.2 Estimand Considerations

The trial compared two moxifloxacin-containing four-month regimens, the isoniazid group and the ethambutol group, with the standard six-month regimen in patients with newly diagnosed pulmonary tuberculosis. The primary objective was to demonstrate the non-inferiority of (i) the isoniazid group versus the control group and (ii) the ethambutol group versus the control group in terms of the between-group difference in the proportion of patients who experienced bacteriologically or clinically defined failure or relapse within 18 months after randomization, had no intercurrent events occurred. The primary comparison of interest was to assess the treatment effect had intercurrent events such as pregnancy and/or reinfection not occurred. The five attributes of the estimand were defined as follows.

(a) Population: Adult patients with newly diagnosed Mycobacterium tuberculosis, not resistant to rifampicin or fluoroquinolones.
(b) Variable: An unfavorable outcome (defined as relapse or treatment failures) at week 78, as derived from the analysis of sputum samples.
(c) Treatments as defined in the following had no intercurrent events occurred:
    (i) Control group: Rifampicin (R), isoniazid (H), pyrazinamide (Z), and ethambutol (E) for eight weeks, followed by 18 weeks of rifampicin and isoniazid.
    Isoniazid group: R, H, Z, and moxifloxacin (M) for 17 weeks, followed by nine weeks of placebo.
    (ii) Control group: Rifampicin (R), isoniazid (H), pyrazinamide (Z), and ethambutol (E) for eight weeks, followed by 18 weeks of rifampicin and isoniazid.
    Ethambutol group: R, M, Z, and E for 17 weeks followed by nine weeks of placebo.
(d) Intercurrent Events: A hypothetical strategy was considered to reflect all intercurrent events, such as exogenous reinfection during treatment and/or follow-up, withdrawal from trial medications due to pregnancy, and changes in treatment for reasons other than treatment failure. Additionally, a supplementary estimand was defined, in which a treatment policy strategy was employed to determine the treatment effect regardless of the intercurrent events occurring.
(e) Population-Level Summary: Difference in proportions for each treatment comparison.

22.2.3.3 Statistical Analysis

In the primary analysis, a two-sided 97.5% Wald confidence interval for the between-group difference in the proportion of patients with an unfavorable outcome was estimated. Non-inferiority was concluded if the upper limit of the confidence interval was smaller than six percentage points. A Bonferroni correction was applied for multiplicity adjustment. Missing responses were assumed to be missing at random, and multiple imputation was used to appropriately account for the uncertainty in the missing data.

A sensitivity analysis was considered for the primary estimand using a missing-not-at-random assumption to explore the robustness of the primary result. The last-mean-carried-forward approach was performed as a sensitivity analysis, which was a reference-based imputation method, and the reference was the patients' randomized arm mean at their last observed time point (Rehal et al., 2023; Leurent et al., 2020; Cro et al., 2020). This approach assumes that patients continued on their randomized arm but that their outcomes stayed at the mean level for their randomized arm at their last observed time point. More details on the reference-based approaches are given in Chap. 15.

22.2.4 Summary and Discussion

Prior to the adoption of the estimand framework, intent-to-treat (ITT) and PP analyses are commonly used in a non-inferiority trial. However, agreement between the ITT and PP results does not guarantee that the conclusion regarding non-inferiority is free from bias (Matilde Sanchez & Chen, 2006; Brittain & Lin, 2005). Under the estimand framework, the estimation should be aligned with the estimand. The causal estimand can be estimated using approaches such as instrumental variables, inverse probability weighting approaches, and other causal inference methods (Morgan et al., 2023; Lou et al., 2019a, b; Dodd et al., 2022; Keene, 2023).

In non-inferiority trials, reference-based approaches should only be used when the underlying assumptions are plausible (Rehal et al., 2023). Tipping point analysis is another useful method for conducting sensitivity analysis (Lou et al., 2019a, b; Hollis, 2002; White et al., 2020).

22.3 Complex Innovative Designs

22.3.1 Background

Complex innovative designs (CID) in clinical trials refer to a range of innovative and novel trial designs, including adaptive, Bayesian, and other complex approaches. The U.S. FDA recognized the importance of CIDs and issued several guidelines to provide direction in this area, including FDA (2019) on adaptive designs, FDA (2022) on the master protocols, and FDA (2020) on interacting with the FDA on CIDs. Likewise, the National Medical Products Administration (NMPA) in China published a guideline on adaptive designs (NMPA, 2021), and the European Medicines Agency (EMA) published a guidance document on complex clinical trials (EMA, 2022); see also Sect. 11.4 for related guidance by the ICH. These guidelines aim to facilitate the development and evaluation of novel trial designs that can expedite the approval process for new drugs and biologics. While there is no precise definition of CID due to the evolving nature of innovation, these guidelines serve as valuable resources for sponsors and applicants engaging in complex trial designs.

The ICH E9(R1) guideline introduced the estimand framework whenever a treatment effect is estimated or a hypothesis related to a treatment effect is tested, whether related to efficacy or safety. This therefore applies in particular to complex innovative designs. Although estimands are becoming the standard practice for standard randomized clinical trials, there is still a lack of experience in applying the estimand framework to these innovative trial designs. Collignon et al. (2022) discussed in detail the implementation of the estimand framework for different types of CIDs, including:

- Adaptive clinical trial designs that allow for prospectively planned modifications to one or more aspects of the trial based on interim analysis of accumulating data from patients in the trial.
- Master protocol designs that include multiple sub-studies with different objectives and involve coordinated efforts to evaluate one or more treatments in one or more diseases or disease subtypes under a common master protocol. Such trials may include adaptive design elements and include basket, umbrella, and platform designs.

In this section, we follow Collignon et al. (2022) and provide a summary of important factors to consider when describing estimands for various types of complex innovative trials. Additionally, we present a case study to illustrate the implementation of the estimand framework for a basket trial design.

Table 22.1 Differences and similarities among the estimands when adding or selecting investigational treatments in a master protocol design. Adapted from Collignon et al. (2022)

Attributes	Proposals
Treatment	Different for each treatment arm
Population	Same
Variable	Usually the same
Intercurrent event	Population-related intercurrent events would be similar, whereas treatment-related intercurrent events may vary
Population-level summary	Usually the same

22.3.2 *Estimand and Innovative Design*

To motivate the subsequent considerations, consider an example trial aiming to study the impact of a marketed drug in three related niche indications. In this scenario, the scientific objective(s) are clear, and given the drug's known safety profile, it could be considered for a phase III program. This program might involve several randomized trials run in parallel, each having an objective to investigate the treatment effect in a specific disease and requiring a dedicated discussion of the estimand for each objective.

These principles remain unchanged when conducting a basket trial, where patients with different nonoverlapping subpopulations (e.g., distinct cancer types with the same genetic alteration) are enrolled. In such cases, each sub-trial objective requires a separate estimand. These estimands will differ due to the distinct diseases and patient populations targeted, despite their relatedness. Table 22.1 provides further differences between the estimands in terms of their attributes.

Once the estimands for the three indications are defined, an appropriate analysis approach can be considered. For example, if sufficient similarity between the diseases is plausible, a hierarchical model (Neuenschwander et al., 2016) aligned with the target estimand could be used. Sensitivity analysis will be crucial to examine the assumptions underlying the chosen analysis approach, including the hierarchical model.

In contrast, if the primary scientific question is about efficacy in the overall population, subsequent discussions on estimands and analysis approaches for individual subpopulations may follow as secondary objectives. This approach could be reasonable when the three related niche indications can be treated as one overall disease.

22.3.3 *Estimand Considerations by Type of Adaptation*

In this section, we discuss the application of the estimand framework by type of adaptation.

22.3.3.1 Adding or Selecting Investigational Treatments

Careful planning of any clinical trial includes following the general estimand framework from the ICH E9(R1) guideline. This is particularly true for adaptive designs, which include adding or selecting investigational treatments in an interim analysis as part of the adaptation step. For such designs, all candidate estimands (i.e., for each treatment-control comparison) should be properly described in the trial protocol. Note that adding a new treatment arm while the trial is ongoing involves introducing a new trial objective, specifically comparing the new treatment with the control. This requires the inclusion of an additional estimand in the protocol, along with a careful discussion of its attributes, in addition to typical components of trial planning (see Sect. 11.4 in this book).

Table 22.1 summarizes the extent to which the estimand attributes can be different among the estimands. Clearly, the treatment attribute is different for each estimand. The other attributes are usually the same, although the variable (and thus the population-level summary) could vary with the drug, as different treatments could target different aspects of the disease. In addition, intercurrent events may be different if they are associated with a specific treatment. It is possible for certain intercurrent events to occur exclusively with one investigational treatment but not with the control or another investigational treatment. Therefore, each estimand associated with a specific investigational treatment should account for these unique intercurrent events.

As an example of a treatment-related intercurrent event, consider a scenario where one of the investigational treatments is a biologic, such as a targeted anticancer agent or an immunotherapy. These biologic drugs can trigger immune responses leading to the formation of antidrug antibodies (ADAs). The presence of ADAs may impact the efficacy or safety of the drug, but they may also bind to regions of the protein that have no clinical effect. Given that ADA positivity is treatment-induced, appears after randomization, and has the potential to influence the interpretation of outcomes, it can be considered an intercurrent event according to the ICH E9(R1) guideline. Importantly, this intercurrent event is specific to the biological treatment, assuming the other treatments are non-biologic.

In contrast, population-specific intercurrent events may exhibit similarities across different treatment arms. For instance, the occurrence of brain metastases is more prevalent in patients with specific cancer types like lung cancer or melanoma, necessitating specialized treatment approaches. These intercurrent events are considered population-specific, thereby requiring similar strategies across all treatment arms.

22.3.3.2 Adding or Selecting Patient Populations

Basket trials are a type of clinical trial that assesses the efficacy of a specific treatment in multiple disease types based on a shared molecular characteristic or genetic alteration. These trials provide insights into targeted therapies for specific patient

Table 22.2 Differences and similarities between the estimands when adding or selecting patient populations in a master protocol design. Adapted from Collignon et al. (2022)

Attributes	Proposals
Treatment	Same
Population	Different across disease types
Variable	May vary across disease types
Intercurrent event	Population-related intercurrent events would be different, whereas treatment-related intercurrent events would be the same
Population-level summary	May vary across disease types

populations and identify new treatment options for rare diseases. Basket trials allow for comparisons of treatments in different settings within a single trial.

In a basket trial, each indication generally has its own estimand. New disease types may be added during the trial, requiring additional estimands. In cases where separate comparisons for each disease type are not feasible, pooling the populations may be considered, but disease-related estimands may still be relevant. Overall, basket trials offer flexibility in comparing treatments across different settings, and the selection of estimands is crucial to properly address the specific objectives of the trial.

Table 22.2 outlines the differences and similarities among estimands across different diseases or subtypes. It is evident that the treatment attribute is usually the same across different disease types, while the populations will be different. The variable (and thus the population-level summary) may vary across disease types. For instance, for one tumor type, the variable of interest might be overall survival, providing insights into the effectiveness of the drug in prolonging survival in that particular population. While in another tumor type within the same basket trial, the variable of interest might be the overall response rate, offering information on the drug's ability to induce tumor shrinkage or complete remission in that specific population. Similar to what has been discussed previously, population-specific intercurrent events would differ, while treatment-related intercurrent events would be the same across the tumor types. The population-level summary would be adjusted based on the variable and the population. For instance, the hazard ratio is often used as the population-level summary for overall survival, which quantifies the relative effect of the treatment on survival by indicating whether the risk of the event is higher or lower in the investigational arm compared to the control arm. On the other hand, the odds ratio is commonly used as the population-level summary for the overall response rate, which provides an estimate of the relative likelihood of response in the investigational arm compared to the control arm.

22.3.3.3 Other Types of Adaptations

There are other types of trial design modifications often encountered during the drug development process that cannot be classified into the previous categories and which will not be discussed here.

- Sample size adaptation based on interim data to increase the chance of fulfilling the trial objective. This adaptive design is related to the estimation process rather than the trial objective, and therefore, it does not impact the trial's estimand. However, the integrity, scientific validity, and reliability of the trial should be carefully considered.
- Adaptations to patient allocation that adjust the future randomization ratio based on patient response to treatments, allowing more patients to receive the better treatment during the trial. This adaptive design is not related to the trial objective, and therefore, it is not reflected in the trial's estimand.

22.3.4 Statistical Analysis

As stated in Section A.5.1 of the ICH E9(R1) guideline, "an estimand for the effect of treatment relative to a control will be estimated by comparing the outcomes in a group of subjects on the treatment to those in a similar group of subjects on the control." For a given estimand, an aligned method of analysis, or estimator, should be implemented that is able to provide an estimate on which a reliable interpretation can be based.

In CIDs with an adaptive design, the selection of estimands at an interim analysis using accumulating data from the ongoing trial poses additional challenges to define reliable estimators, confidence intervals, and hypothesis tests. Especially if the selection of the estimand depends on information internal to the trial, estimators that do not account for the selection may be biased. Estimation becomes even more challenging if the estimand changes in an ongoing trial, such as when there is a change in the control arm. Unplanned changes to the estimand strategy or the estimation strategy (within the same strategy for addressing intercurrent events) at an interim analysis may compromise the trial and are discouraged.

As in any clinical trial, the selection of estimands must be closely examined in conjunction with an evaluation of their feasibility. This evaluation aims to determine whether valid estimation methods are attainable, even when considering the chosen estimand along with potential adaptive adjustments. When no valid estimator can be identified for a specific estimand, it may necessitate multiple iterations involving the formulation of key research questions and the assessment of the feasibility of estimation. In addition to defining the primary estimator, it is imperative to outline a plan for sensitivity analysis, which serves the purpose of assessing the robustness of the estimators concerning the underlying assumptions. One aspect of CIDs that stands out as operationally advantageous is to better harmonize different sub-studies under one master protocol. However, it is important to consider time trends and external factors that may impact the estimation for each sub-trial. To illustrate the complexities of CIDs, consider the scenario where the recruitment pace varies among sub-studies. In cases where one sub-trial advances more rapidly, the protocol or analysis plan should proactively specify whether an early, separate analysis is permissible for this expeditiously recruited sub-trial. In the event that such a provision allows for one or two sub-studies to undergo early analysis, it becomes crucial to establish predefined rules governing the potential adaptation of estimand definitions for the remaining sub-studies, contingent upon recommendations from an independent data monitoring committee (IDMC). Simultaneously, corresponding estimations must also be updated in accordance with these predefined rules. Notice that even when estimand definitions pertain to distinct sub-studies, the overarching trial's integrity and analytical details should be comprehensively addressed within the broader trial framework. Another illustrative example pertains to the handling of missing data, which may exhibit varying patterns across different sub-studies. In specific disease domains, some sub-trial patients may experience a more pronounced impact from seasonal factors compared to others. Consequently, conducting sensitivity analyses for missing data handling becomes a distinct necessity, and these analyses must be executed separately for each individual sub-trial. This ensures a thorough and nuanced examination of missing data patterns within the context of each sub-trial's unique characteristics.

22.3.5 *Case Study*

Chen et al. (2023) addressed important considerations for master protocol studies utilizing external controls, including some discussions on estimands. An essential aspect emphasized is the clear definition of the clinical question and objective for each sub-trial within the master protocol. To ensure comparable arms, the proper definition and prospective use of covariates are crucial. In their example, the covariates aid in matching patients in the master protocol with those in the external control. The identifiability of the causal estimand heavily relies on the assumptions made about the data and treatment effect. Consequently, it is recommended to conduct sensitivity analyses to assess the robustness of estimators under different assumptions and modeling choices. This process ensures accurate and reliable estimation of treatment effects within master protocols reliant on external controls.

In a separate context, Parker et al. (2023) discussed the statistical analysis plan for a platform trial. Their case study demonstrated the application of the estimand framework. In recognizing the absence of an ideal estimand, they thoroughly explained their process of selecting the estimand for the primary analysis. This included evaluating performance criteria and varying assumptions regarding the treatment effect to assess the robustness of their findings.

The examples above underscore the necessity for a clear specification of the estimands and a careful consideration of their attributes in CIDs. Likewise, considerations on the analysis play a pivotal role in achieving accurate and reliable estimation of the treatment effects. In the following, we provide a comprehensive case study that demonstrates the practical implementation of the estimand framework in a basket trial. We consider a phase III program to assess the safety and efficacy of a marketed product in a new indication with three disease subtypes. For confidentiality reasons, we cannot disclose the details about the disease and the investigational product. Some aspects of the case study have been simplified and changed for the purpose of this section.

One option is to conduct three parallel, randomized trials, each aiming to investigate the treatment effect in a particular disease subtype, together with a dedicated estimand discussion. For this phase III program, we decided on the alternative option of conducting a basket trial under a common master protocol. That is, patients are enrolled into the trial and subsequently randomized within each of the three sub-studies to either the investigational product or the comparator for each of the three disease subtypes, all under a common trial protocol. The main advantages of this option are simpler trial logistics and better data quality, as patients are enrolled concurrently at the same centers.

Conducting a basket trial arguably leads to the same trial objectives as if three separate trials were conducted, and a dedicated discussion for each of the three related estimands should take place. According to the ICH E9(R1) guideline, an estimand is a precise description of the treatment effect and should reflect strategies to address intercurrent events occurring during the trial conduct for each disease subtype, as they could impact the interpretation of the trial results. The justification for the proposed primary estimand in this trial is that it will capture both the effect of the investigational product and the effect of additional background and rescue medications, mirroring the conditions in clinical practice.

The primary estimand for each sub-trial is described by the following attributes:

(a) Population

Patients suffering from disease subtype 1, 2, or 3, meeting sub-trial-related inclusion/exclusion criteria, and receiving background therapy at a locally approved dose level.

(b) Variable

- Subtype 1: Change from baseline to primary efficacy assessment score 1 at primary time point 1.
- Subtype 2: Change from baseline to primary efficacy assessment score 2 at primary time point 2.
- Subtype 2: Change from baseline to primary efficacy assessment score 3 at primary time point 3.

Note that the assessment scores and time points of assessment can be different between the three sub-studies.

(c) Treatment

Investigational product or comparator, plus background and allowed rescue medication, as needed. Note that the investigational product and the comparator are the same across all three sub-studies. Also, the dose of the allowed background medication for disease treatment must remain stable during the trial.

(d) Intercurrent Events and Their Strategies

- Discontinuation of initially assigned study treatment due to adverse events, use of prohibited medications, or lack of efficacy: Patients will be encouraged to stay in the trial, but no further treatment is offered (treatment policy strategy).
- Discontinuation of initially assigned study treatment due to other reasons: Interest lies in the treatment effect had patients taken the assigned treatment up to the final time of assessment (hypothetical strategy).
- Intake of prohibited medications without resulting in treatment discontinuation will be ignored (treatment policy strategy).
- Technical challenges with conducting the primary efficacy assessment, or missed treatments due to unavoidable external reasons such as the coronavirus disease (COVID-19) pandemic: Interest lies in the treatment effect had patients not missed their treatment or missed the primary efficacy assessments due to technical challenges (hypothetical strategy).

(e) Population-Level Summary

- Subtype 1: Difference in mean change from baseline in primary efficacy parameter 1 between treatments.
- Subtype 2: Difference in mean change from baseline in primary efficacy parameter 2 between treatments.
- Subtype 3: Difference in mean change from baseline in primary efficacy parameter 3 between treatments.

The aim was to estimate the treatment effect of comparing the investigational product against the comparator for each of the three sub-trial populations. The testing strategies for the primary and secondary endpoints were prespecified and considered separately for each sub-trial, using a (two-sided) significance level of 0.05 within each sub-trial.

Retrieved dropout (RDO) data collected after study treatment discontinuation is used for the main analysis, following the prespecified intercurrent events addressing methods as listed below. For all three sub-studies, the primary analysis accounts for intercurrent events 1 through 4 from above, as explained in the following:

- RDO data collected after study treatment discontinuation are used for the main analysis. If there is insufficient RDO data, missing data is multiply imputed based on a copy-reference for the investigational product arm and under a missing-at-random assumption (MAR) for the comparator arm.
- Data collected after the intercurrent event is used as it is.
- Primary variable is treated as missing and multiply imputed under an MAR assumption across all treatment arms, reflecting the hypothetical scenario under consideration.

We conclude this case study discussion with a few remarks. The disease variation across different subtypes is not clear in this new disease field, such as patient characteristics and standard of care treatment options. A basket trial design with separate trial objectives and estimands increases the overall understanding of the disease. The prespecified analysis and conclusion are based on each disease subtype, which provides the flexibility of having the same conclusion as if three separate studies had been conducted in parallel. Estimation of treatment policy estimands for continuous outcomes using off-treatment RDO data based on sequential multiple imputations needs to be cautious as well, as was discussed in Chap. 15 (Sect. 15.2.1 in this book). The observed RDO data might be sparse or not sufficient, which causes additional challenges for the estimated treatment effects (Drury et al., 2023; Guizzaro et al., 2021). Meanwhile, the platform trial design allows the RDO data collection in a consistent pattern or the checking of the imputation assumptions in a more robust way.

An interim analysis is planned once the primary analysis for the first two disease subtypes is completed. At the time of the interim analyses, the enrollment of patients in the third disease subtype is expected to be ongoing. The interim analysis could potentially stop the trial earlier if the treatment is deemed futile based on the available information across all disease subtypes. Additionally, it provides the possibility of early efficacy stopping or sample size adaptation for the third disease subtype. An appropriate multiplicity adjustment is needed to account for this adaptation.

Since the three subtypes are part of one disease with different disease triggers, one might also consider assessing the efficacy in the pooled trial population. However, the challenge was that no primary endpoint could be used for an overall population assessment. Therefore, estimand attributes other than intercurrent events have to be considered separately for each disease subtype. One master trial protocol will have the platform for the three separate cohorts to be handled consistently in operational setup and analysis strategy-wise. The cross-subtype comparison in a master protocol will be clearer and straightforward.

22.4 Multiregional Clinical Trials

22.4.1 Background

According to the ICH E17 guideline, a multiregional clinical trial (MRCT) is the preferred approach for development programs conducted across multiple regions with the goal of supporting regulatory submissions for an investigational treatment (ICH, 2018). The feasibility of conducting an MRCT and of including an additional region is based on the assumption that the treatment effect is applicable to the entire target population, particularly across all regions involved in the trial. This assumption should be supported by prior knowledge of the disease, the drug's mechanism of action, potential effects of ethnic factors on treatment response across regions, and any data from early exploratory trials of the investigational treatment.

In general, MRCTs aim to address two key clinical questions: First, assessing the trial drug's efficacy in the overall population, and second, evaluating the consistency of the treatment effect across regions (i.e., confirming that the overall drug effect is applicable across all regions). This is critical when the study treatment shows benefit in the overall population but must also avoid adverse outcomes in specific regions. Differences between clinical questions for the overall population and regional populations may lead to differences in estimands. In this section, we will explore these potential differences in estimands between the overall and regional populations.

22.4.2 Estimand Considerations

We discuss the differences of the five estimand attributes as follows.

(a) Population

The overall population typically encompasses all patients meeting the inclusion/exclusion criteria, while the regional population specifically refers to all patients who meet the inclusion/exclusion criteria within a specific region. Clearly, the regional population is a subset of the overall population. However, due to heterogeneity between different regional populations, regional populations may have different distributions of ethnic factors (intrinsic or extrinsic) compared to the overall population. Additionally, these ethnic factors may be predictive factors affecting the treatment effect of the study treatment in the regional population. A notable example is the epidermal growth factor receptor (EGFR) mutation, targeted by EGFR inhibitors with a higher prevalence in Southern Asia, indicating significant regional variability in activating EGFR mutations (Graham et al., 2018). As another example, in the platelet inhibition and patient outcomes study, the differing treatment effects observed between the United States and other regions were attributed to higher aspirin usage in the United States (Held et al., 2011).

It is important to distinguish the population attribute of the estimand from the observed sample in a clinical trial. Quite often, the regional distribution of predictive factors in a clinical trial sample may not be similar to that of the overall sample due to a small sample size in the region, even though the distributions of the predictive factors in the target population are comparable across regions.

(b) Variable

The primary objective of an MRCT is to assess the study treatment's efficacy in the overall population. Therefore, variables reflecting the treatment outcomes should be the same across regions to ensure consistent interpretation of the trial's success or failure. However, challenges arise in diseases like Crohn's, where regulatory agencies may diverge in their choices of the primary variable.

One example is the SIERRAS trial, where Roxadustat was compared with epoetin alfa for anemia treatment in end-stage renal disease patients on dialysis (Charytan et al., 2021). Here, the primary endpoint differed for the FDA and other agencies: For the FDA, it was the mean hemoglobin change from baseline averaged over Weeks 28–52; for other agencies, it was averaged over Weeks 28–36. Note that the ICH E17 guideline discourages the use of different primary variables in different regions.

Although there is no difference in the assessment of objective variables, such as death, we also need to consider possible differences in assessment methods and standards for variables that require subjective judgment. Additionally, from a safety perspective, adverse event reporting in different regions may also be influenced by local clinical practices.

(c) Treatment

A treatment may refer to a single intervention, a combination of interventions, or a comprehensive plan involving a complex sequence of interventions. In principle, all therapies or drugs involved in the treatment should be as consistent as possible across all regions, but there may be some differences due to variations in medical or regulatory practices. These differences may include control treatments not approved for the studied indication in different regions (Nakashima et al., 2011), approved dose regimens of study treatments that vary across regions (Malinowski et al., 2008; Zhou et al., 2019), and differing subsequent treatment plans and background therapy during treatment (Manitz et al., 2022).

(d) Intercurrent Events and Strategies

In a directed acyclic graph (DAG), nodes (vertices) are random variables with directed edges (arrows) and no directed cycles. It could be used to understand the causal network linking region, ethnic factors, intercurrent events, and treatment effect.

In a causal DAG, the lack of an arrow from one node to another could be interpreted as the absence of a direct causal effect from one to another relative to the other variables on the graph, and any variable is a cause of its descendants.

Figure 22.1 displays a DAG with five nodes, R, T, V, E, and M, corresponding to region, treatment effect, two types of ethnic factors, and intercurrent events. According to the ICH E5 guideline (ICH, 1998a), the difference in treatment effects between regions could be explained by ethnic factors, either intrinsic or extrinsic, and the region itself could be considered as a surrogate of the ethnic factors (Wittes, 2012). Therefore, there is no direct effect from region R to treatment effect T, but through two types of ethnic factors, V and E, respectively. One type of factor V characterizes the population living in each region; it acts as a confounder when it is predictive and distributed differently between regions. Meanwhile, the other type of ethnic factors, E, such as environmentally related factors, is determined by the region R; it acts as a mediator between regions. Although many ethnic factors could not be clearly classified, intrinsic factors are more often related to the first type, while extrinsic factors are related to the latter.

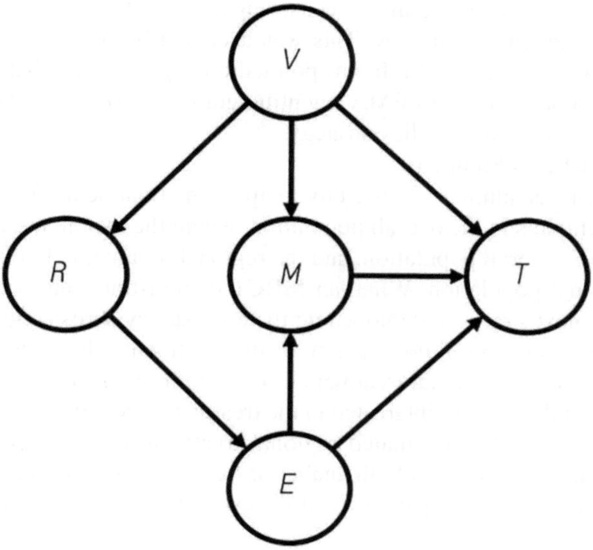

Fig. 22.1 A DAG including region (R), ethnic factors (V and E), intercurrent events (M), and treatment effect (T) in an MRCT

Both intrinsic and extrinsic factors could also have an impact on the occurrence of intercurrent events M. And intercurrent events would affect either the interpretation or the existence of the measurements associated with the clinical question of interest. In summary, treatment effects T may vary across regions due to the difference in prevalence of intrinsic and extrinsic predictive factors and incidence of intercurrent events across regions.

The incidence of different types of intercurrent events should be considered when we assess the treatment effects between regions. Although the ICH E17 guideline recommends unifying the requests from different regulatory agencies in one trial, there may still exist clinical questions of local interest.

For example, the SIERRAS trial provides an example that different regulatory agencies may recommend different strategies for addressing intercurrent events, even though it is not clearly specified in the statistical analysis plan (Charytan et al., 2021). The use of rescue therapy was considered as an intercurrent event in the SIERRAS trial. In the United States, a treatment policy strategy was used for the rescue therapy. Outside the United States, a hypothetical strategy was adopted such that the hemoglobin values after the initiation of the rescue therapy were set to missing up to 6 weeks (or 8 weeks if during the evaluation period).

Another example is the S-TRAC trial, in which adjuvant sunitinib was evaluated in high-risk renal-cell carcinoma after nephrectomy (Ravaud et al., 2016). The initiation of subsequent anticancer therapy was identified as an intercurrent event, though it was not clearly specified under the estimand framework. The primary analysis of S-TRAC treated the initiation of subsequent anticancer therapy with a hypothetical strategy leading to censoring at the last disease assessment prior to the new anticancer therapy. This was accepted by the FDA but not by the EMA (Ravaud et al., 2016). It was pointed out by the EMA that the censoring rules were not in line with EMA scientific guidelines (Party, 2012), which recommended a treatment policy strategy.

(e) Population-Level Summary

A population-level summary is used to compare the treatment effect between different treatments in the overall population, where the overall treatment effect is based on the overall population, and the regional treatment effects are based on each regional population. When an MRCT demonstrates an overall treatment effect, the next step is to demonstrate the consistency across regions. If we are interested in the overall consistency of the treatment effect, we need to show that the estimated regional treatment effects are in favor across all regions. On the other hand, if we are interested in the treatment effect in a certain region, we need to compare this estimated regional treatment effect with the estimated overall treatment effect. In both analyses, we need to use the same population-level summaries for comparability of the estimated treatment effects.

22.4.3 Discussion

MRCTs have become a common approach for simultaneous global drug development. Employing the estimand concept is beneficial both in designing MRCTs and in formulating strategies for regions participating in these trials. Besides addressing the primary clinical questions in an MRCT, sponsors should engage in dialogue with local regulators. This communication is key to understanding region-specific clinical questions and aligning on benefit-risk evaluations. The estimand framework, vital for precisely defining clinical questions of interest, will be useful to meet regional requirements.

22.5 Treatment Switching

22.5.1 Background

Treatment switching is a common intercurrent event in oncology clinical trials. This refers to the initiation of a new anticancer treatment after discontinuation of the assigned study treatment and prior to observing the endpoint of interest (Manitz et al., 2022). Crossover is the special case of treatment switching where patients in the control group can switch to the investigational treatment after some prespecified clinical event (i.e., after progression).

In confirmatory oncology trials, the primary efficacy analysis traditionally compares overall survival (OS) benefit between treatments as they are initially randomized, regardless of whether treatment switching occurs and any subsequent therapy. With the use of treatment switching, the interpretation of trial results becomes more complicated.

When patients in a clinical trial switch treatment, it confounds the evaluation of the benefits and risks of the initially allocated treatment. Patients who switch treatment often differ in baseline characteristics or disease statuses from those who remain on their initial treatment.

However, treatment switching is also relevant in therapeutic areas beyond oncology. To simplify, the following discussion focuses on estimands for overall survival in superiority oncology clinical trials involving treatment switching.

The Oncology Estimand Working Group (see Sect. 6.4 in this book for details) identified three scenarios for treatment switching based on whether the subsequent anticancer treatment is consistent with clinical practice (Manitz et al., 2022).

- Scenario 1: Patients on both arms can switch to subsequent therapies reflecting clinical practice. In a randomized trial of investigational treatment versus control treatment, it is expected that patients in both groups receive subsequent treatment, which is consistent with clinical practice after terminating treatment. At this time, the clinical question of interest is to assess the OS benefit of investigational treatment, plus any subsequent treatment, compared to control treatment, plus any subsequent treatment.
- Scenario 2: Control arm patients can switch treatment to the investigational treatment approved as next-line therapy. If the investigational treatment has been approved (or is expected to be approved soon) as a next-line therapy, patients in the control arm can switch to receive investigational treatment as next-line therapy after progression. If most patients switch from the control arm, the comparison of treatment and control can be seen as the evaluation of OS benefit between the study treatment as the current-line therapy and the next-line therapy.
- Scenario 3: Control arm patients can cross over to not-yet-approved investigational treatments. If the investigational treatment shows promising results in early trials and there is a high unmet medical need in the target population, switching (crossover) from the control arm to the treatment arm after disease progression is allowed. However, in this case, treatment switching does not reflect clinical practice. At this time, a hypothetical scenario may be of interest to clinicians and patients associated with assessing the OS benefit of the investigational treatment compared to the control arm if there was no crossover opportunity.

22.5.2 Considerations for Estimand with Treatment Switching

Prior to selecting a strategy for addressing treatment switching, it is important to clearly define what constitutes a treatment switching event in the context of the trial. For instance, treatment switching may involve switching to a specific subsequent therapy, the investigational treatment (from the control arm), or a class of therapies. Moreover, the timing of treatment switching, whether after progression or at any point, influences the choice of the strategy and the analysis approach. Table 22.3 outlines four different estimands. These are derived from combinations of strategies applied to different treatment switching events in a hypothetical oncology trial, focusing on OS as the endpoint. Table 22.3 identified three types of treatment switching events, where crossover refers to switching from the control arm to the investigational treatment.

Estimand 1 employs a treatment policy strategy for all three types of treatment switching, including the start of subsequent therapy at any time and crossover before and after progression for the control arm. This estimand considers all three types of treatment switching as reflecting the current or upcoming clinical practice and thus uses the treatment policy strategy to evaluate the efficacy of the investigational treatment in the presence of subsequent therapies and crossover from the control arm to the treatment arm. In confirmatory trials, the treatment policy estimand for OS is generally accepted by the regulatory agencies as the primary estimand. The analysis can be conducted by the standard proportional hazard Cox model following the ITT principles.

Estimand 2 uses a hypothetical strategy for all three types of treatment switching. This estimand targets the OS benefit of investigational treatment versus control treatment, assuming no subsequent therapy or crossover to the investigational treatment occurred.

Estimand 3 uses a hypothetical strategy for crossover at any time. This is reasonable when addressing treatment switching that does not reflect clinical practice. For example, if the investigational treatment has not been approved as a next-line standard treatment but a standard of care for subsequent therapy does exist, applying a hypothetical strategy only for crossover while using a treatment policy strategy for approved subsequent anticancer therapy may reflect the clinical practice better than Estimand 2. Therefore, during the trial planning phase, the project team should identify different types of treatment switching and assess whether they reflect the current clinical practice.

Estimand 4 applies a hypothetical strategy for crossover, even occurring at the point of progression. Sometimes an investigational treatment is permitted only after trial patients show disease progression. If assigned to the control arm, crossover to the investigational arm prior to progression can be considered to reflect the actual clinical practice.

Table 22.3 Examples of estimands with treatment switching

Estimand for OS		Estimand 1: Assuming subsequent therapies represent clinical practice	Estimand 2: Assuming that patients would not receive subsequent anticancer therapy	Estimand 3: Assuming that patients would not crossover to investigational arm at any time	Estimand 4: Assuming that patients would not crossover to investigational arm at progression
Population		Patients meet inclusion/exclusion criteria			
Variable		Overall survival			
Treatment		Investigational treatment, plus any subsequent therapies versus control, plus any subsequent therapies (including the investigational treatment)	Investigational treatment versus control	Investigational treatment, plus any subsequent therapies versus control, plus any subsequent therapy (excluding the investigational treatment)	Investigational treatment, plus any subsequent therapies versus control, plus any subsequent therapy (excluding investigational treatment after progression)
Intercurrent events (IEs) and strategies	Start of subsequent therapy at any time	Treatment policy	Hypothetical	Treatment policy	Treatment policy
	Crossover to investigational treatment at any time (excluding progression)	Treatment policy	Hypothetical	Hypothetical	Treatment policy
	Crossover to investigational treatment at progression	Treatment policy	Hypothetical	Hypothetical	Hypothetical
Population-level summary		HR			
Estimation		Cox model using ITT approach	Inverse probability censoring weighting (IPCW) Robins & Finkelstein, 2000) model	HR from a RPSFT model using adjusted survival times (Robins & Tsiatis, 1991); bootstrapped confidence intervals; IPCW methods could also be used	HR from two-stage method using reconstructed survival times (Latimer et al., 2020); IPCW and RPSFT methods could be used

We refer to the references for a thorough explanation of the analysis methods and appropriate sensitivity analyses to investigate robustness of the underlying assumptions (Watkins et al., 2013)
Note: *HR* hazard ratio, *RPSFT* rank-preserving structural failure time, *IPCW* inverse probability of censoring weights

22.5.3 Discussion

Methodological complexities make it inadvisable to use simplistic estimation methods, like censoring or excluding patients who switch treatment, whether they are individual patients or entire trial sites. When patients are censored at the time of treatment switching, the analysis results mainly depend on the assumption of independence between treatment switching and outcome (i.e., censoring at random). If this assumption does not hold, the estimation of the treatment effect by simply censoring the treatment switching is no longer accurate.

If the treatment switching (crossover) deviated from the typical clinical practice, it might be a good choice to adopt a hypothetical strategy to assume patients had not switched and subsequently conduct the appropriate analysis method to adjust the estimation of the efficacy for treatment switching. Although the analysis method is not the focus of this section, Table 22.3 provides the illustrative examples. Other methods that are not mentioned in this section could also be applied, per the choice of the estimand. The appropriateness of these methods depends on the assumption and the availability of the information to be collected, which should be further evaluated by sensitivity analysis. For a more detailed introduction and discussion of the methods, refer to Watkins et al. (2013).

Treatment switching before progression may introduce significant confounding factors. In open-label trials, this issue is pronounced as patients in the control arm might withdraw informed consent and switch to the investigational treatment once they are aware of their group assignments. If such confounding is anticipated, measures should be implemented to restrict switching conditions and mitigate this risk. One approach is to allow patients to switch only after progression, thereby preserving the validity of the data prior to progression.

Another related intercurrent event is the use of concomitant medications, intended to mitigate adverse reactions from treatment. Even if such medications are not anticancer treatments, they may still impact the efficacy of the treatments in cancer trials. In cancer trials, a treatment policy strategy is usually applied to concomitant medications, as it offers valuable insights for future clinical practice. It is important to carefully define the concomitant medications and distinguish them from subsequent treatments.

In this section, we have illustrated the estimand of the treatment switching using the OS in oncology trials as an example, while these estimands are not limited to the oncology studies and can be extended to other therapeutic areas. However, it should be noted that the estimation method described in this section is only applicable for the time-to-event endpoint. For other types of endpoints, an appropriate estimation method should be selected to match their corresponding estimand.

22.6 Estimands in Decentralized Clinical Trials

22.6.1 Background

Decentralization is a clinical trial design strategy that uses patient-centric means, outside of a centralized clinical site, to encourage participation in the trial (Sharma, 2015). Examples of these patient-centric means include collecting laboratory samples by a nurse from the patient's home, mailing the treatment to patients, conducting remote visits by videoconferencing, or measuring the patient's outcomes using their wearable devices.

Decentralized studies, with their patient-centric components for information collection, have been a long-standing interest of clinical researchers to remove the barrier of access to research clinical sites and promote broader patient participation in clinical trials (National Academies of Sciences, 2019). Confinements due to the COVID-19 pandemic accelerated the trends of experimentation and implementation of decentralization measures such as online advertising, e-consent, videoconferencing for trial visits, and use of local laboratories for outcomes collection (Loucks et al. 2021; Dorsey et al., 2020; Alemayehu et al., 2022). In the past two years, several regulatory guidance documents during the COVID-19 pandemic or beyond discussed decentralization (FDA, 2023a, b; EMA, 2021; SwissMedic, 2021).

Adding decentralized means to an investigator's design toolbox broadens how he/she can engage and interact with patients. This expansion of design choices beyond clinical site-based ones enlarges the set of possible questions or estimands that can be pursued in clinical trials. It makes it possible to target new estimands that were previously challenging or impossible to target with more conventional designs.

Moreover, decentralizing components that were previously centralized can either alter the estimand or the properties of an estimator. Discussing these alterations at the planning stage can help align the design with the intended research goals.

22.6.2 Decentralization and Estimands

As a design choice, decentralizing a component should consider alignment to the target estimand or question (Izem et al., 2024). Expanding the design options beyond on-site components can increase the potential set of estimands investigators could target. For example, if the indicated population is geographically dispersed away from research sites, then the population may be hard to reach by traditional clinical trials, and having a decentralized design using local sites or at-home participation can make this population attribute easier to target. Similarly, if the expected treatment delivery in clinical practice is decentralized (e.g., insulin pump device titrated to continuous glucose monitoring in the management of diabetes), then incorporating this decentralization in the trial is more aligned with the treatment attribute. Finally, measuring the benefit and risk of new or existing therapies can collect novel patient-centric assessments using decentralized measures, thereby targeting novel variable attributes of the estimand. Decentralizing the follow-up component can also lead to a new set of intercurrent events, such as loss of connectivity, device malfunction, or absence from home, to consider and plan for in the design. Thus, targeting novel estimands is a great motivation for decentralization and may require discussions with relevant stakeholders to establish fitness for purpose and fitness for use. The use of the estimand framework was discussed by Izem et al. (2024) when decentralization is considered. It provides a helpful workflow and a set of considerations, attribute by attribute. These tools can guide investigators at the design and planning stages to consider the added value of decentralization to the target estimands. They illustrate the use of the framework and this workflow in a case study (Izem et al., 2024).

22.6.3 Decentralization and Estimation

Whether the decentralization components target a novel estimand or the same estimand as previously conducted clinical trials, decentralization can impact several properties of the estimators. Those estimator properties can be better or worse depending on the decentralization component and the target estimand. When multimodal strategies are used (some centralized and some decentralized) in hybrid designs, then questions are not only about which strategy may have better properties but also about whether the two are equivalent or could be used jointly.

For example, a more convenient recruitment procedure in clinical trials could reach a broader patient population quicker than a controlled clinical trial and thereby shorten trial timelines and generalize findings more easily to a diverse target population. However, outcomes in a more diverse population may be more variable, thereby requiring a larger sample size to detect a meaningful treatment effect than a controlled trial. In addition, a trial with flexible follow-up and fewer visits with investigators than more controlled clinical trials could lead to a different treatment adherence pattern. The adherence could be worse if patients preferred in-person interactions or better if patients were failing to show up to scheduled on-site visits because they were less convenient. Also, off-site laboratory measurements may be more frequent and timelier but less accurate than an on-site standardized measure. Patient-reported questionnaires filled out at home could have smaller recall bias but a higher rate of missingness than the typical questionnaires given at the site at set visits. Therefore, assessing the potential impact of decentralization on each attribute of the estimand and the estimator needs to be tailored to the question. Going through the impact of each estimand attribute can help with planning and navigating complex design trade-offs.

22.7 Concluding Remarks

The advent of the ICH E9(R1) guideline encourages us to approach trial design under a more scientific framework. This chapter illustrates these trends across several specific trial designs, ranging from traditional non-inferiority and equivalence trials, multiregional clinical trials, and complex innovative designs to complex treatment regimens and emerging decentralized clinical trials. However, experiences with the use of the estimand framework in these designs are limited. Moreover, knowledge of these designs, including complex innovative designs, consistency evaluation in MRCTs, and decentralized clinical trials, is continuously evolving. We will undoubtedly encounter more problems and new challenges in the future as our experiences and knowledge continue to accumulate. We hope the considerations discussed in this chapter will help you apply the ICH E9(R1) guideline to these designs, develop new ideas for better use of the estimand framework, and ultimately find the best approach for these trial designs.

References

Alemayehu, D., Hemmings, R., Natarajan, K., & Roychoudhury, S. (2022). Perspectives on virtual (remote) clinical trials as the "new Normal" to accelerate drug development. *Clinical Pharmacology and Therapeutics, 111*, 373–381.

Brittain, E., & Lin, D. (2005). A comparison of intent-to-treat and per-protocol results in antibiotic noninferiority trials. *Statistics in Medicine, 24*, 1–10.

Charytan, C., Manllo-Karim, R., Martin, E. R., Steer, D., Bernardo, M., Dua, S. L., Moustafa, M. A., Saha, G., Bradley, C., Eyassu, M., & Leong, R. (2021). A randomized trial of roxadustat in anemia of kidney failure: SIERRAS study. *Kidney International Reports, 7*, 1829–1839.

Chen, J., Yuan, S., Yung, G., Ye, J., Tian, H., & Lin, J. (2023). Considerations for master protocols using external controls. *arXiv preprint arXiv*:2307.05050.

Collignon, O., Bretz, F., Pinheiro, J., & Bornkamp, B. (2022). Estimands and complex innovative designs. *Clinical Pharmacology & Therapeutics, 6*, 1183–1190.

Cro, S., Morris, T. P., Kenward, M. G., et al. (2020). Sensitivity analysis for clinical trials with missing continuous outcome data using controlled multiple imputation: A practical guide. *Statistics in Medicine, 39*, 2815–2842.

Dodd, M., Feilding, K., Carpenter, J. R., Thompson, J. A., & Elbourne, D. (2022). Statistical methods for non-adherence in non-inferiority trials: Useful and used? A systematic review. *BMJ Open, 12*, e052656.

Dorsey, E. R., Kluger, B., & Lipset, C. H. (2020). The new Normal in clinical trials: Decentralized studies. *Annals of Neurology, 88*, 863–866.

Drury, T., Abellan, J. J., Best, N., White, I. R. (2023). Estimation of treatment policy estimands for continuous outcomes using off treatment sequential multiple imputation. https://browse.arxiv.org/pdf/2308.10857.pdf.

EMA (2021). Guidance to sponsors on how to manage clinical trials during the COVID-19 pandemic. https://health.ec.europa.eu/system/files/2022-02/guidanceclinicaltrials_covid19_en_1.pdf

EMA (2022). Complex clinical trials—Questions and answers Version 2022-05-23 https://health.ec.europa.eu/system/files/2022-06/medicinal_qa_complex_clinical-trials_en.pdf

FDA (2016). Guidance for industry: Non-inferiority clinical trials to establish effectiveness. https://www.fda.gov/media/78504/download.

FDA (2019). Guidance for industry: Adaptive designs for clinical trials of drugs and biologics. https://www.fda.gov/media/78495/download

FDA (2020). Interacting with the FDA on complex innovative trial designs for drugs and biological products. https://www.fda.gov/media/130897/download

FDA (2022). Master protocols: efficient clinical trial design strategies to expedite development of oncology drugs and biologics. https://www.fda.gov/media/120721/download

FDA (2023a). Decentralized clinical trials for drugs, biological products, and devices. https://www.fda.gov/media/167696/download

FDA (2023b). FDA guidance on conduct of clinical trials of medical products during COVID-19 Public Health Emergency. https://www.fda.gov/regulatory-information/search-fda-guidance-documents/fda-guidance-conduct-clinical-trials-medical-products-during-covid-19-public-health-emergency

Gillespie, S. H., Crook, A. M., McHugh, T. D., Mendel, C. M., Meredith, S. K., Murray, S. R., Pappas, F., Phillips, P. P. J., & Nunn, A. J. (2014). Four-month moxifloxacin-based regimens for drug-sensitive tuberculosis. *New England Journal of Medicine, 371*, 1577–1587.

Graham, R. P., Treece, A. L., Lindeman, N. I., Vasalos, P., Shan, M., Jennings, L. J., & Rimm, D. L. (2018). Worldwide frequency of commonly detected EGFR mutations. *Archives of Pathology & Laboratory Medicine, 2*, 163–167.

Guizzaro, L., Pétavy, F., Ristl, R., & Gallo, C. (2021). The use of a variable representing compliance improves accuracy of estimation of the effect of treatment allocation regardless of discontinuation in trials with incomplete follow-up. *Statistics in Biopharmaceutical Research, 13*, 119–127.

Held, C., Åsenblad, N., Bassand, J. P., Becker, R. C., Cannon, C. P., Claeys, M. J., Harrington, R. A., Horrow, J., Husted, S., James, S. K., & Mahaffey, K. W. (2011). Ticagrelor versus clopidogrel in patients with acute coronary syndromes undergoing coronary artery bypass surgery: Results from the PLATO (platelet inhibition and patient outcomes) trial. *Journal of the American College of Cardiology, 6*, 672–684.

Hollis, S. (2002). A graphical sensitivity analysis for clinical trials with non-ignorable missing binary outcome. *Statistics in Medicine, 21*, 3823–3834.

ICH (1998a). E5(R1) Ethnic factors in the acceptability of foreign clinical data. https://database.ich.org/sites/default/files/E5_R1__Guideline.pdf.

ICH(1998b).E9Guidanceforindustry.Statisticalprinciplesforclinicaltrials.https://www.ema.europa.eu/en/documents/scientific-guideline/ich-e-9-statistical-principles-clinical-trials-step-5_en.pdf

ICH (2018). E17 General principles for planning and design of multiregional clinical trial guidance for industry. https://database.ich.org/sites/default/files/E17_Guideline.pdf.

ICH (2019). E9(R1) addendum on estimands and sensitivity analysis in clinical trials to the guideline on statistical principles for clinical trials. https://www.ema.europa.eu/en/documents/scientific-guideline/ich-e9-r1-addendum-estimands-sensitivity-analysis-clinical-trials-guideline-statistical-principles_en.pdf

ICH (2021). ICH E9(R1) training materials. https://database.ich.org/sites/default/files/E9%28R1%29%20Training%20Material%20-%20PDF_0.pdf

Izem, R., Zuber, E., Daizadeh, N., Bretz, F., Sverdlov, O., Edrich, P., Branson, J., Degtyarev, E., Sfikas, N., & Hemmings, R. (2024). Decentralized clinical trials: Scientific considerations through the lens of the Estimand framework. *Therapeutic Innovation & Regulatory Science, 58*, 495–504.

Keene, O. (2023). Adherence, per-protocol effects, and the estimands framework. *Pharmaceutical Statistics, 22*, 1141–1144.

Latimer, N. R., White, I. R., Tilling, K., & Siebert, U. (2020). Improved two-stage esti-mation to adjust for treatment switching in randomized trials: G-estimation to address time-dependent confounding. *Statistical Methods in Medical Research, 29*, 2900–2918.

Leurent, B., Gomes, M., Cro, S., Wiles, N., & Carpenter, J. R. (2020). Reference-based multiple imputation for missing data sensitivity analyses in trial-based cost-effectiveness analysis. *Health Economics, 29*, 171–184.

Lou, Y., Jones, M. P., & Sun, W. (2019a). Assessing the ratio of means as a causal estimand in clinical endpoint bioequivalence studies in the presence of intercurrent events. *Statistics in Medicine, 38*, 5214–5235.

Lou, Y., Jones, M. P., & Sun, W. (2019b). Estimation of causal effects in clinical endpoint bioequivalence studies in the presence of intercurrent events: Noncompliance and missing data. *Journal of Biopharmaceutical Statistics, 29*, 151–173.

Loucks, T. L., Tyson, C., Dorr, D., Garovic, V. D., Hill, J., McSwain, S. D., Radovick, S., Sonnenberg, F. A., Weis, J. A., & Brady, K. T. (2021). Clinical research during the COVID-19 pandemic: The role of virtual visits and digital approaches. *Journal of Clinical and Translational Science, 5*, e102.

Lynggaard, H., Keene, O. N., Mütze, T., & Rehal, S. (2024). Applying the estimand framework to non-inferiority trials. *Pharmaceutical Statistics, 23*(6), 1156–1165.

Malinowski, H. J., Westelinck, A., Sato, J., & Ong, T. (2008). Same drug, different dosing: Differences in dosing for drugs approved in the United States, Europe, and Japan. *The Journal of Clinical Pharmacology, 8*, 900–908.

Manitz, J., Kan-Dobrosky, N., Buchner, H., Casadebaig, M. L., Degtyarev, E., Dey, J., Haddad, V., Jie, F., Martin, E., Mo, M., & Rufibach, K. (2022). Estimands for overall survival in clinical trials with treatment switching in oncology. *Pharmaceutical Statistics, 1*, 150–162.

Matilde Sanchez, M., & Chen, X. (2006). Choosing the analysis population in non-inferiority studies: Per protocol or intent-to-treat. *Statistics in Medicine, 25*, 1169–1181.

Mo, Y., Lim, C., Watson, J. A., White, N. J., & Cooper, B. S. (2020). Non-adherence in non-inferiority trials: Pitfalls and recommendations. *BMJ, 370*, m2215.

Morgan K. E., White I. R., Leyrat C. Stanworth S., & Kahan B. C. (2023). Applying the estimands framework to non-inferiority trials: guidance on choice of hypothetical estimands for non-adherence and comparison of estimation methods. https://doi.org/10.48550/arXiv.2312.00494.

Nakashima, K., Narukawa, M., Kanazu, Y., & Takeuchi, M. (2011). Differences between Japan and the United States in dosages of drugs recently approved in Japan. *The Journal of Clinical Pharmacology, 4*, 549–560.

National Academies of Sciences (2019). Virtual clinical trials: Challenges and opportunities: Proceedings of a workshop. https://nap.nationalacademies.org/catalog/25502/virtual-clinical-trials-challenges-and-opportunities-proceedings-of-a-workshop.

Nauta, J. (2024). Estimand for non-inferiority influenza vaccine immunogenicity trials. *Vaccine, 42*, 840–843.

Neuenschwander, B., Wandel, S., Roychoudhury, S., & Bailey, S. (2016). Robust exchangeability designs for early phase clinical trials with multiple strata. *Pharmaceutical Statistics, 2*, 123–134.

NMPA (2018). Statistical guideline on bioequivalence studies. https://www.nmpa.gov.cn/zhuanti/ypqxgg/ggzhcfg/20181029173101911.html

NMPA (2021). Guideline on adaptive designs for clinical trials. https://www.cde.org.cn/zdyz/domesticinfopage?zdyzIdCODE=4409e51a403a911757af6caf3ecef129

Parker, R. A., Weir, C. J., Pham, T. M., White, I. R., Stallard, N., Parmar, M. K., Swingler, R. J., Dakin, R. S., Pal, S., & Chandran, S. (2023). Statistical analysis plan for the motor neuron disease systematic multi-arm adaptive randomized trial (MND-SMART). *Trials, 1*, 1–15.

Party, O. W. (2012). Guideline on the evaluation of anticancer medicinal products in man. *Oncology*.

Polverejan, E., & Dragalin, V. (2020). Aligning treatment policy Estimands and estimators—A simulation study in Alzheimer's disease. *Statistics in Biopharmaceutical Research, 12*, 142–154.

Ratitch, B., Bell, J., Mallinckrodt, C., Bartlett, J. W., Goel, N., Molenberghs, G., O'Kelly, M., Singh, P., & Lipkovich, I. (2020). Choosing Estimands in clinical trials: Putting the ICH E9(R1) into practice. *Therapeutic Innovation & Regulatory Science, 2*, 324–341.

Ravaud, A., Motzer, R. J., Pandha, H. S., George, D. J., Pantuck, A. J., Patel, A., Chang, Y. H., Escudier, B., Donskov, F., Magheli, A., & Carteni, G. (2016). Adjuvant sunitinib in high-risk renal-cell carcinoma after nephrectomy. *New England Journal of Medicine, 23*, 2246–2254.

Rehal, S., Cro, S., Phillips, P. P. J., Fielding, K., & Carpenter, J. R. (2023). Handling intercurrent events and missing data in non-inferiority trials using the estimand framework: A tuberculosis case study. *Clinical Trials, 20*, 497–506.

Robins, J. M., & Finkelstein, D. M. (2000). Correcting for noncompliance and dependent censoring in an AIDS clinical trial with inverse probability of censoring weighted (IPCW) log-rank tests. *Biometrics, 56*(3), 779–788.

Robins, J. M., & Tsiatis, A. A. (1991). Correcting for noncompliance in randomized trials using rank preserving structural failure time models. *Communications in Statistics - Theory and Methods, 20*(8), 2609–2631.

Sharma, N. S. (2015). Patient centric approach for clinical trials: Current trend and new opportunities. *Perspectives in Clinical Research, 6*, 134–138.

SwissMedic (2021). Clinical trials on medicinal products—Pandemic by SARS-Cov-2. https://www.swissmedic.ch/swissmedic/en/home/news/coronavirus-covid-19/klv-cov-2-pandemie-2.html

Watkins, C., Huang, X., Latimer, N., Tang, Y., & Wright, E. J. (2013). Adjusting over-all survival for treatment switches: Commonly used methods and practical application. *Pharmaceutical Statistics, 12*, 348–357.

White, I. R., Joseph, R., & Best, N. (2020). A causal modelling framework for reference-based imputation and tipping point analysis in clinical trials with quantitative outcome. *Journal of Biopharmaceutical Statistics, 20*, 334–350.

Wiens, B., & Lipkovich, L. (2020). The impact of major events on ongoing noninferiority trials, with application to COVID-19. *Statistics in Biopharmaceutical Research, 4*, 443–450.

Wittes J. (2012). Why is this subgroup different from all other subgroups? Thoughts on regional differences in randomized clinical trials. *Proceedings of the Fourth Seattle Symposium in Biostatistics: Clinical Trials*, 95–115.

Zhou, L., Higashimori, M., Shen, K., Zhang, Z., Sheng, J., Xu, H., Horiuchi, M., Ichikawa, K., Al-Huniti, N., & Zhou, D. (2019). Oncology therapy drugs in China, Japan, and the United States: Pharmacokinetic characteristics, dose regimens, and development strategies. *Clinical Pharmacology and Therapeutics, 6*, 1303–1320.

Chapter 23
Leveraging the Estimand Framework for Clinical Trial Disruptions

Frank Bretz, Jiawei Wei, and Xiaoling Wei

Abstract Major disruptions like the coronavirus disease (COVID-19) pandemic or the Ukrainian war can lead to significant challenges in the conduct and analysis of clinical trials. This chapter explores how the estimand framework, outlined by the ICH E9(R1) guideline, provides a structured approach to address and mitigate these challenges, ensuring scientific rigor and reliability of trial data amidst unprecedented circumstances. The framework's structured approach facilitates the design and analysis of clinical trials, ensuring that results remain interpretable and relevant. We discuss various risk assessment and mitigation strategies, alongside a detailed exploration of different hypothetical scenarios for estimating treatment effects in disrupted trials. We also cover specific estimand considerations in view of major clinical trial disruptions in disease areas like stroke, oncology, and central nervous system trials, highlighting unique considerations for each. As global public health emergencies, geopolitical conflicts, or other major reasons for trial disruptions continue in the future, structured approaches like the estimand framework can serve as crucial tools for ensuring the continuity and data integrity of clinical trials.

F. Bretz
Advanced Methodology and Data Sciences/Statistical Methodology, Novartis Pharma AG, Basel, Switzerland
e-mail: frank.bretz@novartis.com

J. Wei
Advanced Methodology and Data Sciences/Statistical Methodology, Novartis Institutes for Biomedical Research Co., Shanghai, China
e-mail: jiawei.wei@novartis.com

X. Wei (✉)
Advanced Quantitative Sciences, Novartis Institutes for Biomedical Research Co., Shanghai, China
e-mail: xiaoling.wei@novartis.com

J. Wei et al. (eds.), *Estimands in Clinical Trials*, Springer Series in Pharmaceutical Statistics, https://doi.org/10.1007/978-3-032-02192-2_23

23.1 Introduction

Clinical trial disruptions like the coronavirus disease (COVID-19) pandemic refer to unforeseen events or circumstances that interrupt or impede the normal progression and conduct of a clinical trial. They have the potential to delay or even halt the trial altogether. Clinical trial disruptions can introduce inconsistencies in data collection, missing data, or biases, making it challenging to ensure the integrity and quality of trial data. Mitigating these disruptions and addressing their impact on trial conduct and data integrity is crucial for maintaining the scientific rigor and reliability of impacted clinical trials.

This chapter focuses mainly on the COVID-19 pandemic, as it led to unique challenges and unprecedented clinical trial disruptions on a global scale. In what follows, we explain how the estimand framework (ICH, 2019) helped to address the challenges faced by clinical trials during the pandemic by providing a clear and structured approach to trial design and analysis. The estimand framework helped to ensure that trial results remained interpretable and relevant to the extent possible. It also helped to identify the impact of the pandemic on trial outcomes and provided a basis for making decisions about the validity and reliability of trial results. The considerations presented in this chapter can also be applied to other situations facing clinical trial disruptions.

23.2 Impact of the COVID-19 Pandemic

The novel coronavirus, known as SARS-CoV-2, is a previously unidentified strain of coronavirus that infects humans. On January 30, 2020, the World Health Organization (WHO) declared the outbreak of this virus a global public health emergency. Subsequently, on March 11, 2020, the WHO classified the situation as a pandemic.

The COVID-19 pandemic had a most relevant impact on the conduct of clinical trials for medical products worldwide. Numerous challenges have emerged due to factors such as quarantines, site closures, travel restrictions, disruptions in the supply chain for investigational products, and the possibility of site personnel or patients contracting COVID-19. As outlined by Akacha et al. (2020), among others, these challenges included the following:

- Healthcare systems in many regions were overwhelmed, with medical personnel heavily involved in COVID-19-related activities.
- Government-imposed restrictions directly affected trial monitoring, data collection, and drug supply activities.
- Some patients were hesitant to attend scheduled visits due to concerns about being around sick individuals, traveling, or being in public places.

- Other patients were unable to attend scheduled visits due to health issues related to COVID-19 (e.g., hospitalization or death) or government restrictions (e.g., self-isolation, quarantine, lockdowns).
- Yet other patients needed additional medications to treat COVID-19 symptoms or other health issues related to the confinement situation, which were not anticipated during the trial's design stage.

These challenges led to difficulties in adhering to protocol-specific procedures, including the administration or use of investigational products, adherence to scheduled visits, efficacy assessments, and laboratory/diagnostic testing. Consequently, these disruptions resulted in compromised trial data (e.g., missed assessments, virtual assessments replacing traditional procedures) and posed challenges in interpreting clinical trial results due to systematic biases that can be introduced in various ways (e.g., underrepresentation of patients with certain comorbidities or in specific age groups).

The extent of these challenges depended on factors such as the duration of the COVID-19 pandemic in a specific region, the number of affected patients, the specific disease being studied, and various elements of trial design (e.g., duration and interval of visit schedules). In some cases, the disruptions were so severe that continuing the trial was not feasible. In other cases, trials continued, but the data collected beyond the time of disruption were questionable, presenting methodological challenges.

To illustrate these challenges, consider, for example, the Physio4FMD trial, a randomized controlled trial involving adults with functional neurological disorder, a common cause of disabling neurological symptoms such as weakness and tremor (Marston et al., 2023). The trial's intervention consisted of a specialized physiotherapy protocol, with the control group receiving treatment as usual. Patients had assessments at baseline, 6, and 12 months (the primary variable time point). The primary objective was to assess the efficacy of specialized physiotherapy versus treatment as usual in reducing disability at 12 months post-randomization, as assessed by the physical function questionnaire. The COVID-19 pandemic significantly disrupted the Physio4FMD trial by impeding timely treatment for 33% of patients recruited before March 2020. Consequently, some patients either did not receive their assigned treatment within the intended follow-up period or experienced substantial treatment delays. To adapt to the pandemic, the trial implemented remote assessments, provided online resources, and extended the follow-up period. Additionally, it had to be discussed whether and how its planned statistical analysis had to be modified to account for the pandemic's influence on trial outcomes.

Various approaches have been proposed in the literature to address the challenges posed by the COVID-19 pandemic in assessing the integrity and interpretability of clinical trials. For instance, Meyer et al. (2020) recommended conducting a risk assessment using aggregated and blinded data to evaluate whether trials impacted by the pandemic could yield interpretable results; see also Hemmings (2020) and Collins and Levenson (2020). This risk assessment would benefit from incorporating a forward-looking approach, anticipating potential effects not yet observed but likely to occur, and should be maintained throughout the trial. Corresponding measures are necessary to minimize sources of operational and statistical bias. Key elements include, but are not limited to:

- Determine whether trial modifications are needed to ensure patient safety and maintain trial integrity.
- Identify patients affected by the pandemic and understand the impact on them.
- Decide what additional information should be collected in the trial database, or from trial investigators, to effectively monitor, document, and address pandemic-related issues.
- Balance the advantages of remote data collection or other decentralized trial elements against the risk that a new method of data collection may not be fully exchangeable with the original method.
- Evaluate the extent of missing data and the specific reasons for missingness.
- Determine any changes to planned analyses and analysis population definitions, or additional sensitivity analyses that need to be prespecified prior to unblinding.

Several authors advocated the use of the estimand framework introduced in Part I of this book to address the challenges posed by the COVID-19 pandemic in assessing the integrity and interpretability of clinical trials (Akacha et al., 2020; Meyer et al., 2020). Similarly, when examining the impact of COVID-19 on oncology clinical trials, Degtyarev et al. (2020) argued that the estimand framework introduced in the ICH E9(R1) guideline provides a structured and transparent language to discuss the pandemic's effects. Cro et al. (2020) outlined a four-step strategy for addressing missing data in ongoing randomized trials during the pandemic, accounting for disruptions arising from the aforementioned factors. Also, Kahan et al. (2020) discussed several challenges in the context of trials of treatments for patients hospitalized with COVID-19 and made suggestions for how estimands should be defined for key variables.

Regulatory guidance for addressing the impact of the COVID-19 pandemic on clinical trials has been released by various agencies (MHRA, 2020; EMA, 2020a; FDA, 2021). Bacchieri et al. (2020) advocated a risk and mitigation actions plan for clinical trials during the COVID-19 pandemic, based on the European Medicines Agency (EMA) (EMA, 2020b) and FDA (2021) guidelines and building on the estimand framework. Their proposal provides advice to evaluate how the different aspects of clinical trials should be handled to mitigate the impact of the pandemic on data management, statistics, and medical writing activities, maintaining the required quality standards. Finally, Leahy et al. (2020) discussed the impact of the pandemic on health technology assessments, as it might affect the estimation of the treatment effect, costs, life-years, utilities, discontinuation rates, and methods of evidence synthesis and extrapolation. As the authors argued, the pandemic left large deficits in the budgets of many jurisdictions, so that funding for other treatments, in particular new treatments, may have become more constrained than previously expected.

23.3 Estimand Considerations

According to the ICH E9(R1) guideline, an estimand is described through a precise specification of five attributes: treatment, population, variable, intercurrent events, and population-level summary (Chap. 2). These attributes should align with the objectives of the clinical trial and encompass the definition of each attribute, along with suitable strategies for addressing intercurrent events.

As argued by Van Lancker et al. (2023), in most cases, the original research question remained unchanged even after the emergence of the COVID-19 pandemic. However, the unforeseen intercurrent events caused by COVID-19 introduced uncertainty into the original trial questions, requiring sponsors to consider how to account for them. Not adapting to the original estimand implies a treatment policy approach for all unforeseen intercurrent events. However, in the presence of intercurrent events related to operational challenges due to the COVID-19 pandemic, it seems reasonable to frame the clinical questions of interest using a hypothetical estimand strategy (Meyer et al., 2020; Akacha et al., 2020). The relevance and acceptability of a hypothetical estimand strategy may be less clear when intercurrent events are related to health status, such as death due to COVID-19 in a cardiovascular trial where death is an outcome of interest. Van Lancker et al. (2023) discussed in detail different estimand strategies to address intercurrent events related to the pandemic. Specifically, they presented and explored three hypothetical strategies that vary in their assumed hypothetical scenarios and populations; see also Qu and Lipkovich (2021).

The first estimand discussed by Van Lancker et al. (2023) focuses on the treatment effect within the overall patient population, including those recruited before, during, and after the pandemic. In this scenario, individuals can suffer from COVID-19 infections from the time of the outbreak but without experiencing administrative and operational challenges caused by the pandemic. In this hypothetical world, there are no COVID-19-related lockdowns, administrative restrictions, withdrawals from the trial medication, or non-adherence due to pandemic-related reasons. Therefore, intercurrent events associated with operational and administrative challenges resulting from the pandemic can be addressed using this hypothetical strategy. However, individuals may still get COVID-19, while others may receive vaccinations. These COVID-19 health-related intercurrent events, which could potentially lead to withdrawals from or interruptions of the trial medication, can be managed using a treatment policy strategy.

The second estimand focuses on the treatment effect in a patient population within a post-pandemic world, where society and the healthcare system have adapted to living with COVID-19. This is a somewhat practical definition because variations within this population are possible, taking into account factors like different levels of vaccination, infection rates, and other relevant variables at the time of recruitment. As before, a hypothetical setting is considered where patients can get COVID-19 infections but without experiencing administrative and operational challenges. This estimand thus differs from the first estimand through the choice of the population attribute: The first estimand considers the overall patient population, including individuals recruited before, during, and after the pandemic, whereas the second estimand focuses specifically on the patient population in a post-pandemic world. As before, COVID-19 health-related intercurrent events can be addressed using the treatment policy strategy.

The third estimand focuses on the treatment effect in a world where COVID-19 does not exist, thus being associated with the original objective of the trial. All COVID-19-related events would be addressed using a hypothetical strategy. Specifically, the hypothetical scenario of interest involves examining what would have happened if patients who withdrew from the randomized trial medication due to pandemic-related reasons had instead remained on the randomized treatment. Similarly, it explores the situation where patients who experienced interruptions to the trial medication due to pandemic-related reasons had instead continued on the randomized treatment without any interruptions. Lastly, it considers a scenario where patients who were infected with the COVID-19 virus or received treatment or vaccination for COVID-19 had instead not been infected, treated, or vaccinated. When defining this estimand, the focus is on the patient population that was actually recruited during the pre-pandemic period.

The second estimand above appears relevant for the design of future trials, as it is reasonable to assume that future medical practices may differ slightly from pre-pandemic times, even with the majority of the population vaccinated and high levels of immunity. However, when a substantial proportion of subjects were recruited and treated prior to or during the pandemic, the first estimand might often be a pragmatic choice. Note that the estimands introduced above are not an exhaustive list of estimands that could be relevant in the context of COVID-19 and its associated intercurrent events. For instance, given the emergence of new COVID-19 variants, the treatment policy strategy might be relevant in addressing intercurrent events such as discontinuation of COVID-19-related treatments.

Regardless of the chosen estimand, it is critical that the targeted outcome can be reliably estimated with justifiable assumptions and plausible sensitivity analyses. If this is not possible, such as due to limited understanding of the disease or drug for imputing missing or hypothetical data, an alternative estimand should be chosen. Specifically, in cases with a large number of intercurrent events related to COVID-19, the treatment policy approach may be more suitable for reliable estimation than a hypothetical strategy.

23.4 Considerations on Estimation

General considerations on estimation under the estimand framework are covered in Part IV of this book. More specifically, considerations on analyzing different types of variables are covered in Chaps. 15–18, and the principles discussed in these chapters remain applicable to estimation problems that are specific to the COVID-19 pandemic. For each estimand, an aligned method of analysis, or estimator, should be implemented that is able to provide an estimate on which a reliable interpretation can be based. As a starting point to guide the choice of the estimator, key assumptions regarding the occurrence of the intercurrent events and their consequences on the outcome (including on its missingness) should be specified. After a main estimator is defined for an estimand, sensitivity estimator(s) need to be defined for the same estimand, stating how the assumptions differ from those of the main estimator. To be noted, the amount of missing data is likely to be substantially increased for trials impacted by the COVID-19 pandemic, and pandemic-related missingness needs to be handled appropriately in the context of each estimand and analysis method. Van Lancker et al. (2023) pointed out that all estimation methods discussed in their article depend sensitively on the amount of missing data. While no thresholds for the proportion of missing data can be specified above which an analysis becomes invalidated, the authors note that the performance characteristics depend on the validity of the underlying assumptions regarding the unobserved data. Therefore, it is crucial to thoughtfully consider and select plausible assumptions, and conducting sensitivity analyses is essential to assess the robustness of results under alternative missing data assumptions; see also Meyer et al. (2020).

Various authors have published specific analysis approaches that account for pandemic-related intercurrent events or have conducted extensive simulation studies. For example, Van Lancker et al. (2023) discussed potential estimators for the different (hypothetical) estimands outlined above. More specifically, they reviewed various estimation methods using approaches for handling missing data, such as likelihood-based analysis and multiple imputation, as well as simple and augmented inverse probability weighting. Along similar lines, Lasch and Guizzaro (2022) presented a simulation study to compare different estimators for an estimand that includes hypothetical strategies for COVID-related intercurrent events. Guo et al. (2020) discussed statistical issues related to changes in the patient population due to protocol modifications during the pandemic. Wiens and Lipkovich (2020) presented simulations to study the performance of several multiple imputation strategies compared with traditional nonresponder imputation and observed case analyses when the primary variable is binary in the context of non-inferiority trials impacted by the pandemic. Jin et al. (2021) proposed a modified reference-based imputation and tipping point analysis in the presence of missing data due to the pandemic. Finally, Vansteelandt (2023) highlighted in a commentary that whenever possible, analyses of randomized clinical trials should protect the Type I error rate at a prespecified significance level when testing the null hypothesis of no treatment. He further argued that if intercurrent events occur at equal rates in both arms of the trial, then standard analyses targeting the treatment policy estimand, thus ignoring intercurrent events, will protect the null hypothesis of no treatment effect.

23.5 Specific Disease Areas

In certain disease areas, specific estimand considerations might apply in view of the pandemic. In the following, we review exemplarily some considerations that apply to stroke, oncology, and central nervous system clinical trials and go beyond the considerations presented in Part II of this book.

23.5.1 *Stroke Clinical Trials*

Yassi et al. (2021) emphasized the need for a carefully planned approach to ensure the appropriate conduct of stroke trials during the pandemic and to maintain patient safety. The authors illustrated how the estimand framework could help ensure the proper planning, conduct, and interpretation of stroke clinical trials in the face of clinical trial disruptions. For example, the COVID-19 pandemic might have impacted the trial population of interest on many levels: In many jurisdictions, patients with stroke were reluctant or unable to seek acute medical care due to hospitals being overwhelmed with COVID-19 patients, which may have led to the initial randomized trial population being different from the final trial population. Yassi et al. (2021) further pointed out that in addition to the trial population, COVID-19 can also affect the variable measurements of the trial. Apart from the effects on functional or surrogate variables as a direct result of a COVID-19 infection, limitations imposed during the pandemic may have prevented the collection of a variable in the trial if a patient could not be assessed onsite or collected by remote assessment or telemedicine. The biological interactions between COVID-19 infections and stroke may have also confounded the natural history of stroke or the interpretation of treatment effects. The authors recommended that investigators should prespecify the practical strategies to mitigate the potential impact of the pandemic on the trial, categorizing them into two factors: those related to suspected or confirmed COVID-19 infections and those related to the logistical impacts of the pandemic. In addition, the authors presented a hypothetical trial example to illustrate how the estimand framework can be used to provide a statistical contingency strategy within stroke research trials impacted by the pandemic. It is important to recognize that an intercurrent event can be addressed using various strategies, and selecting the most appropriate strategy for a given trial depends on the trial's overall clinical and scientific objectives.

23.5.2 *Oncology Clinical Trials*

Degtyarev et al. (2020) identified key intercurrent events due to COVID-19 in oncology clinical trials: death due to COVID-19 infection, treatment discontinuation due to COVID-19 infection, and treatment discontinuation for reasons unrelated to COVID-19 infection. Focusing on time-to-event endpoints, they also suggested strategies for addressing these intercurrent events, depending on their relationship to malignancy and treatment and the interpretability of data after them. The authors argued that the objective of clinical trials in a pandemic-free world remains of interest, as clinical trials that started before the pandemic were designed with the intention of informing clinical practice in a world without a pandemic. Degtyarev et al. (2020) therefore argued in favor of a hypothetical strategy, in line with the original trial objectives. If, however, the frequency of intercurrent events was low, treating them with the treatment policy strategy might provide an approximate response to the original objective of the clinical trial. Degtyarev et al. (2020) also provided recommendations for the analysis of time-to-event endpoints under different estimand strategies. When using a hypothetical estimand strategy, the relative effect can be estimated through simple censoring at the intercurrent event for estimating hazard-based quantities (e.g., hazard ratio) when assuming the absence of informative censoring. If informative censoring cannot be excluded (e.g., patients are censored at the start of new therapy after discontinuation that could be attributed to disease), methods such as inverse probability of censoring weights might be preferred. The authors also discussed the impact on other important variables in oncology clinical trials. For example, they acknowledged that no ideal approach seems available for estimating a hypothetical estimand of the objective response rate and discussed various approaches.

Sridhara et al. (2022) provided a summary of discussions among oncologists, patient advocates, and experts from international regulatory agencies, academicians, and representatives of the pharmaceutical industry on how best to incorporate lessons learned during the COVID-19 pandemic into the design of future oncology trials. It was pointed out that some changes, such as decentralized informed consent and the use of local laboratories for routine blood tests, can be incorporated into future clinical trials and are unlikely to bias treatment effect estimates (see also Sect. 22.6 in Chap. 22 of this book). Increased adoption of decentralization in oncology trials will also depend on the extent to which heterogeneity (populations, treatment modalities, variables, frequency of testing, etc.) is taken into account at the trial planning stage, and the estimand framework is acknowledged as being useful in this regard. The discussions also highlighted the importance of flexibility to reduce patients' burden, which can facilitate access to and participation in oncology clinical trials and increase the representativeness of patients in the trial setting.

23.5.3 Central Nervous System Clinical Trials

Mészáros et al. (2023) conducted a survey examining the strategies proposed by sponsors and supported by regulators for the implementation of the estimands framework in central nervous system clinical trials. The authors searched scientific advice letters issued by the EMA between 2017 and 2022. Strategies proposed and recommended were summarized by category of intercurrent events, and the rationale for the choices was analyzed qualitatively. While this survey did not focus specifically on trials impacted by the pandemic, a total of five trials were reported that included 10 pandemic-related intercurrent events. In most cases, the regulatory-relevant strategy recommended for estimating the treatment effect in central nervous system clinical trials was the hypothetical strategy. However, in one trial, the impact of the pandemic on missed doses was differentiated into two distinct intercurrent events, contingent upon the quantity of doses that had been missed. For the intercurrent event associated with a lower number of missed doses, a treatment policy strategy was endorsed.

The survey findings underscore a tendency toward endorsing the hypothetical approach to reflect the treatment effect in a world without the acute effects of the early waves of the COVID-19 pandemic. This endorsement is often accompanied by the recommendation that the intercurrent events had to be unequivocally and solely attributable to the pandemic, rather than, for instance, the health status of the patients.

23.6 Implications for Future Clinical Trial Disruptions

So far, we have focused on the COVID-19 pandemic, although clinical trial disruptions can arise from various sources, including but not limited to:

- External Factors: Events such as natural disasters, pandemics (e.g., COVID-19), political conflicts (e.g., the Ukraine war), or regulatory changes can significantly disrupt the trial's operations and pose challenges to data collection, patient recruitment, and overall trial conduct.
- Site-related Issues: Site closures, staff unavailability, or limitations in resources at trial sites can disrupt the smooth execution of the trial. These issues can hinder patient recruitment, adherence to the trial protocol, and data collection.
- Supply Chain Disruptions: Delays or interruptions in the availability or delivery of investigational products, study materials, or laboratory supplies can impact the trial's progress. These disruptions can lead to deviations from the planned trial procedures and affect data quality.

Trial disruptions make it challenging to ensure trial integrity and trial quality. Many sponsors have already developed standardized metrics of trial operational status, such as rates of missed visits, discontinuations from treatment and study, protocol deviations, and adverse events, to reinforce a consistent approach to risk monitoring and assessment. Such metrics are useful to identify trials that are more acutely impacted by disruption in the future. To minimize the trial disruption impact, different considerations for future trials might be helpful. For example, Van Lancker et al. (2023) proposed some insights for future trials in view of the past COVID-19 pandemic to target the relevant treatment effect to be estimated. In the following, we adopt their proposals for future clinical trial disruptions.

- Trial Population: Inclusion/exclusion criteria for future clinical trials should specify pandemic status and other risk factors. This means the eligibility criteria should be clear on any restrictions, which may depend on the target disease (e.g., restrictions on COVID-19-infected patients during the past COVID-19 pandemic). Patient factors, including the geographical area of the trial, racial diversity of the patient population, underlying disease conditions, and trial duration, might be considered here.
- Primary Variable(s): The primary variables of new trials should reflect clinical practice and be able to measure clinical benefits. In some cases, the disruption may affect the reliability of primary variable measurements due to site closures, staff unavailability, or limitations in resources at trial sites. Surrogate variables that can reliably measure clinical benefits may be needed, such as estimates at landmark time points or earlier time points rather than later time points. In accordance with local regulations and depending on operational capabilities, phone calls, virtual contacts (e.g., teleconsultations), or home visits by site staff or off-site healthcare professionals may substitute in-person visits for certain assessments. This arrangement would last for the duration of the disruption until it is safe for patients to return to the site.
- Treatment: Considering the possibility of patients being affected by a public health emergency and requiring medication, it is crucial to clearly define the scope of treatment interest, particularly whether any additional medications become integral to the treatment plan. Moreover, disruptions to trials may lead to issues with drug supply, including delays or interruptions in the availability of investigational products. In cases where trial disruptions limit or prevent on-site study visits, the direct delivery of study treatment to a patient's home might be allowed, in accordance with local regulations. This approach may be considered if the investigator deems an on-site visit by the patient impractical or unsafe and believes that administering the study treatment at home, even without an on-site visit, is in the best interest of the patient's health.
- Intercurrent Events: New trials may encounter various challenges arising from patient exposure to public health emergencies, geopolitical conflicts, or other disruptions. These challenges could include regional administrative travel restrictions and health impacts on patients affected by the public health crisis. Consequently, identifying relevant intercurrent events, such as disruption-related restrictions and the use of concomitant medications during such disruptions, along with developing strategies to manage these events, will be crucial for addressing the scientific questions at hand. Considering diverse strategies for managing intercurrent events related to disruptions, as well as other types of intercurrent events, will be essential.

23.7 Concluding Remarks

The COVID-19 pandemic had a significant impact on the conduct of clinical trials globally. The pandemic-related operational challenges, such as site closures, travel limitations, and interruptions to the supply chain for the investigational product, or from health-related challenges such as COVID-19 infections, led to unforeseen intercurrent events that affect either the interpretation or the existence of the measurements associated with the clinical question of interest. The estimand framework provides a rigorous basis to discuss potential pandemic-related trial disruptions and to embed these disruptions in the context of trial objectives and design elements.

Regarding the scientific objectives and estimands, several authors have argued that a hypothetical estimation strategy for intercurrent events related to operational challenges seems to be plausible, although the hypothetical scenario needs to be well described, as described in Sect. 23.3. The relevance and acceptability of a hypothetical estimand strategy seem to be less clear for intercurrent events related to health status, such as death due to COVID-19, in a cardiovascular outcome trial where death is by itself an outcome of interest. It is critical that one can estimate the outcome of interest under reasonable and plausible assumptions. If this does not appear to be possible (e.g., limited understanding of the disease or the drug to impute/predict missing or hypothetical data), alternative estimands should be chosen. Note that the relevance of a clinical trial question may have shifted due to the varying impact of the COVID-19 pandemic and the evolving understanding by various stakeholders. As always, the choice of an appropriate estimand (and agreed analysis approaches) is ultimately a cross-functional discussion between all stakeholders (sponsors, regulatory authorities, etc.).

This chapter focuses on how the estimand framework could be utilized to navigate the challenges posed by the COVID-19 pandemic, particularly in view of efficacy-related clinical questions. As advocated by Buchanan et al. (2023), however, the estimand framework has also enhanced the ability to account for the confounding effects of post-randomization events due to the pandemic that could skew the perceived safety profile of a drug. Nilsson et al. (2020) provided guidance on how safety analyses and reporting of clinical trial safety data could be modified in view of the COVID-19 pandemic. They also acknowledged that when assessing the potential impact of COVID-19 on safety analyses, safety planning could be updated using the estimand framework (as outlined, for example, in Sect. 21.3 of Chap. 21 in this book). Wang et al. (2023) also discussed the potential use of safety estimands to address the impact of pandemic-related intercurrent events on safety assessments. They pointed out that the pandemic might also affect the observation of certain adverse event outcomes and their population summary. COVID-19 infections could increase the occurrences of adverse events such as fever or cough and therefore pose challenges to obtaining an accurate population-level summary. Under the estimand framework, the while on treatment estimand could be used to split the adverse events that occurred before or after the COVID-19 infection so that one can have an accurate definition of treatment-emergent adverse events or COVID-19-related adverse events.

While the focus on COVID-19 in clinical trials has diminished, the practices established during the pandemic have led to an increased interest in new standards for designing and conducting clinical trials, such as remote visits or home administration of treatments. The COVID-19 pandemic has also provided insights into how trial disruptions, whether due to public health emergencies, geopolitical situations, or other major reasons, can be addressed in the future. In the context of unforeseen intercurrent events caused by such disruptions, which can impact either the interpretation or the availability of measurements related to the clinical question of interest, the estimand framework emerges as a valuable tool.

References

Akacha, M., Branson, J., Bretz, F., Dharan, B., Gallo, P., Gathmann, I., Hemmings, R., Jones, J., Xi, D., & Zuber, E. (2020). Challenges in assessing the impact of the COVID-19 pandemic on the integrity and interpretability of clinical trials. *Statistics in Biopharmaceutical Research, 12*(4), 419–426.

Bacchieri, A., Rossi, A., & Morelli, P. (2020). Risk and mitigation actions for clinical trials during COVID-19 pandemic (RiMiCOPa). *Contemporary Clinical Trials Communications, 20*, 100682.

Buchanan, J., Li, M., Hendrickson, B. A., Bhargava, P., & Roychoudhury, S. (2023). Assessing adverse events in clinical trials during the era of the COVID-19 pandemic. *Journal of Biopharmaceutical Statistics, 33*(4), 466–475.

Collins, S., & Levenson, M. (2020). Comment on "statistical issues and recommendations for clinical trials conducted during the COVID-19 pandemic.". *Statistics in Biopharmaceutical Research, 12*(4), 412–413.

Cro, S., Morris, T. P., Kahan, B. C., Cornelius, V., & Carpenter, J. (2020). A four-step strategy for handling missing outcome data in randomized trials affected by a pandemic. *BMC Medical Research Methodology, 20*, 1.

Degtyarev, E., Rufibach, K., Shentu, Y., Yung, G., Casey, M., Englert, S., Liu, F., Liu, Y., Sailer, O., Siegel, J., Sun, S., Tang, R., & Zhou, J. (2020). Assessing the impact of COVID-19 on the clinical trial objective and analysis of oncology clinical trials—Application of the Estimand framework. *Statistics in Biopharmaceutical Research, 12*(4), 427–437.

EMA (2020a). Points to consider on implications of coronavirus disease (COVID-19) on methodological aspects of ongoing clinical trials. Available at: https://www.ema.europa.eu

EMA (2020b), International regulators provide guiding principles for COVID-19 clinical trials [Internet], Available at: https://www.ema.europa.eu

FDA (2021). FDA guidance on conduct of clinical trials of medical products during COVID-19 public health emergency: Guidance for industry, investigators, and institutional review boards. Available at: https://www.fda.gov

Guo, T., Chen, C., Chiang, C., Chen, C., & Hsiao, C. (2020). Operational experiences in China and statistical issues on the conduct of clinical trials during the COVID-19 pandemic. *Statistics in Biopharmaceutical Research, 12*(4), 438–442.

Hemmings, R. (2020). Under a black cloud glimpsing a silver lining: Comment on statistical issues and recommendations for clinical trials conducted during the COVID-19 pandemic. *Statistics in Biopharmaceutical Research, 12*(4), 414–418.

ICH (2019). International Council for Hamonisation Topic E9(R1) on Estimands and sensitivity analysis in clinical trials. Available at: https://www.ich.org

Jin, M., Liu, R., & Robieson, W. (2021). Modified reference based imputation and tipping point analysis in the presence of missing data due to COVID-19. *Contemporary Clinical Trials, 110*, 106575.

Kahan, B. C., Morris, T. P., White, I. R., Tweed, C., Cro, S., Dahly, D., Pham, T. M., Esmail, H., Babiker, A., & Carpenter, J. (2020). Treatment estimands in clinical trials of patients hospitalized for COVID-19: Ensuring trials ask the right questions. *BMC Medicine, 18*, 1.

Lasch, F., & Guizzaro, L. (2022). Estimators for handling COVID -19-related intercurrent events with a hypothetical strategy. *Pharmaceutical Statistics, 21*(6), 1258–1280.

Leahy, J., Hickey, C., McConnell, D. J., Cassidy, O., Trela-Larsen, L., Barry, M., Tilson, L., & McCullagh, L. (2020). Coronavirus disease 2019: Considerations for health technology assessment from the National Centre for Pharmacoeconomics Review Group. *Value in Health, 23*(11), 1423–1426.

Marston, L., Novere, M. L., Ricciardi, F., Nazareth, I., Carson, A., Edwards, M. J., Goldstein, L. H., Marsden, J., Noble, H., Reuber, M., Stone, J., Hunter, R., & Nielsen, G. (2023). COVID-19 and the Physio4FMD trial: Impact, mitigating strategies and analysis plans. *Contemporary Clinical Trials Communications, 33*, 101124.

Mészáros L., Lasch F., Delafont, B., & Guizzaro L. (2023) Strategies for addressing intercurrent events in CNS trials. Available at https://ssrn.com/abstract=4516200

MHRA (2020) Guidance on minimizing disruptions to the conduct and integrity of clinical trials of medicines during COVID-19. Available at: https://www.gov.uk

Meyer, R. D., Ratitch, B., Wolbers, M., Marchenko, O., Quan, H., Li, D., Fletcher, C., Li, X., Wright, D., Shentu, Y., Englert, S., Shen, W., Dey, J., Liu, T. T., Zhou, M., Bohidar, N. R., Zhao, P., & Hale, M. (2020). Statistical issues and recommendations for clinical trials conducted during the COVID-19 pandemic. *Statistics in Biopharmaceutical Research, 12*(4), 399–411.

Nilsson, M., Crowe, B., Anglin, G., Ball, G., Munsaka, M., Shahin, S., & Wang, W. (2020). Clinical trial drug safety assessment for studies and submissions impacted by COVID-19. *Statistics in Biopharmaceutical Research, 12*(4), 498–505.

Qu, Y., & Lipkovich, I. (2021). Implementation of ICH E9 (R1): A few points learned during the COVID-19 pandemic. *Therapeutic Innovation & Regulatory Science, 55*(5), 984–988.

Sridhara, R., Barksdale, E., Marchenko, O., Jiang, Q., Ando, Y., Bloomquist, E., Coory, M., Crouse, M., Degtyarev, E., Framke, T., Freidlin, B., Gerber, D. E., Gwise, T., Josephson, F., Hess, L., Kluetz, P. G., Li, D., Mandrekar, S. J., Posch, M., et al. (2022). Cancer clinical trials beyond pandemic: report of an American Statistical Association Biopharmaceutical Section Open Forum Discussion. *Statistics in Biopharmaceutical Research, 15*(2), 444–449.

Van Lancker, K., Tarima, S., Bartlett, J., Bauer, M., Bharani-Dharan, B., Bretz, F., Flournoy, N., Michiels, H., Parra, C. O., Rosenberger, J. L., & Cro, S. (2023). Estimands and their estimators for clinical trials impacted by the COVID-19 pandemic: A report from the NISS Ingram Olkin forum series on unplanned clinical trial disruptions. *Statistics in Biopharmaceutical Research, 15*(1), 94–111.

Vansteelandt, S. (2023). Comment on 'Estimands and their estimators for clinical trials impacted by the COVID-19 pandemic: A report from the NISS Ingram Olkin forum series on unplanned clinical trial disruptions'. *Statistics in Biopharmaceutical Research, 15*(1), 112–115.

Wang, X., Yang, P., Yuan, S., & Wang, W. W. B. (2023). Application of estimand framework in ICH E9 (R1) to safety evaluation. *Journal of Biopharmaceutical Statistics, 33*(4), 476–487.

Wiens, B. L., & Lipkovich, I. (2020). The impact of major events on ongoing noninferiority trials, with application to COVID-19. *Statistics in Biopharmaceutical Research, 12*(4), 443–450.

Yassi, N., Hayward, K. S., Campbell, B. C., & Churilov, L. (2021). Use of the Estimand framework to manage the disruptive effects of COVID-19 on stroke clinical trials. *Stroke, 52*(11), 3739–3747.

Index

J. Wei et al. (eds.), *Estimands in Clinical Trials*, Springer Series in Pharmaceutical Statistics, https://doi.org/10.1007/978-3-032-02192-2

E

F

G

MIX
Papier aus verantwortungsvollen Quellen
Paper from responsible sources
FSC® C105338

If you have any concerns about our products,
you can contact us on
ProductSafety@springernature.com

In case Publisher is established outside the EU,
the EU authorized representative is:
Springer Nature Customer Service Center GmbH
Europaplatz 3, 69115 Heidelberg, Germany

Printed by Libri Plureos GmbH
in Hamburg, Germany